SEXUALLY
TRANSMITTED
DISEASES

Second Edition

Companion Handbook

NOTICE

SEXUALLY

TRANSMITTED

DISEASES

Second Edition

Companion Handbook

Adaora A. Adimora, M.D., M.P.H.
Clinical Assistant Professor of Medicine
Division of Infectious Diseases
Department of Medicine
School of Medicine
The University of North Carolina at Chapel Hill

Holli Hamilton, M.D.
Research Assistant Professor
Division of Infectious Diseases
Department of Medicine
School of Medicine
The University of North Carolina at Chapel Hill

King K. Holmes, M.D., Ph.D.
Director
Center for AIDS and STD
Professor of Medicine and Adjunct Professor of
  Microbiology and Epidemiology
University of Washington
Seattle, Washington

P. Frederick Sparling, M.D.
Chairman and J. Herbert Bate Professor of
  Medicine and Microbiology and Immunology
Department of Medicine
School of Medicine
The University of North Carolina at Chapel Hill

McGraw-Hill, Inc.
Health Professions Division
New York St. Louis San Francisco Auckland Bogotá Caracas
Lisbon London Madrid Mexico City Milan Montreal New Delhi
Paris San Juan Singapore Sydney Tokyo Toronto

This book is printed on acid-free paper.

SEXUALLY TRANSMITTED DISEASES
Second Edition
COMPANION HANDBOOK

1234567890 DOC DOC 9876543

ISBN 0-07-000380-7

This book was set in Times Roman by ComCom.

The editors were J. Dereck Jeffers and Steven Melvin.

The production supervisor was Clare Stanley.

The cover was designed by E. Schultheis.

The project was supervised by Editorial Services of New
England, Inc.

R.R. Donnelley & Sons was the printer and binder.

Library of Congress Cataloging-in-Publication Data

Sexually transmitted diseases. Companion handbook / Adaora A. Adimora
. . . [et al.].—Second edition.
    p.   cm.
  Updated, rev., and expanded ed. of: Sexually transmitted diseases /
editors, King K. Holmes . . . [et al]. 2nd ed. c1990.
  Includes bibliographical references and index.
  ISBN 0-07-000380-7
  1. Sexually transmitted diseases.   I. Adimora, Adaora A.
  [DNLM: 1. Sexually Transmitted Diseases. WC 140 S5192 1994]
RC200.S49   1994
616.95′1—dc20
DNLM/DLC
or Library of Congress   93-2394
                                                                   CIP

To Paul and Alegro Godley with thanks for their unfailing patience and support

AAA

To Ernest

HH

Contents

Preface   xi

PART I   EPIDEMIOLOGY OF SEXUALLY TRANSMITTED DISEASES

Chapter 1   Epidemiology of Sexually Transmitted Diseases   1

PART II   SYSTEMATIC APPROACH TO THE PATIENT WITH SEXUALLY TRANSMITTED DISEASE

Chapter 2   Clinical and Laboratory Approach to the Patient   10

PART III   SEXUALLY TRANSMITTED AGENTS

Section 1: Bacteria

Chapter 3   Gonococcal Infections in the Adult   25

Chapter 4   *Chlamydia Trachomatis* Infections in the Adult   41

Chapter 5   Lymphogranuloma Venereum   56

Chapter 6   Syphilis in the Adult   63

Chapter 7   Chancroid and *Haemophilus Ducreyi*   87

Chapter 8   Donovanosis   93

Section 2: Viral Infections

Chapter 9   Clinical Manifestations of HIV Infection in Adults in Industrialized Countries   99

Chapter 10   Primary Care of Patients with HIV Infection   124

Chapter 11   Genital Herpes   135

Chapter 12   Cytomegalovirus as a Sexually Transmitted Infection   155

Chapter 13   Genital Human Papillomavirus Infection   162

Chapter 14   Molluscum Contagiosum   175

Chapter 15   Viral Hepatitis   180

Section 3: Ectoparasites

Chapter 16   Human Lice   200

Chapter 17   Scabies   204

Section 4: Protozoan Infections

Chapter 18   *Trichomonas Vaginalis* and Trichomoniasis   212

Chapter 19   Vulvovaginal Candidiasis   223

PART IV: APPROACH TO COMMON CLINICAL SYNDROMES

Chapter 20   Lower Genital Tract Infections in Women: Cystitis, Urethritis, Vulvovaginitis, and Cervicitis   233

Chapter 21   Bacterial Vaginosis   245

Chapter 22   Pelvic Inflammatory Disease   254

Chapter 23   Urethritis in Males   271

Chapter 24   Epididymitis   281

Chapter 25   Sexually Transmitted Proctitis and Diarrheal Disease   291

Chapter 26   Genital Ulcer Adenopathy Syndrome   309

Chapter 27   Arthritis Associated with Sexually Transmitted Diseases   319

PART V   SEXUALLY TRANSMITTED DISEASES IN REPRODUCTION, PERINATOLOGY, AND PEDIATRICS

Chapter 28   Sexually Transmitted Diseases in Pregnancy   335

Chapter 29   Gonococcal Diseases in Infants and Children   352

Chapter 30   Chlamydial Infections in Infants   359

Chapter 31   Congenital Syphilis   365

Chapter 32   Child Sexual Abuse and Sexually Transmitted Diseases   378

PART VI   COUNSELING PATIENTS WITH STDS

Chapter 33   Patient Education and Counseling and Other
Strategies for Prevention of Sexually Transmitted
Diseases   387

Chapter 34   HIV Counseling and Testing   398

PART VII   SEXUAL ASSAULT AND STDS

Chapter 35   Sexual Assault and STDs   409

Index   413

Preface

This book is primarily intended for use by clinicians and public health professionals in the evaluation and treatment of patients with sexually transmitted diseases. Therapeutic recommendations are based on the Centers for Disease Control (CDC) Sexually Transmitted Diseases Treatment Guidelines. Much of the text and almost all tables and figures were taken from the second edition of *Sexually Transmitted Diseases* on which this book is based. This text, however, has been updated, revised, and expanded to reflect research advances and changes in medical practice since the release of the parent text.

We gratefully acknowledge the contributions of the CDC and the original authors of *Sexually Transmitted Diseases,* second edition.

Epidemiology of Sexually Transmitted Diseases

The overall trends in STD morbidity during the AIDS era can be summarized succinctly:

1. Greatly reduced rates of the classic STDs (e.g., gonorrhea, syphilis, chancroid) in nearly every industrialized country except the United States, presumably due to effective public health programs and changing sexual behavior. The incidence of viral STDs, such as genital herpes, seems to have stabilized in many countries after two decades of rapid increase, but so far, dramatic declines have not been reported.
2. Continued hyperendemic spread of STDs in Africa, Asia, Oceania, Latin America, and the Caribbean with little evidence of declining rates, and even some evidence of increasing rates in these developing regions during the AIDS era—highlighting the need for intensified AIDS-STD control efforts.
3. A surprising resurgence of heterosexual syphilis and chancroid in the United States, and hyperendemic gonorrhea in poor inner city and rural populations, all three diseases closely associated with the crack cocaine epidemic of the late 1980s and the 1990s.

The goal of this chapter is not to summarize the epidemiology of individual sexually transmitted diseases (STDs) in more detail but rather to develop an overall perspective of their epidemiology. We are particularly interested in the importance of demographic and sociocultural change and in the behavioral determinants of STDs.

STD TRANSMISSION DYNAMICS

Persistence of a sexually transmitted disease in a human population requires that the pathogen infect a person who is capable of transmitting infection to another susceptible host who is in turn capable of further transmission. This property, the reproductive rate R_0, is the number of infections a transmitter spreads in a fully susceptible population. At equilibrium, R_0 equals 1. When R_0 is greater than 1, the prevalence of infection rises in the population; when R_0 is less than 1, disease prevalence falls. Three variables determine the reproductive rate of infection in a population: the average probability of transmitting infection from an infected individual to a susceptible person, or the efficiency of transmission (β); the average rate of acquisition of new sexual partners *(c)*; and the average duration of infectiousness *(D)*. Thus, the following model reflects STD transmission dynamics in a population:

$$R_0 = \beta c D^1$$

These variables can seldom be measured directly. Epidemiologists have therefore used as proxies a variety of other variables, such as "risk factors" and "risk markers," to determine risk and explain patterns of disease transmission.

RISK FACTORS AND RISK MARKERS

In STD epidemiology the terms *risk factor, risk marker,* and *determinant* have been used interchangeably without much attention to the existence of a causal link between the relevant attribute or exposure and the disease. Many of the traditional STD risk factors appear to be correlates of the probability of encountering an infected partner, whereas others may influence the probability of infection if exposed, or the probability of disease if infected (Table 1-1). Since the causal link between demographic variables and STDs is probably explained by coincidental differences in sexual behavior and/or disease prevalence, such variables are perhaps most accurately referred to as *risk markers* or *risk indicators.* For example, single marital status and inner-city residence fall into this category.

Other variables, such as sexual behaviors and health care behaviors, are directly related to the probability of exposure to STDs, to

TABLE 1-1. Risk Markers and Risk Factors for Sexually Transmitted Diseases

Risk markers	Risk markers or risk factors	Risk factors
Marital status	Age	Sexual behaviors*
Race	Gender	Number of partners
Residence	Smoking	Rate of acquiring new partners
Rural/urban	Alcohol	Casual partners
Socioeconomic	Drug abuse	Sex preference
Status	Other STDs	Sexual practices
	Lack of	Health care behaviors
	circumcision	No use of barriers and
	Contraceptive	microbicidal agents
	method	Late consultation for
		diagnosis, treatment
		Nonreferral of partners
		Noncompliance with therapy
		Douching

*The essential risk factor for acquiring an STD is exposure to an STD; some of these risk factors are current surrogates for such exposure. Better surrogates are needed. Several practices (e.g., rectal intercourse) can be additional risk factors for infection, given exposure.

Poor health care behaviors are risk factors either for acquiring an STD or for developing complications of an STD.

infection following exposure, or to complications once infection occurs, and can be referred to as *true risk factors.* Sexual behavior is the key determinant for incidence of incurable viral STDs, whereas both sexual and health care behaviors are important determinants of the incidence of bacterial STDs.

The major sexual behavioral risk factors for STDs appear to include a large number of sexual partners, high rates of acquiring new sexual partners within specific time periods, high rates of partner change, contact with casual sexual partners, sexual orientation, and specific sexual practices. These variables represent attempts to estimate β and c.

Health care behaviors which can reduce the risk of acquiring or transmitting STDs include use of condoms for prophylaxis, early consultation for diagnosis and treatment, compliance with therapy, and partner referral. Absence of such behaviors can be regarded as a risk factor for STDs.

Several other variables could function both as risk markers and as risk factors, or are difficult to classify as one or the other at present (Table 1-1). For example, age and gender are certainly risk markers, indirectly related to risk of STDs as correlates of sexual behavior and of disease prevalence in sex partners. However, age and gender may also directly influence host susceptibility. For example, the prevalence of cervical ectopy is higher in young women than in older women, and ectopy may influence susceptibility to certain STD pathogens such as *Chlamydia trachomatis* and HIV. Regarding gender-specific risk, the risk of infection per exposure during vaginal intercourse may be greater for the female than for the male with respect to several STD pathogens such as *Neisseria gonorrhoeae, C. trachomatis,* hepatitis B virus, and HIV, although evidence remains inconclusive. Alcohol and drug abuse can perhaps be referred to as *risk modifiers,* since they produce situational modification of sexual behavior or health care behavior.

Another way of conceptualizing the terms *risk markers, risk modifiers,* and *risk factors* is to envision a long chain of steps along a causal pathway that ultimately leads to infection and disease. Those factors that occur at an early step in the pathway, and which are most remote from the disease outcome (e.g., being born in an inner city), are only indirectly related to an STD outcome and represent markers of risk of STD. In contrast, events that occur farther along the causal pathway, proximate to the disease outcome (e.g., unprotected receptive anorectal sex) represent causal risk factors, directly related to the disease outcome. Clinical epidemiologists tend to focus on identifying the most proximate, direct, causal risk factors; but there remains a need to understand and improve the underlying, more indirect factors that contribute to STD incidence.

STDs as Risk Factors for Other STDs

Many known interactions occur among different infectious diseases. The growing evidence that certain STDs (genital ulcer diseases, gonorrhea, chlamydial infection, trichomoniasis) function as risk factors for transmission of HIV infection is extremely important in and of itself. Furthermore, HIV infection and immunosuppression appear to alter the natural history of many STDs (e.g., herpes, human papillomavirus infection, chancroid) in ways that probably enhance their transmission. These phenomena raise other questions about potential interactions. For example:

1. HIV and Human Papillomavirus (HPV)—Does HIV infection "reactivate" genital or anal HPV infection? Does HIV infection increase the risk of genital or anal dysplasia or cancer among those with HPV infection? If so, is this related to or independent of level of immunosuppression?
2. Vaginal flora and other STDs—Is the normal H_2O_2-producing *Lactobacillus*-dominated vaginal flora protective against other STD pathogens? Does bacterial vaginosis with absence of H_2O_2-producing vaginal flora increase susceptibility to other genital infections?
3. *N. gonorrhoeae, C. trachomatis,* and "polymicrobial pelvic inflammatory disease"—Does gonococcal or chlamydial salpingitis "pave the way" for tubal infection by vaginal organisms of lesser virulence?
4. Herpes simplex virus (HSV) and other genital ulcers—Does HSV, by producing recurrent genital epithelial ulceration, present a risk factor for acquiring other genital epithelial infection, such as chancroid?

Assessing one STD as a cofactor for another STD presents difficult methodological problems, since the sexual exposures leading to one infection are those which directly lead to exposures to the other STDs. Case-control studies which adequately adjust for confounders, such as sexual behaviors, are difficult to design. Cohort studies which allow assessment of the temporal relationships between a first and second STD, and intervention trials (e.g., prevention of one STD to reduce the risk of another STD) represent possible ways to assess such interactions.

Drug Use and STDs

Alcohol and marijuana use have been linked with high-risk sexual behavior in many societies, and heroin use has been associated with prostitution in most industrialized countries. However, the crack cocaine epidemic, which became apparent in North America in the mid-1980s, was temporally and dramatically linked with resurgent syphilis, chancroid, and gonorrhea in communities that were hit hardest by the crack epidemic, and the phenomenon of exchanging sex for cocaine. Cocaine use has been directly linked with various STDs, including HIV infection, in more than a dozen case-control studies.

Contraception

Patterns of contraception use markedly influence the transmission and sequelae of STDs. Barrier methods such as the diaphragm with spermicide probably offer some protection, particularly against organisms transmitted mainly between the columnar or transitional epithelium of the urethra and the cervix (e.g., *C. trachomatis, N. gonorrhoeae*). Condoms, used properly, offer strong protection against these organisms, as well as partial protection against those which commonly infect the stratified squamous epithelium of the vulva and penis, such as HSV and HPV. Oral contraceptive use has been associated with increased risk of cervical infection with *C. trachomatis,* and perhaps with increased risk of cervical infection with *N. gonorrhoeae,* but with decreased risk of severe pelvic inflammatory disease among women who do acquire cervical chlamydial infection.

Current global public health efforts to increase condom use to prevent transmission of STDs including HIV are targeted at large proportions of the sexually active population which do not use condoms, particularly in developing countries. However, interest is growing in targeted promotion of condom use for those at highest risk of STDs (such as prostitutes, clients of prostitutes, and people with many casual sex partners), which may be a more practical and cost-effective approach to STD prevention.

Dimensions of Sexual Behavior

As noted earlier, sexual behavior has been recognized as the major risk factor for STDs for some time, but our understanding of its relevant components has changed considerably over the past two decades. The AIDS epidemic has been the most important factor in both highlighting the need for more systematic information on sexual behavior and facilitating an unprecedented increase in infection-related studies of sexual behavior. Behavioral intervention has again, for the first time since penicillin, become the most important approach to STD control.

The term *sexual behavior* involves many components: sexual experience and activity, age at sexual debut, current and lifetime number of sex partners, frequency of sexual intercourse, consistency of sexual activity, mode of recruitment of sexual partners, duration of sexual unions, and types of sexual practice. The conjoint distribution of these component variables in the population determines aggregate exposure to the risk of STDs. However, the specific relationship between each of these variables and STD risk, and the distribution of these variables across population subgroups, have not yet been determined.

Some individuals are at risk for STDs because of their own sexual behaviors; these persons have a relatively high likelihood of being infected and of transmitting STD to new partners, and perhaps are best described by the term *high-frequency transmitters* or *core group members.* Poor health care behavior (for example, failure to seek treatment while remaining sexually active with symptoms of STD) is another important feature of high-frequency transmitters.

Other persons are at risk for STDs because of the sexual behaviors of their partners; while their probability of acquiring infection could be high, their likelihood of infecting others is relatively low, since they do not have many sexual partners. This second category can be described as *receivers.* Although data are limited and there is probably great variation between societies, gender differences in reported sexual behaviors suggest that in many societies most women are more likely to be receivers.

The nonlinear increase in STD risk with increasing numbers of sexual partners is well documented. The possibility of STD risk due to one's partner's behavior and the nonlinear nature of the relationship between number of sex partners and STD risk highlight the importance of two other dimensions of sexual behavior: choice of partners and contact with core groups of high-STD-risk individuals.

Whether one has sexual relationships with high-frequency transmitters is determined by who one's sex partners are and, indirectly, by how one chooses one's sex partners. A nondiscriminating approach to sex partner recruitment increases the probability of sexual contact with members of high-risk core groups and thus of exposure to STDs. The nature of sex partner recruitment has only recently emerged as a research topic, and very few data are available concerning it. Better understanding of modes of partner recruitment in population subgroups will help explain some of the variability in STD risk.

DEMOGRAPHIC AND SOCIAL CORRELATES OF STDs

At the beginning of the 1990s, inner-city, poor, minority populations of developed countries, particularly the United States, and the populations of many developing countries (especially their urban communities) appear to have similar profiles with respect to STD as a public health problem. Interestingly, these populations are also alike with respect to several demographic, sociopolitical, and economic characteristics which are associated with high levels of STD incidence.

First, both developing countries and inner-city minority populations are primarily composed of young people, with relatively high and increasing proportions of the total population belonging to sexually active adolescent and young-adult age groups. In the United States the proportion of the white population in the sexually active age groups has been declining since the mid-1980s, but in contrast, the proportion of the black and Hispanic populations in these age groups is still increasing. Thus these nonwhite populations of the United States, unlike the white population, have age pyramids which are similar to those of developing countries and conducive to increasing STD incidence.

Second, both developing countries and inner-city minority populations are characterized by rapid demographic change. Developing countries in general have high population growth rates resulting from the combination of continuing high fertility rates and low and/or declining mortality rates. In addition, these countries have high rates of urbanization and population movement. Inner-city urban populations of developed countries are also marked by high physical mobility. In some cities, such as New York, this geographic mobility appears to have been accelerated by deterioration of certain critical social services, such as fire control.

Rapid economic change is another characteristic common to inner cities of the developed world and to whole societies of the developing world. The transition from agricultural self-sufficiency to dependence on income from wage labor, which has occurred in most developing countries, is one of the best-known examples of rapid economic change in society. This economic evolution has caused structural transformations of the most basic kind. The changes being introduced into inner-city communities of the United States through the sale of drugs, especially crack cocaine, are described by observers in similar terms. During the course of drug trade large sums of money change hands very rapidly, often through very young teenagers, and radically alter the social structure of these communities.

Third, unstable power hierarchies of developing countries and inner-city minority populations result in rapid political change. The frequency of civil wars, coups, and border disturbances, and the extensive need for police and military presence to ensure peace in everyday life, are indicators of lack of political stability in many countries of the third world. Similarly, frequent violence in inner-city communities in the United States is an indicator of the tentative nature of power hierarchies in these communities. The disruptive effects of unemployment, drug use, and drug trade on the stability of these communities are visible.

The rapid demographic, economic, and political changes in these populations result in a social situation where levels of transience and marginality are high, the normative structure is destabilized, and social disintegration reigns. In these social systems, the basic patterns of need, dependency, and opportunity structures reinforce inequality-based social exchanges. Institutions like prostitution and drug trade emerge as adaptive responses to the existing sociopolitical structures and function as social factors which enhance the spread of STDs.

CHALLENGES FOR THE FUTURE

Successful control of STDs in the coming decades should be reflected by a fall in the prevalence of disease. The most effective strategies will therefore be those which most efficiently reduce the components of the reproductive rate of infection, R_0. As noted earlier, these variables include β, the efficiency of transmission; $c,$ the average rate of acquisition of new sex partners; and $D,$ the duration of infectiousness. STD control will require a multifaceted approach.

Transmission efficiency may be reduced through strategies such as condom use; improved diagnosis and treatment of STDs to reduce the efficiency of transmission of HIV; and adoption of safer sex practices (for example, avoidance of high-risk behaviors such as receptive anal intercourse with persons who are not known to be free of HIV infection).

The rate of acquisition of new infected sexual partners may be decreased by delaying sexual debut, reducing number of partners, and altering partner selection methods. Changes in these behaviors will in many cases require fundamental changes in societal norms, which may be difficult to effect.

A reduction of the duration of infectiousness of persons with treatable bacterial STDs, such as chancroid, gonorrhea, and syphilis, will decrease the prevalence of these diseases. Reducing the duration of infectiousness will require improvements in access to health care, with expansion of STD clinic hours and increased staffing by clinicians to accommodate more patients, together with a greater role of primary care clinicians in providing STD services; improvement in quality of care to allow proper diagnosis and treatment; and targeted health education to promote early symptom recognition and treatment.

Implementation of these strategies will require substantial resources. Since health care resources are limited, public health programs must appropriately target their intervention efforts. STD control efforts should focus on specific high-risk groups—so-called core transmitters—whose high rates of partner change and prolonged duration of infectivity promote STD transmission in the population.

REFERENCE

1. Anderson RM: The transmission dynamics of sexually transmitted diseases: The behavioral component, in Wasserheit JN et al (eds): *Research issues in Human Behavior and Sexually Transmitted Diseases in the AIDS Era.* Washington, DC, American Society for Microbiology, 1991

ADDITIONAL READING

Anderson RM: The transmission dynamics of sexually transmitted diseases: The behavioral component, in Wasserheit JN et al (eds): *Research Issues in Human Behavior and Sexually Transmitted Diseases in the AIDS Era.* Washington, DC, American Society for Microbiology, 1991

Brunham RC: The concept of core and its relevance to the epidemiology and control of sexually transmitted diseases. *Sex Transm Dis* 18:67, 1991

Brunham RC, Plummer FA: A general model of sexually transmitted disease epidemiology and its implications for control. *Med Clin North Am* 74:1339, 1990

Granath F et al: Estimation of a preference matrix for women's choice of male sexual partner according to rate of partner change, using partner notification data. *Math Biosci* 107:341, 1991

Kassler WJ, Cates WJ: The epidemiology and prevention of sexually transmitted diseases. *Urol Clin North Am* 19:1, 1992

Kault DA, Marsh LM: Modeling AIDS as a function of other sexually transmitted disease. *Math Biosci* 103:17, 1991

Mertens TE et al: Epidemiological methods to study the interaction between HIV infection and other sexually transmitted diseases. *AIDS* 4:57, 1990

Padian NS et al: The effect of number of exposures on the risk of heterosexual HIV transmission. *J Infect Dis* 161:883, 1990

Padian NS et al: Risk factors for acquisition of sexually transmitted diseases and development of complications, in Wasserheit JN et al (eds): *Research Issues in Human Behavior and Sexually Transmitted Diseases in the AIDS Era.* Washington, DC, American Society for Microbiology, 1991

Padian NS et al: Female-to-male transmission of human immunodeficiency virus. *JAMA* 266:1664, 1991

Quinn TC et al: Evolution of the human immunodeficiency virus epidemic among patients attending sexually transmitted disease clinics: A decade of experience. *J Infect Dis* 165:541, 1992

For a more detailed discussion, see Aral SO, Holmes KK: Epidemiology of Sexual Behavior and Sexually Transmitted Diseases, Chap. 2, p. 19; and Rothenberg RB: Analytic Approaches to the Epidemiology of Sexually Transmitted Diseases, Chap. 3, p. 37, in STD-2.

| **Clinical and Laboratory Approach to the Patient**

Medicine is an art as well as a science. The practice of clinical medicine is as diverse as its practitioners. Clearly there is no single, optimal method for conducting the history and physical examination. Some themes, however, are common to most clinicians. The goal of this chapter is to provide basic guidelines which clinicians may use in their initial evaluation of patients with sexually transmitted diseases (STDs).

TAKING THE HISTORY

The goal of the history in the evaluation of STDs is to obtain information concerning symptoms and past events which will assist in diagnosis and treatment. Such information is usually obtained directly from the patient but may also be gleaned from the medical record or surrogate historians, such as sexual partners, family members, or friends. Critical information includes reason for consultation, symptoms and signs noted by the patient, past medical history—especially history of other STDs—allergies and current medications, and assessment of behavior which increases risk of acquiring or transmitting STDs.

Most patients seek assistance because of disturbing symptoms, but a substantial proportion are asymptomatic and request evaluation because they have been exposed to an STD or simply desire a "checkup" to ensure that they are free of infection.

Sexually transmitted pathogens produce a variety of clinical manifestations. The most common complaints include penile or vaginal discharge, vaginal itching, genital ulcers, dysuria, and pelvic and abdominal pain. Careful questioning is often necessary to help direct the physical examination and assist with differential diagnosis of diseases that are not sexually transmitted and require alternative therapy. For example, patients with pelvic inflammatory disease (PID) and those with appendicitis both generally present with lower abdominal pain. However, PID is often associated with irregular vaginal bleeding and may be treated with antibiotics alone, while appendicitis usually requires surgery. In addition, multiple STDs may coexist. Historical evidence sometimes suggests the presence of multiple pathogens.

Although most persons with STDs are young and have little past medical history, information concerning past illnesses should be sought, as it may aid diagnosis and determination of likelihood of compliance. HIV disease and other immunocompromising conditions, for example, can alter the presentation of syphilis, scabies, PID, and other STDs. A history of past STD is also important.

Persons who have had previous STDs may be more likely to have one in the future. Moreover, recurrent STDs suggest ongoing high-risk behavior and failure to adopt safer sexual practices.

Risk assessment helps determine the risk of exposure to infection and also helps tailor safer sex and other counseling messages for maximum efficiency. Persons who do not engage in oral sex have little risk of acquiring gonococcal pharyngitis, while those who practice receptive anal intercourse may contract proctitis and are at higher risk for acquiring HIV infection. Individual counseling should take into consideration the patient's sexual practices. Many clinicians, however, find it difficult to take a sexual history.

The most difficult part of taking a sexual history is introducing the subject in a way that will prompt the most truthful response from the patient. Obviously, the attitude of the health care provider will affect his or her ability to help establish such a setting. The sexual history is sometimes avoided until the very end of the history-taking process. In doing so, the clinician signals the patient that the examiner is uncomfortable with the subject. Close-ended questions such as "I assume that you are only having sex with your wife?" will severely limit the accuracy of information. The best approach is to obtain the sexual history in the context of the overall social history. Thus, you can begin with a statement to the effect that "In order to provide you with optimal care, there are a number of areas of your personal habits and practices that I need to understand and be aware of. These include the use of any nonprescription drugs or alcohol, any special diets you have been on, sexual practices, and foreign travel." Such an introductory statement alerts the patient to your interest in his or her sexual practices and places that concern within the overall context of an open and honest clinician–patient relationship.

It is usually necessary to inquire about specific practices, as well as the broad categories of homo- and heterosexual orientation. Asking, "Do you have sex only with men, only with women, or with both?" will establish the presence or absence of same-sex activity. Questions regarding specific sexual practices with same and/or opposite sex partners should follow. Specific practices may be associated with specific infections or traumatic problems (Table 2-1). Because patients frequently use the vernacular terms and may be unfamiliar with medical terminology, the lay term or terms for each practice are included in parentheses.

PHYSICAL EXAMINATION OF THE GENITAL TRACT

Males

We suggest that the physical examination proceed according to an orderly sequence as outlined in Table 2-2. Proceeding in this fashion

TABLE 2-1. Specific Sexual Practices and Possible Associated Disease Problems

Sexual practice (street terms)	Disease problems listed in approximate order of frequency	Sexual practice (street terms)	Disease problems listed in approximate order of frequency
Close body contact	Pediculosis pubis Scabies Fungal infections	Anal intercourse, receptive (Does your partner put his penis into your rectum?)	Traumatic proctitis Rectal gonorrhea Anal condylomata acuminata HIV/AIDS Molluscum contagiosum (rare) Nonspecific proctitis (chlamydia and others) Anorectal herpes simplex virus Anorectal syphilis Hepatitis B Rectal trichomoniasis (?) Lymphogranuloma venereum Anorectal granuloma inguinale Anorectal chancroid Cytomegalovirus infection Anorectal candidiasis
Masturbation (jacking off, beating off)	Physical abrasions Conjunctivitis		
Douches, lubricants	Allergic reactions Rectal fatty tumors		
Amyl nitrite, butyl nitrite (poppers)	Amyl and butyl nitrite burns; contact dermatitis		
Fellatio, receptive (Do you suck your partner's penis?)	Physical abrasions Oral gonorrhea Oral herpes simplex virus (especially type 2) Nongonococcal pharyngitis (chlamydia and others) Oral condylomata acuminata		

12

Fellatio, receptive (continued)	Syphilis Hepatitis B Enteric infections Lymphogranuloma venereum Oral donovanosis (granuloma inguinale) Oral chancroid	Anilingus (oral-anal intercourse) (Do you rim or do scat?)	Enteric infections Shigellosis Campylobacter fetus Enterotoxigenic *Escherichia coli* Hepatitis A, B, non-A non-B Amebiasis Giardiasis Salmonellosis *Enterobius vermicularis* *Strongyloides stercoralis* Oral infections Oral warts Oral gonorrhea Syphilis Lymphogranuloma venereum Oral donovanosis Oral chancroid Oral or rectal HIV/AIDS (?) Herpes simplex virus Anorectal meningococcal infection
Fellatio, insertive (Does your partner suck your penis?)	Physical abrasions Bites Genital herpes simplex virus (especially type 1) Nongonococcal urethritis Gonococcal urethritis Meningococcal urethritis		
Anal intercourse, insertive (Do you put your penis into your partner's rectum?)	Nongonococcal urethritis Gonococcal urethritis Genital herpes simplex virus Molluscum contagiosum Condylomata acuminata Syphilis Trichomoniasis		

(continued)

13

TABLE 2-1. Specific Sexual Practices and Possible Associated Disease Problems *(continued)*

Sexual practice (street terms)	Disease problems listed in approximate order of frequency	Sexual practice (street terms)	Disease problems listed in approximate order of frequency
Anal intercourse, insertive *(continued)*	Epididymitis and/or prostatitis Fungal infections Lymphogranuloma venereum Donovanosis (granuloma inguinale) Chancroid Cytomegalovirus (?) Hepatitis B HIV/AIDS	Fist and/or finger fornication, receptive (Have you been fist-fucked?)	Enteric infections
		Toys and/or apparatus (cock rings, dildoes, leather, tit clamps, etc.)	Allergic reactions to metal, plastic, rubber Friction dermatitis Physical torsions Varicoceles Peyronie's disease Fungal infections Lost rectal foreign bodies Testicular strangulation
		Sadomasochism (piercing, bondage) (Are you into S/M, piercing, or bondage?)	Lacerations Cutaneous infections Trauma HIV/AIDS
		Group sex	*See* Anilingus (above)

SOURCE: After DG Ostrow, A Obermaier, in Sexually Transmitted Diseases in Homosexual Men, DG Ostrow (ed). New York, Plenum, 1983.

TABLE 2-2. Routine STD Examination of the Male

General appearance
Skin
Abdominal examination
Groin
  Hernia
  Adenopathy
Genitalia
  Penis
    Prepuce
    Urethral meatus
    Shaft
Scrotum
    Testis
    Vas
    Epididymis
Rectal examination
  Tone
  Fissure, hemorrhoids, or mass lesions
  Prostate examination
Laboratory studies
  Stool guaiac
  Urethral smear
  Urinalysis
  Other

---

has two advantages. First, there is an orderly sequence to the examination that limits the opportunity for errors of omission in a busy clinical situation. Second, there is minimal need for the patient to move. The examination may be initiated by having the patient sit on the examining table. If necessary, head and neck examination and percussion and auscultation of the chest may be done with the patient in this position. Next, the patient is asked to lie supine. Cardiovascular examination, if indicated, may be conducted with the patient in this position, and attention is directed to the abdominal examination. The patient is then asked to stand for examination of the groin and genitalia. Finally, the patient is asked to turn and bend over, placing his elbows on the examining table, for the rectal and prostate examination. There is minimal need for the patient to move from position to position if the examination is done in this order. Figures 2-1 and 2-2 illustrate the male reproductive system.

Groin

While the patient is lying supine on the examining table, the groin, or inguinal region, should be examined for the presence of adenopathy. The patient is then asked to stand, and the inguinal

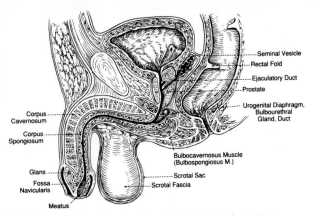

FIG. 2-1. Sagittal section of pelvis and male reproductive system.

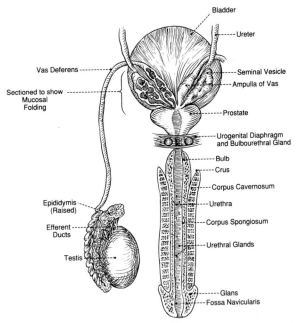

FIG. 2-2. Coronal section of male pelvis and urethra viewed posteriorly.

16

area is again examined for the presence of hernia by direct palpation of the area and again by insertion of the index finger through the neck of the scrotum following the spermatic cord. Both examinations are done with the patient standing quietly and again while he is straining.

Penis

Patients should refrain from voiding, if at all possible, prior to examination because signs of urethritis may not be apparent if the patient has recently voided. In fact, in symptomatic patients who do not have objective evidence of urethritis on examination or on the urethral smear, we suggest repeating the examination before the first urination of the day.

The skin should be examined first. A good light source and a hand lens is strongly recommended. In patients undergoing evaluation for condylomata or in sexual contacts of patients with condylomata, an acid "wash" should be applied after the initial evaluation. This is done by soaking gauze pads in 3 to 5% acetic acid. The gauze is then applied to the skin of the scrotum and penis and left in place for 5 min before the examination is repeated. The patient should then be examined with a magnifying lens in search of "flat warts."

Attention is then directed to examination of the penis. In uncircumcised patients, the foreskin should be retracted to rule out phimosis with an obstructing small opening. This maneuver may reveal balanitis, condylomata, and, occasionally, tumor, as the cause of a foul discharge. The glans and inner surface of the foreskin should be inspected to rule out presence of ulcers, vesicles, or warts. The location of the meatus is determined, and the urethra is examined for presence of spontaneous discharge.

The shaft of the penis and the urethra are palpated for evidence of induration. Induration is often secondary to infection, stricture (or scarring), or, rarely, tumor, abscess, or foreign body inserted by the patient. The urethra should be "milked," or stripped, beginning at the bulbous urethra (located at the perineal body, behind the scrotum in the midline) and proceeding to the meatus. This is necessary for evaluation for urethritis and may yield discharge at the meatus.

Scrotum

The scrotum and its contents are examined next. The testis is the most anterior intrascrotal structure. It should be palpated for masses, and any masses found should be transilluminated. On occasion, the testis may twist within the scrotum, compromising its blood supply. This is termed testicular torsion and is one cause of acute scrotal pain and swelling.

Immediately posterior to the testis is the epididymis, which should be carefully palpated for size, tenderness, and induration. Induration usually results from infection, as primary epididymal tumors are rare. During acute infection, the testis and epididymis are often indistinguishable, since both structures are involved in the inflammatory process. Tenderness is exquisite; swelling may be impressive and accompanied by an acute inflammatory hydrocele.

The spermatic cord at the neck of the scrotum should be palpated between the thumb and index finger. The solid, ropelike vas is usually identified easily and may be followed to its junction with the tail of the epididymis. Varicoceles represent collections of dilated veins and are usually present on the left side of the scrotum. They are best demonstrated with the patient standing and feel "like a bag of worms."

Rectum and Pelvic Organs

Inspection may reveal the presence of external hemorrhoids, rectal fissures, or fistulas. Internal examination is performed by inserting a well-lubricated, gloved index finger into the anal canal. The sphincter tone is evaluated, and the canal is examined for undue tenderness or induration. Presence of induration, rectal stenosis, or mass lesions may indicate the need for additional studies, such as anoscopy or proctoscopy.

With the patient bent over the examining table, the prostate and seminal vesicles are palpated through the anterior rectal wall. Normally, the prostate gland is smooth, somewhat mobile, and nontender. The consistency is rubbery and resembles the tip of the nose. Differential diagnosis of a firm area in the prostate includes cancer, calculi, infarction, granulomatous prostatitis, and nodular benign hyperplasia. Above the prostate it may be possible to feel soft, tubular seminal vesicles extending obliquely beneath the base of the bladder. Usually, clear presence of seminal vesicles on rectal examination indicates a pathologic process.

Females

In the female patient who presents to the STD clinic, few portions of the physical examination will yield as much information as the pelvic examination. Symptomatic pathologic lesions abound, and unsuspected pathologic lesions are found in a significant proportion of relatively asymptomatic women.

Rapport with the patient is always important in the physical examination but is especially critical in the female pelvic exam. Evidence of concern for the patient's concerns at the initial interview

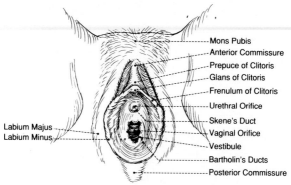

Mons Pubis
Anterior Commissure
Prepuce of Clitoris
Glans of Clitoris
Frenulum of Clitoris
Urethral Orifice
Skene's Duct
Vaginal Orifice
Vestibule
Bartholin's Ducts
Posterior Commissure

Labium Majus
Labium Minus

FIG. 2-3. External genitalia.

will help provide needed rapport. Some specific suggestions to establish and maintain rapport are as follows. Prior to the examination always wash your hands where the patient can see you. Unless you are checking for incontinence, have the patient void before the examination, as a full bladder is uncomfortable and inhibits the examination. Obtain urine for analysis and/or culture if indicated. Recognize that the dorsal lithotomy position is one of vulnerability. The patient's comfort may be improved by elevating the backrest, suggesting that the patient wear her shoes so that the stirrups do not cause discomfort, and providing a drape if desired. The speculum should be kept warm in a warming drawer or warmed with water just before the examination. All the equipment should be present in the examination room, which should be private and quiet.

You should tell the patient what you are doing at each step. It will help her anxiety if she is told of normal structures and normal findings during the examination. A mirror should be available to demonstrate specific findings to the patient, as the more involved she becomes in her own care the more apt she is to return for subsequent visits and necessary treatments. We recommend that the examination proceed in an orderly sequence.

You may begin by having the patient sit on the examining table. If indicated, head and neck examination and inspection, palpation, percussion, and auscultation of the chest and breast may be done in this position. Next, the patient is asked to lie supine. Skin, extremity, breast, cardiovascular, and abdominal examination may be conducted in this position, if indicated. Attention is then directed to the pelvic examination.

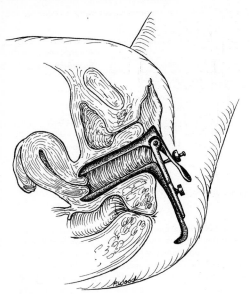

FIG. 2-4. Position of vaginal speculum.

External Genitalia and Perineum

The examination begins with palpation of the inguinal nodes and inspection of the mons pubis and the external genitalia. The pubic hair should be examined for nits indicative of lice infestation.

The labia are separated, and the vaginal introitus is inspected (see Fig. 2-3). Redness signifies an irritation which may be due to infection with *Candida, Trichomonas vaginalis,* herpes simplex virus (HSV), or certain bacteria (e.g., toxic shock syndrome, streptococcal cellulitis). A homogeneous white or gray discharge at the introitus is suggestive of bacterial vaginosis. Small tender fissures in the mucous membrane should arouse suspicion of genital herpes, as many genital HSV occurrences do not form classic ulcerations. Pigmented or nodular areas on the vulva may be due to human papillomavirus infection or carcinoma in situ. Pigmented areas may also be benign nevi or malignant melanomas. Suspicious areas should be removed by excisional biopsy for histologic inspection. The inspection for such lesions should include the frenulum and clitoris.

The urethra with its associated periurethral (Skene's) glands should be palpated and milked by gentle finger pressure from above downward. If infection or a urethral diverticulum is present, a small amount of discharge may be evident at the urethral meatus or at the orifices of Skene's glands.

The greater vestibular glands (of Bartholin) are located at approximately 5 and 7 o'clock on the face of the posterior fourchette. When these regions are explored with gentle pressure between the thumb and forefinger, the normal gland cannot be palpated and the region is not tender. However, an infected gland is extremely tender. If any palpable mass is discovered in this area in a perimenopausal or menopausal woman, it should be removed for histologic examination, as the incidence of carcinoma increases with age.

Vagina, Cervix, Uterus, and Adnexal Structures

Speculum examination and collection of specimens for microscopy and culture A warm speculum should be inserted into the vagina and opened to reveal the cervix. It should be inserted at an angle directed toward the hollow of the sacrum (Fig. 2-4). With the speculum in place, specimens may be obtained for pH determination and wet mount examination of vaginal fluid; vaginal fluid Gram stain and selected cultures, if indicated; and endocervical Gram stain and cultures and Papanicolaou (Pap) smear. If there are no

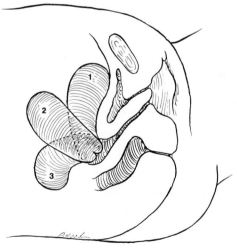

FIG. 2-5. Positions of the uterus: (1) anteverted, (2) midposition, and (3) retroflexed.

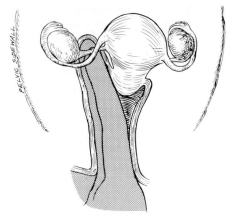

PELVIC SIDEWALL

FIG. 2-6. Preparation for bimanual pelvic examination: placement of vaginal fingers (shaded).

symptoms or signs of vaginal discharge or inflammation, no tests of vaginal fluid are usually done. If such symptoms or signs exist, a specimen of the vaginal discharge should be tested on pH paper to determine the vaginal pH, which is normally 4.5 or less. A vaginal pH above 4.5 suggests bacterial vaginosis or trichomoniasis. Care should be taken to avoid mixing vaginal discharge with cervical mucus for determination of vaginal fluid pH, since cervical mucus has a pH of about 7.0. Vaginal discharge should also be mixed with saline for microscopic examination for motile trichomonads and clue cells; and with 10% potassium hydroxide for detection of a fishy, amine-like odor, characteristic of bacterial vaginosis; and for microscopic detection of fungal elements. A Gram stain of a thinly smeared slide of vaginal discharge is useful for confirming the diagnosis of bacterial vaginosis. With rare exceptions (e.g., toxic shock syndrome), bacterial cultures of vaginal fluid are not useful. However, for detection of *Candida* or *T. vaginalis,* vaginal cultures are more sensitive than microscopic examination of vaginal fluid, especially in the absence of abnormal discharge.

For Pap smear, separate samples should be obtained from the ectocervix including the transformation zone, using an Ayer's spatula; and from the endocervix, using a cytobrush.

Specimens for gonorrhea culture and for diagnosis of chlamydia by culture or antigen detection test are next taken from the endocervix. A specimen of the endocervical mucus can also be inspected for color [yellow indicates increased numbers of polymor-

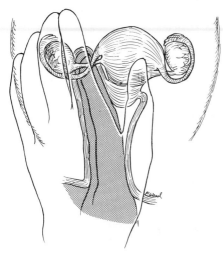

FIG. 2-7. Bimanual examination: comparing position of vaginal fingers (shaded) and abdominal hand.

phonuclear (PMN) leukocytes], and used to prepare a Gram-stained smear for microscopic enumeration of PMN leukocytes in cervical mucus and for detection of gonococci.

While the speculum is still in place, colposcopy can be performed before and after applying dilute (3%) acetic acid and/or dilute Lugol's solution of the cervix. Colposcopy enables one to better visualize cervical, vaginal, and vulvar abnormalities such as dysplasia or infection with human papillomavirus, as well as cervical ulcers caused by HSV, or "strawberry cervix" caused by *T. vaginalis*.

Bimanual examination After removal of the speculum, the first two fingers of the vaginal examining hand are lubricated and inserted into the vagina. This should cause no discomfort other than the sensation of needing to void. The cervix should be palpated and moved. Both it and the attached uterine body should be freely mobile without pain. The body of the uterus is next located by applying suprapubic pressure with the abdominal hand to keep the uterus in the pelvic cavity. The two fingers of the examining vaginal hand should outline the uterus in its entirety. This is usually easy if the uterus is anterior. If it is in a mid or posterior retroflexed position, it will be more difficult to locate and may be best palpated on rectovaginal examination (Fig. 2-5). After the size, shape, position, mobility, consistency, and contour of the uterus are noted, it is moved to one side and the fingers of the examining hand are inserted into the right lateral vaginal fornix as far as possible (Fig. 2-6). The abdominal hand produces pressure on the right lower abdomen and the fingers of the vaginal hand are swept to the side to evaluate the adnexal structures consisting of the tube, ovary, round and cardinal ligaments, and the pelvic sidewall (Fig. 2-7). Only the ovaries should be palpable in the normal examination. Often they are not felt. A normal ovary in a menstruating woman measures approximately $3 \times 3 \times 2$ cm. Any enlargement above 5 to 6 cm is an abnormal finding. Both pelvic sidewalls should be evaluated for enlarged lymph nodes. Tenderness of any of the pelvic structures is noted.

Rectovaginal Examination

After the patient is informed of the procedure, a well-lubricated middle finger is placed in the rectum, and the index finger is simultaneously placed in the vaginal vault. The rectal finger evaluates the entire rectal wall for nodularity or polyps. It is then placed against the cervix, which is felt through the rectal and vaginal wall. Pressure from the abdominal hand brings the uterus down so its entire posterior surface can be palpated with the rectal finger. This is the best method to examine the posterior wall of the uterus if it is in the mid or posterior position in the pelvis.

Throughout the pelvic examination a mental image of the pelvic organs should be formed, noting size, shape, consistency, mobility, contour, and tenderness. These observations should be accurately documented in the record.

LABORATORY EXAMINATION

Laboratory studies are dictated by the differential diagnosis generated by the patient's history and physical findings. Please refer to the appropriate chapters for details.

For a more detailed discussion, see Ostrow DG: Homosexual Behavior and Sexually Transmitted Diseases, Chap. 6, p. 61; Graney DO, Krieger JN: Anatomy and Physical Examination of the Male Genital Tract, Chap. 10, p. 95; and Graney DO, Vontver LA: Anatomy and Physical Examination of the Female Genital Tract, Chap. 11, p. 105, in STD 2.

MICROBIOLOGY

Neisseria gonorrhoeae (gonococci; GC) are the etiologic agent of gonorrhea. GC are gram-negative diplococci, nonmotile and non-spore-forming, which characteristically grow in pairs with adjacent sides flattened.

Techniques have been developed which allow differentiation among strains. The auxotype technique classifies strains according to their ability to grow without certain amino acids or other specific nutrients. Certain auxotypes are biologically and clinically important. One strain, for example, which requires arginine, hypoxanthine, and uracil (AHU−), is associated with multiple other properties, including resistance to killing by normal human serum; propensity for causing asymptomatic male urethral infection; and increased likelihood of causing bacteremia. Strains can also be differentiated by serotyping schemes based on antigenic differences in gonococcal outer membrane protein I.

Gonococci do not tolerate drying; clinical specimens usually must be plated onto appropriate media as soon as they are obtained. Alternatively, specimens may be put into transport media, where the organisms can survive for up to 24 h until they are plated on definitive culture media. Growth is optimal at 35 to 37°C in a 5% CO_2 atmosphere. The organisms require a complex growth medium, which is usually provided in the form of either chocolate agar or similar complex agar. Selective media containing antibiotics is used for culturing sites (such as the cervix, pharynx, or rectum) colonized by less fastidious organisms that would otherwise outgrow the gonococci and obscure their presence.

ANTIMICROBIAL SUSCEPTIBILITY

Compared with other gram-negative bacteria, GC are quite sensitive to antibiotics. However, during the past few decades there has been a gradual selection for antibiotic-resistant strains.

Several independent chromosomal mutations have resulted in a gradual increase in prevalence and extent of resistance to penicillin. In addition, many GC have acquired plasmids which encode for the production of β-lactamase (penicillinase-producing *Neisseria gonorrhoeae,* or PPNG).

Resistance to tetracycline also has increased in recent years. This resistance is due either to the additive effects of several chromosomal mutations or to acquisition of a previously undescribed tetracycline-resistance plasmid.

Spectinomycin resistance has become more common in areas where this antibiotic has been used frequently.

No resistance, however, has yet been reported to ceftriaxone.

EPIDEMIOLOGY

The incidence of gonorrhea varies with age and is highest among young, sexually active people. Eighty-two percent of reported cases in the United States in 1987 occurred in patients aged 15 to 29 years. Demographic risk factors for gonorrhea include low socioeconomic status, urban residence, early onset of sexual activity, unmarried marital status, and a history of past gonorrhea. In the 1980s, illicit drug use and prostitution also appeared to become increasingly associated with increased risk of gonorrhea, syphilis, and probably other sexually transmitted diseases (STDs) as well.

The efficiency of gonorrhea transmission is dependent on anatomic sites exposed as well as number of exposures. The risk of acquiring urethral infection for a man following a single episode of vaginal intercourse with an infected woman is estimated to be about 20 to 30 percent. The single-exposure transmission rate from male to female is higher (about 60 to 80 percent) than that from female to male, in part because of retention of the infected ejaculate within the vagina. The risk of transmission by other types of sexual contact is less well defined. Gonorrhea transmission through insertive or receptive rectal intercourse presumably is relatively efficient. Transmission of pharyngeal infection during fellatio and cunnilingus has been documented and is thought to be rare, although conflicting data exist. In women, use of hormonal contraception may increase risk of acquiring gonorrhea, and use of spermicides and/or the diaphragm clearly has a protective influence. Transmission by fomites or through nonsexual contact is extremely rare but may account for rare cases of gonorrhea in infants.

The prevalence of gonorrhea within communities appears to be sustained by continued transmission by asymptomatically infected persons and also by "core group" transmitters who are more likely than members of the general population to become infected and transmit gonorrhea to their sex partners. Core group members tend to be clustered in geographic areas (usually within inner cities). Members are often persons with repeated episodes of gonorrhea, those who fail to abstain from sex despite the presence of symptoms or knowledge of recent exposure, and patients who practice high-risk behaviors such as illegal drug use, prostitution, or prostitute patronage. At present, gonorrhea control efforts are heavily invested in the concept of vigorous pursuit and treatment of infected core-group members and asymptomatically infected individuals.

CLINICAL MANIFESTATIONS OF UNCOMPLICATED INFECTION

Urethral Infection in Men

Urethritis is the most common manifestation of GC infection in men (Fig. 3-1). The incubation period can range from 1 to more than 14 days, but most men develop symptoms within 2 to 5 days. The predominant symptoms are dysuria or urethral discharge which is often grossly purulent and accompanied by variable degrees of edema and erythema of the urethral meatus. About one-quarter of patients develop only a scant or minimally purulent exudate that is grossly indistinguishable from that of nongonococcal urethritis, and a minority never develop overt signs or symptoms of urethritis.

Without treatment, the usual course of GC urethritis is spontaneous resolution. Complications, however, include epididymitis, acute or chronic prostatitis, posterior urethritis, seminal vesiculitis,

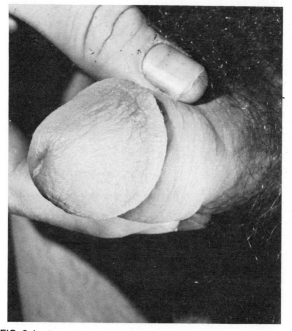

FIG. 3-1. Purulent urethral discharge and penile edema in a patient with gonococcal urethritis.

and infections of Cowper's and Tyson's glands. These are now rare in industrialized societies.

Urogenital Infection in Women

The endocervix is the primary site of GC infection in women. Although urethral colonization is present in most patients, it is uncommon in the absence of endocervical infection, except in hysterectomized women, in whom the urethra is the primary site of infection.

The incubation period in women is more variable than in men, but most women who develop local symptoms do so within 10 days of infection. The most common symptoms include some combination of increased vaginal discharge, dysuria, intermenstrual uterine bleeding, and menorrhagia.

Physical examination may be normal, but many infected women have cervical abnormalities such as mucopurulent cervical discharge, erythema and edema of the zone of ectopy, and bleeding that is easily induced by gentle endocervical swabbing. Exudate can sometimes be expressed from the urethra, periurethral glands, or Bartholin's duct (Fig. 3-2).

Rectal Infection

The rectal mucosa is infected in 35 to 50 percent of women with GC cervical infection and is the only site of infection in 5 percent of women with gonorrhea. In women, rectal infection is usually asymptomatic and unaccompanied by history of rectal sexual contact; infection is assumed to result from local spread of infected cervical secretions.

The rectum is the only site of infection in 40 percent of homosexually active men and is due to direct inoculation through receptive rectal intercourse.

Symptoms of rectal GC range from minimal anal pruritis, painless mucopurulent discharge, or scant rectal bleeding to symptoms of overt proctitis, including severe rectal pain, tenesmus, and constipation.

External inspection of the anus occasionally shows erythema and abnormal discharge, but anoscopy often reveals mucoid or purulent exudate, erythema, edema, friability, or other inflammatory mucosal changes (see Chap. 25 for a discussion of sexually transmitted proctitis).

Pharyngeal Infection

Among patients with gonorrhea, pharyngeal infection occurs in 3 to 7 percent of heterosexual men, 10 to 20 percent of heterosexual

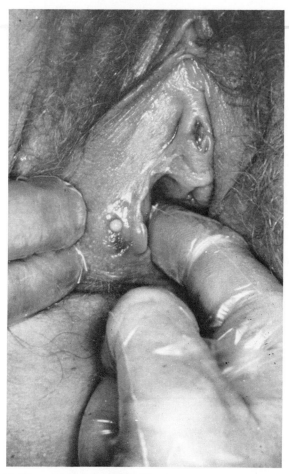

FIG 3-2. Purulent exudate expressed from the Bartholin's gland duct of a woman with gonococcal Bartholin's gland abscess. *(From JA Davies et al., Br J Vener Dis 54:409, 1978.)*

women, and 10 to 25 percent of homosexual men. The pharynx is the sole site of infection in less than 5 percent of patients irrespective of gender or sexual orientation. Infection is usually transmitted to the pharynx by orogenital sexual contact and is more efficiently acquired by fellatio than by cunnilingus. Transmission of gonorrhea from patients with pharyngeal infection to their sex partners is inefficient and relatively rare.

Although pharyngeal GC infection may cause acute pharyngitis or tonsillitis and occasionally is associated with fever or cervical lymphadenopathy, over 90 percent of infections are asymptomatic.

COMPLICATIONS OF LOCAL GONOCOCCAL INFECTION

Local Complications in Men

The most common local complication of GC urethritis in men is epididymitis, which is characterized by unilateral testicular pain and swelling. Most patients with GC epididymitis have overt urethritis when they present.

Other complications include penile lymphangitis, generalized penile edema, urethral strictures, and periurethral abscesses, all of which are rare in the postantibiotic era.

Local Complications in Women

Acute salpingitis or pelvic inflammatory disease (PID) is the most common of all complications of gonorrhea. It occurs in an estimated 10 to 20 percent of women with acute GC infection.

Patients with GC PID usually present with various combinations of lower abdominal pain, dyspareunia, abnormal menses, intermenstrual bleeding, or other complaints consistent with intraabdominal infection.

Physical examination usually reveals lower abdominal, uterine, or adnexal tenderness; cervical motion pain; abnormal cervical discharge; and sometimes an adnexal mass or tuboovarian abscess.

Gram stains of cervical secretions may show gram-negative intracellular diplococci, but the Gram stain is negative in 40 to 60 percent of women with GC PID. Laboratory investigation may reveal fever, leukocytosis, elevation of the erythrocyte sedimentation rate, and increased levels of C-reactive protein.

Infertility and ectopic pregnancy are important long-term sequelae of this syndrome.

Apart from salpingitis, Bartholin's gland abscess is the most common urogenital complication of gonorrhea in women.

SYSTEMIC COMPLICATIONS

Disseminated Gonococcal Infection

Disseminated gonococcal infection (DGI) is the most common systemic complication of acute gonorrhea and occurs in 0.5 to 3 percent of patients with untreated mucosal gonorrhea.

As suggested by the pseudonym *arthritis-dermatitis syndrome,* the most common clinical manifestations of DGI are joint pain and skin lesions. Skin lesions, occurring in 50 to 75 percent of DGI patients, generally present on the distal portions of extremities and usually number fewer than 30. Although the classic skin lesion is a tender, necrotic pustule on an erythematous base, macules, papules, pustules, petechiae, bullae, or ecchymoses are often seen.

Many patients have arthralgia or tenosynovitis early in the disease. Approximately 30 to 40 percent of patients with DGI have frank arthritis. While any joint may be involved, knee, wrist, ankle, or metacarpophalangeal joints are most commonly affected (see Chap. 27).

The syndrome is more common in women than in men. In about half of women with DGI, onset of symptoms occurs within 7 days following menstruation. Several studies have also cited pregnancy and pharyngeal gonorrhea as risk factors. In addition, complement deficiency may predispose individuals to *Neisseria* bacteremia. However, since only a small percentage of DGI patients have complement deficiency syndromes, screening for complement deficiency should only be performed in persons with a second episode of systemic *Neisseria* infection.

Patients with clinical manifestations of DGI are often stratified on the basis of mucosal and blood culture results into proven, probable, and possible DGI. Patients with positive cultures from blood, joint fluid, skin lesions, or otherwise sterile sites (proven DGI) constitute less than 50 percent of DGI cases. In more than 80 percent of DGI patients, *N. gonorrhoeae* may be isolated from anogenital or pharyngeal cultures or from a sexual partner; in the absence of positive blood or other sterile-site cultures, these patients are referred to as having probable DGI. Patients with an appropriate clinical syndrome and the expected response to therapy but with negative cultures are referred to as having possible DGI.

Clinical manifestations arise from bacteremia, but proving infection in patients with DGI is sometimes difficult. The bacteremia associated with DGI is not continuous, and positive blood cultures become less common as the duration of clinical signs and symptoms increases. Overall, only 20 to 30 percent of DGI patients have positive blood cultures. Nearly all gonococci isolated from patients with DGI are serum-resistant but may be inhibited by the concentrations of vancomycin contained in selective media for gonococcal isolation from mucosal sites and by the sodium polyanetholsulfonate anticoagulant used in many blood culture media.

Gonococcal Endocarditis and Meningitis

GC endocarditis is an uncommon complication of GC bacteremia, occurring in an estimated 1 to 3 percent of patients with DGI. Nonetheless, recognition of GC endocarditis among patients with DGI is essential because of the possibility of rapidly progressive valvular damage with life-threatening consequences. The aortic valve is most often infected.

Fewer than 25 cases of GC meningitis have been reported. Case reports of this complication describe patients with typical presentations of acute bacterial meningitis, usually without typical findings of DGI.

LABORATORY DIAGNOSIS

Culture

Isolation of *N. gonorrhoeae* is the diagnostic standard for GC infections. Available antibiotic-containing selective media (e.g., modified Thayer-Martin medium) have diagnostic sensitivities of 80 to 95 percent for promptly incubated specimens, depending in part on the anatomic site cultured (Table 3-1). (Vancomycin-containing selective culture media sometimes fail to support growth of vancomycin-sensitive gonococci. The prevalence of such strains varies among geographic areas.)

For urethral specimens from symptomatic men, selective and nonselective media are equally sensitive because the concentration of gonococci in the urethra usually exceeds that of other flora. In contrast, selective media should be used for culturing the endocervix, rectum, and pharynx, where other less fastidious bacteria often outnumber *N. gonorrhoeae.*

For women, single endocervical cultures on most selective media detect 80 to 90 percent of cervical infections. Urethral cultures should be performed in women with suspected gonorrhea who have undergone hysterectomy. Otherwise, for women, cultures of the urethra, accessory gland ducts, anal canal, and pharynx should be considered optional, depending on symptoms, sites exposed, culture methods employed, and available resources.

Recommended culture sites for men also depend on sexual orientation and anatomic sites exposed. For heterosexual men, culture of urethral exudate alone is usually sufficient. Pharyngeal cultures may also be useful for men with pharyngitis who practice cunnilingus or men who have performed cunnilingus with a woman known to have gonorrhea. Among homosexually active men,

TABLE 3-1. Frequency of Isolation of *Neisseria gonorrhoeae* by Site from Patients with Uncomplicated Gonorrhea*

	N	Total positive number (%)	Only site positive, number (%)
Women	162		
Endocervix		155 (96)	75 (46)
Anal canal		62 (38)	3 (2)
Pharynx		35 (22)	4 (3)
Heterosexual men	177		
Urethra		177 (100)	166 (94)
Pharynx		11 (6)	0
Homosexual men	355		
Urethra		205 (58)	146 (41)
Anal canal		177 (50)	109 (31)
Pharynx		62 (17)	18 (5)

*Analysis limited to patients for whom all indicated sites were cultured; single cultures on modified Thayer-Martin medium were used.
Women who had undergone hysterectomy were excluded.
SOURCE: Data are combined from the following references: data on women and heterosexual men are from HH Handsfield et al, *Sex Transm Dis* 7:1, 1980; data on homosexual men are combined from HH Handsfield et al, *Sex Transm Dis* 7:1, 1980, and WM Janda et al, *JAMA* 244:2060, 1980.

urethral and anal cultures both have high yield, while pharyngeal cultures are positive less often.

Stained Smears

Several dyes have been used to prepare clinical specimens for microscopic examination for gonococci, but Gram's stain has been the most extensively studied. A smear is positive when gram-negative diplococci with typical morphology are identified within or closely associated with polymorphonuclear leukocytes (Fig. 3-3); it is considered equivocal if only extracellular organisms or morphologically atypical intracellular gram-negative diplococci are seen, and negative if no gram-negative diplococci are present. Table 3-2 shows the sensitivity and specificity of gram-stained smears for various categories of genital and rectal infection relative to isolation of *N. gonorrhoeae*.

Urethral smears from men with urethritis are sensitive and specific, but in general, isolation should also be attempted to permit testing for antimicrobial resistance.

Culture is the standard for diagnosis of gonorrhea in women; stained smears should be used as an adjunct to, but not replacement for, culture. Although endocervical smears are less sensitive than

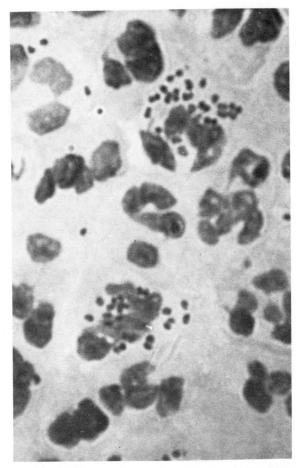

FIG. 3-3. Gram-stained smear showing polymorphonuclear leukocytes with intracellular gram-negative diplococci in urethral exudate from a man with gonococcal urethritis (× 1000).

TABLE 3-2. Sensitivity and Specificity of Gram-Stained Smears for Detection of Genital or Anorectal Gonorrhea

Site and clinical setting	Sensitivity*	Specificity*
Urethra		
Men with symptomatic urethritis	90–95	95–100
Men with asymptomatic urethral infection	50–70	95–100
Endocervix		
Uncomplicated gonorrhea	50–70	95–100
Pelvic inflammatory disease	60–70	95–100
Anorectum		
Blind swabs	40–60	95–100
Anoscopically obtained specimens	70–80	95–100

*Sensitivity = percent of patients with positive cultures who have positive Gram-stained smears. Specificity = percent of patients with negative cultures whose Gram-stained smears also are negative.

The studies showing 95–100% specificity for anorectal smears did not report whether meningococcal infection was distinguished from gonorrhea. Until further data are available, a positive anorectal smear should be considered highly specific for either gonococcal or meningococcal infection.

SOURCE: Data are combined from the following references: HH Handsfield et al, *N Engl J Med* 290: 117, 1974; NF Jacobs, SJ Kraus, *Ann Intern Med* 82:7, 1975; RN Thin, EJ Shaw, *Br J Vener Dis* 55:10, 1979; D Barlow, I Phillips, *Lancet* 1:761, 1978; J Wallin, *Br J Vener Dis* 51:41, 1974; RB Rothenberg et al, *JAMA* 235:49, 1976; ER Wald, *Am J Dis Child* 131:1094, 1977; DC William et al, *Sex Transm Dis* 8:16, 1981; P Deheragoda, *Br J Vener Dis* 53:311, 1977.

those from the urethra, positive endocervical smears are specific and have a high predictive value when obtained from women with signs or symptoms of genital tract infection. Predictive value of smears is lower, however, when they are used for screening asymptomatic women. Pharyngeal Gram stains are both insensitive and nonspecific and are not recommended.

Other Diagnostic Techniques

Although serologic tests and rapid diagnostic techniques (e.g., immunologic or biochemical detection of gonococcal antigens or metabolic products) are under investigation, these modalities are not widely available for clinical use at the present time.

TREATMENT REGIMENS FOR *N. GONORRHOEAE*

The choice of antimicrobial agents for gonorrhea therapy is influenced by a variety of factors. Antibiotic serum levels should be greater than or equal to three times the minimum inhibitory concentration of the infecting strain of *N. gonorrhoeae* for at least 8 h in order to reliably cure uncomplicated infection. Single-dose therapy is preferred for gonorrhea in order to enhance patient compliance. In addition, the choice of antimicrobial agents should reflect local patterns of antimicrobial resistance and the probability that patients with acute GC infection are coinfected with or have recently been exposed to other STD agents. *Chlamydia trachomatis,* for example, coinfects 15 to 25 percent of men and 30 to 50 percent of women with acute urogenital gonorrhea. Until universal testing for chlamydia with quick, inexpensive, and highly accurate tests becomes available, it is generally more cost-effective to treat presumptive chlamydial infections in all persons with gonorrhea. Thus, all regimens outlined below include an empirical course of treatment for chlamydial disease.

Uncomplicated Urethral, Endocervical, or Rectal Infections in Adults

Recommended Regimens
Ceftriaxone 125 mg IM, once *or* **cefixime 400 mg orally, once** *or* **ciprofloxacin 500 mg orally, once** *or* **ofloxacin 400 mg orally, once** *plus* **a regimen effective against possible coinfection with *C. trachomatis,* such as doxycycline 100 mg orally 2 times a day for 7 days.** Ciprofloxacin and ofloxacin are contraindicated for pregnant or nursing women, and for children less than 18 years of age.

Alternative Regimens
For patients who cannot take cephalosporins or quinolones, the preferred alternative is **spectinomycin 2 g IM, in a single dose (followed by doxycycline).**

If infection was acquired from a source proved not to have penicillin-resistant gonorrhea, a penicillin such as **amoxicillin 3 g orally with 1 g probenecid followed by doxycycline** may be used for treatment.

Management of Sex Partners

Persons exposed to gonorrhea within the preceding 30 days should be examined, specimens cultured, and the patients treated presumptively.

Follow-up

Patients treated with any of the regimens recommended above need not return for a follow-up culture ("test of cure"). In many instances, a more cost-effective strategy may be to reexamine with culture 1 to 2 months after treatment ("rescreening"); this strategy will detect both treatment failures and reinfections. Patients should be advised to return for examination if any symptoms persist at the completion of treatment.

Treatment Failures

Persistent symptoms after treatment should be evaluated by culture for *N. gonorrhoeae,* and any gonococcal isolate should be tested for antibiotic sensitivity. Symptoms of urethritis may also be caused by *C. trachomatis* and other organisms associated with nongono-coccal urethritis. Additional treatment for gonorrhea should be **ceftriaxone 125 mg, followed by doxycycline.** Infections occurring after treatment with one of the recommended regimens are commonly due to reinfection rather than treatment failure and indicate a need for improved sex partner referral and patient education.

Pharyngeal Gonococcal Infection

Recommended Regimen
Ceftriaxone 125 mg IM once. Patients who cannot be treated with ceftriaxone should be treated with **ciprofloxacin 500 mg orally as a single dose.** Since experience with this regimen is limited, such patients should be evaluated with repeat culture 3 to 7 days after treatment.

Treatment of Gonococcal Infections in Pregnancy

Pregnant women should be cultured for *N. gonorrhoeae* (and tested for *C. trachomatis* and syphilis) at the first prenatal care visit. In women at high risk of STD, a second culture for gonorrhea (as well as tests for chlamydia and syphilis) should be obtained late in the third trimester.

Recommended Regimen
Ceftriaxone 250 mg IM once plus erythromycin base 500 mg orally 4 times a day for 7 days (erythromycin stearate 500 mg or erythromycin ethylsuccinate 800 mg or equivalent may be substituted for erythromycin base).

Pregnant women allergic to β-lactams should be treated with **spectinomycin 2 g IM once (followed by erythromycin).** Follow-up cervical and rectal cultures for *N. gonorrhoeae* should be obtained 3 to 7 days after completion of treatment.

Disseminated Gonococcal Infection

Hospitalization is recommended for initial therapy, especially for those who cannot reliably comply with treatment, have uncertain diagnoses, or have purulent synovial effusions or other complications. Patients should be examined for clinical evidence of endocarditis or meningitis.

Recommended Initial Regimen
Ceftriaxone 1 g IM or IV every 24 h
Alternative Initial Regimens
Cefotaxime 1g IV every 8h. *or* **ceftizoxime 1g IV every 8h,** *or* **(for patients allergic to betalactam drugs) spectinomycin 2g IM every 12h.**

When the infecting organism is proved to be penicillin-sensitive, parenteral treatment may be switched to **ampillin 1 g every 6 h (or equivalent).**

Patients treated for DGI should be tested for genital *C. trachomatis* infection. If chlamydial testing is not available, the patients should be treated empirically for coexisting chlamydial infection.

Reliable patients with uncomplicated disease may be discharged 24 to 48 h after all symptoms resolve, and complete therapy should be used (for a total of 1 week of antibiotic therapy) with an oral regimen of **cefixime 400g orally twice a day,** *or* **ciprofloxacin 500 mg 2 times a day.** Ciprofloxacin is contraindicated in pregnant and nursing women, and persons less than 18 years of age.

Meningitis and Endocarditis

Meningitis and endocarditis caused by *N. gonorrhoeae* require high-dose IV therapy with an agent effective against the strain causing the disease, such as **ceftriaxone 1 to 2 g IV every 12 h.** Optimal duration of therapy is unknown, but most clinicians treat patients with gonococcal meningitis for 10 to 14 days and with gonococcal endocarditis for at least 4 weeks.

Adult Gonococcal Ophthalmia

Adults and children over 20 kg with nonsepticemic gonococcal ophthalmia should be treated with **ceftriaxone 1 g IM once.** Irrigation of the eyes with saline or buffered ophthalmic solutions may be useful adjunctive therapy to eliminate discharge. All patients must have careful ophthalmologic assessment including slit-lamp examination for ocular complications. Topical antibiotics alone are not sufficient therapy and are unnecessary when appropriate systemic therapy is given. Simultaneous ophthalmic infection with *C.*

trachomatis has been reported and should be considered in patients who do not respond promptly.

PREVENTION

Properly used condoms provide a high degree of protection against acquisition and transmission of gonorrhea and other genital infections. The diaphragm and cervical cap may also reduce transmission and acquisition of endocervical infection. Topical spermicidal and bactericidal agents have been shown recently to reduce the probability of infection by both *N. gonorrhoeae* and *C. trachomatis* in patients using these gels.

ADDITIONAL READING

Balachandran T et al: Single-dose therapy of anogenital and pharyngeal gonorrhoea with ciprofloxacin. *Int J STD AIDS* 3:49, 1992

Bickell NA et al: Human papillomavirus, gonorrhea, syphilis, and cervical dysplasia in jailed women. *Am J Public Health* 81:1318, 1991

Covino JM et al: Comparison of ofloxacin and ceftriaxone in the treatment of uncomplicated gonorrhea caused by penicillinase-producing and non-penicillinase-producing strains. *Antimicrob Agents Chemother* 34:148, 1990

Faro S et al: Effectiveness of ofloxacin in the treatment of *Chlamydia trachomatis* and *Neisseria gonorrhoeae* cervical infection. *Am J Obstet Gynecol* 164:1380, 1991

Gershman KA, Rolfs RT: Diverging gonorrhea and syphilis trends in the 1980s: Are they real? *Am J Public Health* 81:1263, 1991

Goldstein AM et al: Comparison of single-dose ceftizoxime or ceftriaxone in the treatment of uncomplicated urethral gonorrhea. *Sex Transm Dis* 18:180, 1991

Gransden WR et al: 4-Quinolone-resistant *Neisseria gonorrhoeae* in the United Kingdom. *J Med Microbiol* 34:23, 1991

Handsfield HH et al: A comparison of single-dose cefixime with ceftriaxone as treatment for uncomplicated gonorrhea. The Gonorrhea Treatment Study Group. *N Engl J Med* 325:1337, 1991

Ison CA, Easmon CS: Epidemiology of penicillin resistant *Neisseria gonorrhoeae*. *Genitourin Med* 67:307, 1991

Ngeow YF et al: Treatment of gonorrhea with sulbactam/ampicillin. *Sex Transm Dis* 18:192, 1991

Rice RJ et al: Sociodemographic distribution of gonorrhea incidence: Implications for prevention and behavioral research. *Am J Public Health* 81:1252, 1991

Schwarcz SK et al: Crack cocaine and the exchange of sex for money or drugs. Risk factors for gonorrhea among black adolescents in San Francisco. *Sex Transm Dis* 19:7, 1992

Smith BL et al: Evaluation of ofloxacin in the treatment of uncomplicated gonorrhea. *Sex Transm Dis* 18:18, 1991

Upchurch DM et al: Behavioral contributions to acquisition of gonorrhea in patients attending an inner city sexually transmitted disease clinic. *J Infect Dis* 161:938, 1990

Zimmerman HL et al: Epidemiologic differences between chlamydia and gonorrhea. *Am J Public Health* 80:1338, 1990

For a more detailed discussion, see Sparling PF: Biology of *Neisseria gonorrhoeae,* Chap. 13, p. 131; Hook EW III, Handsfield HH: Gonococcal Infections in the Adult, Chap. 14, p. 149, in STD-2.

Chlamydia trachomatis, one of the three species within the genus *Chlamydia,* is an important cause of blindness and sexually transmitted diseases in humans (Table 4-1). This species contains three biovars that have distinctive clinical and biological differences. The trachoma biovar includes strains that cause common human genital tract diseases (urethritis, cervicitis, salpingitis, infant diseases, etc.) and trachoma. The lymphogranuloma venereum (LGV) biovar is related serologically to the trachoma serovar but produces a much more invasive clinical disease.

MICROBIOLOGY

Chlamydiae are obligate intracellular bacteria that lack the ability to synthesize high-energy compounds (such as ATP and GTP). Chlamydiae are distinguished from all other microorganisms on the basis of a unique growth cycle. The cycle alternates between two highly specialized morphologic forms that are adapted to either intracellular or extracellular environments. The infectious particle, the elementary body (EB), is relatively resistant to the extracellular environment but is not metabolically active. This particle attaches to the host cell, enters it, and changes to a metabolically active and dividing form called the reticulate body (RB). The organism then uses host cell substrates to synthesize its own RNA, DNA, and protein. Glycogen accumulates within the inclusions of *C. trachomatis,* reaching levels detectable by iodine stain at 30 to 48 h postinfection. The RBs divide by binary fission from about 8 h to 18 to 24 h after entry into the cell. This is the stage of greatest metabolic activity when the organisms are most sensitive to inhibitors of bacterial metabolic activity. This entire cycle takes place within the phagosome, which undergoes a large increase in size. At some time between 48 and 72 h the cell ruptures, releasing the infectious EBs.

The disease process and clinical manifestations of chlamydial infections probably represent the combined effects of tissue damage resulting from chlamydial replication as well as the inflammatory responses caused by the presence of chlamydiae and necrotic material from the destroyed host cells. Yet, despite the release of hundreds of viable EBs by each inclusion, relatively few nearby cells are infected. Control mechanisms that limit infectivity must therefore exist, but the mechanisms are not clear. Immunity induced by chlamydial infection is not well understood. It is clear that single infections will not result in solid immunity to reinfection. The

TABLE 4-1. Human Diseases Caused by Chlamydiae

Species	Serovar*	Disease
C. psittaci	Many unidentified serovars	Psittacosis
C. pneumoniae	TWAR	Respiratory disease
C. trachomatis	L1, L2, L3	Lymphogranuloma venereum
C. trachomatis	A, B, Ba, C	Hyperendemic blindness trachoma
C. trachomatis	D, E, F, G, H, I, J, K	Inclusion conjunctivitis (adult and newborn), nongonococcal urethritis, cervicitis, salpingitis, proctitis, epididymitis, pneumonia of newborns

*Predominant, but not exclusive, association of serovar with disease.
SOURCE: Schachter J, *N Engl J Med* 298:428, 490, 540, 1978.

immune response may contribute to some of the late sequelae of genital chlamydia infection, including scarring of the fallopian tubes.

EPIDEMIOLOGY

Since the early 1970s, *C. trachomatis* has been recognized as a genital pathogen responsible for an increasing variety of clinical syndromes, many closely resembling infections caused by *Neisseria gonorrhoeae* (Table 4-2). Because few practitioners have access to facilities for isolation of *C. trachomatis,* these infections must usually be diagnosed and treated without benefit of microbiological confirmation. Newer, noncultural diagnostic tests using antigen-detection methods have in part addressed this problem but are not available to many clinicians. Unfortunately, many chlamydial infections, particularly in women, are difficult to diagnose clinically and elude detection because they produce few or no symptoms and because the symptoms and signs they do produce are nonspecific. Incidence of these infections has increased in large part due to inadequate laboratory facilities for their detection and eventual treatment; the nonspecific signs and symptoms of chlamydial infections; the lack of familiarity of clinicians with these infections; and the lack of resources directed toward screening of high-risk patients, contact tracing, and treatment of infected partners.

The prevalence of chlamydial urethral infection in men ranges from 3 to 5 percent of asymptomatic men seen in general medical

TABLE 4-2. Clinical Parallels Between Genital Infections Caused by *N. gonorrhoeae* and *C. trachomatis*

Site of infection	Resulting clinical syndrome	
	N. gonorrhoeae	*C. trachomatis*
Men:		
Urethra	Urethritis	NGU, PGU
Epididymis	Epididymitis	Epididymitis
Rectum	Proctitis	Proctitis
Conjunctiva	Conjunctivitis	Conjunctivitis
Systemic	Disseminated gonococcal infection	Reiter's syndrome
Women:		
Urethra	Acute urethral syndrome	Acute urethral syndrome
Bartholin's gland	Bartholinitis	Bartholinitis
Cervix	Cervicitis	Cervicitis, cervical metaplasia
Fallopian tube	Salpingitis	Salpingitis
Conjunctiva	Conjunctivitis	Conjunctivitis
Liver capsule	Perihepatitis	Perihepatitis
Systemic	Disseminated gonococcal infection	Reactive arthritis

settings to 15 to 20 percent of all men seen in STD clinics (Fig. 4-1). Prevalence and site of mucosal infection as judged by positive culture appear to be strongly correlated with both age and sexual orientation. Several studies have revealed a higher prevalence of urethral infection due to chlamydia among heterosexual men than among male homosexuals. However, chlamydial infection is a cause of proctitis among homosexual men who practice receptive rectal intercourse without condom protection. Prevalence has generally been higher in nonwhites than in whites. Evidence of chlamydial infection has been infrequent in sexually inexperienced populations.

Prevalence of chlamydial infection among women has ranged from 3 to 5 percent in asymptomatic women to over 20 percent in women seen in STD clinics (Fig. 4-2). Demographic factors associated with an increased risk of chlamydial isolation in several studies include young age, nonwhite race, single marital status, and use of oral contraceptives. The proportion of sexually active women with positive cervical cultures for *C. trachomatis* has been highest for women aged 15 to 21 and declines strikingly thereafter, while the prevalence of serum antibody increases with age until about 30 years, when it plateaus at approximately 50 percent. Sexually inexperienced populations rarely exhibit chlamydial cervical infections.

The incidence of *C. trachomatis* genital infection in both men and

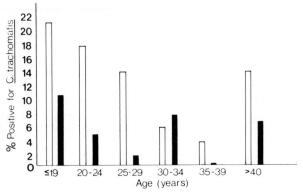

FIG. 4-1. Prevalence of *C. trachomatis* urethral infection by age in men attending an STD clinic. *Open bars* = heterosexual men; *solid bars* = homosexual or bisexual men.

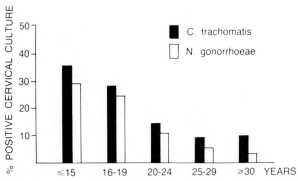

FIG. 4-2. Prevalence of *C. trachomatis* and *N. gonorrhoeae* cervical infection by age in women attending an STD clinic. *Open bars* = *N. gonorrhoeae; solid bars* = *C. trachomatis.*

women is uncertain because the infection produces no specific symptoms and is often asymptomatic, is seldom confirmed micro-biologically, and is rarely reported. Transmissibility is also under-stood poorly. Preliminary studies suggest that chlamydial infection may be associated with slightly lower transmission rates than gonorrhea, although the differing lengths of incubation and differing efficiency of isolation of these two agents may at least partly explain these results.

CLINICAL MANIFESTATIONS

Clinical manifestations of genital infections caused by *C. trachomatis* closely parallel those due to *N. gonorrhoeae* (Table 4-2). Both organisms preferentially infect columnar or transitional epithelium of the urethra, with extension to the epididymis; the endocervix, with extension to the endometrium, salpinx, and peritoneum; and the rectum. Both organisms can produce extensive subepithelial inflammation, epithelial ulceration, and scarring. *Chlamydia trachomatis,* with the exception of LGV biovars, rarely produces systemic manifestations.

INFECTIONS IN MEN

Urethritis

Evidence suggests that *C. trachomatis* causes 35 to 50 percent of nongonococcal urethritis (NGU) in heterosexual men. Chlamydia-positive and chlamydia-negative NGU cannot be differentiated on the basis of signs or symptoms. Both usually present with dysuria and mild to moderate whitish or clear urethral discharge. Examination reveals no abnormalities other than the discharge in most cases; associated adenopathy, focal urethral tenderness, and meatal or penile lesions suggest herpetic urethritis. Gonorrhea usually presents after a 3- to 10-day incubation period with a white to yellow-green urethral discharge, whereas chlamydial infection produces milder urethritis and has a longer (7- to 21-day) incubation period.

Both *C. trachomatis* and gonococcal urethral infection may be asymptomatic. Many men with asymptomatic chlamydial urethral infection have persistent urethral leukocytosis [≥ four polymorphonuclear leukocytes (PMNs) per 1000× field] on Gram stains of urethral secretions or persistent pyuria in a first-void urine, indicating ongoing inflammation.

Interestingly, postgonococcal urethritis in heterosexual men, like NGU, frequently results from *C. trachomatis* infection. These patients probably acquire gonorrhea and chlamydial infection simultaneously but, due to the longer incubation period of *C. trachomatis,* develop a biphasic illness if their original gonorrhea is treated with an agent that does not eradicate chlamydia. It is possible that gonococcal infection causes reactivation of latent chlamydial infection, although this is still speculative. Coinfection with these two agents occurs in 15 to 35 percent of heterosexual men with gonorrhea but rarely in homosexual men.

Epididymitis and Prostatitis

Chlamydia trachomatis causes most cases of what was previously termed idiopathic epididymitis in young, heterosexually active males. Clinically, chlamydial epididymitis presents as unilateral scrotal pain, swelling, tenderness, and fever in a young male who often has associated chlamydial urethritis, though the urethritis may be asymptomatic. Men with chlamydial epididymitis improve rapidly with tetracycline treatment, supporting the causal role of *C. trachomatis*. The role of chlamydia in nonbacterial prostatitis, however, remains unclear.

Proctitis

Both LGV and non-LGV immunotypes can produce proctitis in persons who practice receptive anal intercourse. Non-LGV immunotypes produce milder infections than LGV, and range from asymptomatic infection to symptomatic proctitis resembling gonococcal proctitis with rectal pain and bleeding, mucous discharge, and diarrhea. Most *C. trachomatis*–infected patients have abnormal numbers of PMNs in their rectal Gram stain, and on sigmoidoscopy, those with symptoms are found to have friable rectal mucosa.

Reiter's Syndrome

Both Reiter's syndrome (urethritis, conjunctivitis, arthritis, and characteristic mucocutaneous lesions) and reactive tenosynovitis or arthritis without the other components of Reiter's syndrome have been related to genital infection with *C. trachomatis*. Microimmunofluorescent antibody assays indicate that preceding or concurrent infection with *C. trachomatis* is present in more than 80 percent of men with the syndrome (see Chap. 27).

Like postenteric *(Salmonella, Shigella, Yersinia)* arthritides, sacroiliitis, and spondylitis, Reiter's syndrome occurs with increased frequency in patients with the HLA-B27 haplotype. The HLA-B27 haplotype appears to confer a 10-fold increased risk of developing Reiter's syndrome.

INFECTIONS IN WOMEN

Cervicitis

While many women with chlamydia isolated from the cervix have no signs or symptoms of infection, at least a third have local signs. Most commonly found are mucopurulent discharge (37 percent of women) and hypertrophic ectopy (19 percent). *Hypertrophic ectopy* refers to an area of cervical ectopy that is edematous, congested, and bleeds easily. Women with these signs of chlamydial cervicitis yield greater numbers of chlamydial inclusion–forming units on primary isolation in tissue culture than women who have chlamydial infection without cervicitis.

The prevalence of *C. trachomatis* infection appears greater in women with cervical ectopy than in those without ectopy. Ectopy may predispose women to chlamydial infection by exposing a greater number of susceptible columnar epithelial cells, making infection more likely upon exposure. Alternatively, ectopy may increase the shedding of *C. trachomatis* from the cervix, or *C. trachomatis* infection of the cervix may cause ectopy. Oral contraceptives have also been associated with increased risk of cervical chlamydial infection, probably because their use promotes ectopy; the increased risk appears limited to oral contraceptive users with ectopy.

Clinical recognition of chlamydial cervicitis depends upon a high index of suspicion and a careful cervical examination. Findings suggestive of chlamydial infection include easily induced endocervical bleeding, mucopurulent cervical discharge, and edema of an area of ectopy. The differential diagnosis of mucopurulent discharge from the endocervical canal in a young, sexually active woman includes chlamydial infection; gonococcal endocervicitis; and endometritis of various causes, including IUD-induced inflammation. Gram stain of appropriately collected mucopurulent endocervical discharge from patients with chlamydial endocervicitis usually shows greater than 30 PMNs per 1000× field, and only occasional bacteria. Similarly, the observation of purulent (yellow or green) cervical discharge on a cervical swab correlates with the presence of chlamydial and/or gonococcal infection. Unfortunately, the majority of women with chlamydial infection cannot be distinguished from uninfected women by clinical examination or by these simple tests.

Nearly all women with endocervical chlamydial infections have or develop antibodies to *C. trachomatis.* Only 20 to 30 percent exhibit IgM antibody at the time of diagnosis, however, suggesting that many newly diagnosed cervical infections in women are not recent but long-lived. Sequential culturing of samples from untreated women has demonstrated that chlamydial infection may persist for weeks or months without development of symptoms, or may spontaneously resolve.

Urethritis

Screening studies in STD clinics suggest that among women from whom specimens from both the cervix and urethra were cultured for *C. trachomatis,* 50 percent are positive at both sites and 25 percent at either site alone. Available evidence implicates *Chlamydia* as an important cause of dysuria in young, sexually active women with pyuria and no bacteriuria or other urinary pathogens. Although urethral symptoms may develop in women with chlamydial infection, the majority of female STD clinic patients with urethral chlamydial infection do not have dysuria or frequency. Even in women with symptomatic chlamydial urethritis, signs of urethritis (urethral discharge, meatal redness, or swelling) are infrequent. Nevertheless, the presence of mucopurulent cervicitis in a woman with dysuria and frequency should suggest concomitant chlamydial urethritis.

Chlamydia trachomatis urethritis should be suspected in young, sexually active women with dysuria, frequency, and pyuria, especially if they have had a new sex partner within the last month or a sex partner with NGU. Other correlates of chlamydial urethral syndrome include duration of dysuria of more than 7 to 10 days, lack of hematuria, lack of suprapubic tenderness, and use of birth control pills. An abnormal urethral Gram stain showing greater than or equal to 10 PMNs per oil-immersion field in women with dysuria but without coliform bacteriuria supports the diagnosis of chlamydial urethritis. However, this finding is also seen in women with gonococcal or trichomonal infection of the urethra.

Bartholinitis

Like gonococci, *C. trachomatis* may produce an exudative infection of Bartholin's ducts. Purulent infections of Bartholin's ducts may thus be due to chlamydial infection, either alone or with concurrent gonococcal infection.

Endometritis

Histologic evidence of endometritis is present in nearly one-half of patients with chlamydial mucopurulent cervicitis and can be demonstrated in nearly all patients with chlamydial salpingitis. Chlamydial cervicitis probably spreads through the endometrial cavity to reach the fallopian tubes. Intrapartum fever and late postpartum endometritis are associated with untreated antenatal *C. trachomatis* infection.

Salpingitis

The proportion of acute salpingitis cases due to *C. trachomatis* varies geographically and with the population studied. As discussed in Chap. 22, many cases of chlamydial salpingitis are associated with mild or absent symptoms or signs, despite progressive tubal scarring, resulting in ectopic pregnancy or infertility.

Perihepatitis (Fitz-Hugh-Curtis Syndrome)

Perihepatitis occurring after or with salpingitis has long been a recognized complication of gonococcal infection. Recent studies suggest that chlamydial infection may be more commonly associated with perihepatitis than is *N. gonorrhoeae*. Perihepatitis should be suspected in young, sexually active women who develop right upper-quadrant pain, fever, nausea, or vomiting. Evidence of salpingitis may or may not be present.

DIAGNOSIS

When to Use Diagnostic Testing

All women suspected of having *C. trachomatis* genital infections on the basis of symptoms, signs, or exposure history (including women with suspected mucopurulent cervicitis, endometritis, pelvic inflammatory disease, acute urethritis, or acute proctitis, as well as women whose male partners have gonorrhea or NGU) should have specific diagnostic testing. The diagnosis of many of these conditions is difficult to establish on clinical grounds alone, and the presence of a positive chlamydial test is thus of great value in confirming the suspected diagnosis. Although women in these categories should be empirically treated with tetracycline or doxycycline without awaiting test results, a specific confirmation of *C. trachomatis* infection clarifies the diagnosis, improves the patient's understanding of her illness, probably enhances medication compliance, and facilitates management of sexual partners.

Second, unrecognized *C. trachomatis* infections should be identified by appropriate screening of women in high-risk groups. Such groups include all women attending STD clinics or other clinics (family planning clinics, juvenile detention centers, and abortion clinics, for example) where the prevalence of infection exceeds 10 to 12 percent. Physicians should screen women who have specific risk factors associated with chlamydial infections: adolescent age, a new sexual partner, multiple sexual partners, racial or ethnic groups found to be at high risk in the local setting, and signs of cervicitis.

In men, given both the relative paucity of serious complications that arise from *C. trachomatis* infections and the considerably greater proportion of infections that can be accurately diagnosed on clinical grounds alone, both specific diagnostic testing and screening for *C. trachomatis* infections should be given a lower priority than in women when resources limit the numbers of tests that can be done. However, knowledge of the role of *C. trachomatis* in NGU has prognostic implications and other benefits for men even though most infected men with symptoms or signs of urethritis can be treated empirically with tetracycline before the test results are known.

Up to one-third of heterosexual men with *C. trachomatis* urethral infection attending STD clinics lack symptoms of urethritis, and a case can be made for routine screening tests for *C. trachomatis* in such clinics to identify these persons. Alternatively, such men could be screened for increased numbers of PMNs in first-voided urine specimens with leukocyte esterase testing, or for increased PMNs (e.g., greater than or equal to five per 1000× field) on Gram-stained urethral smear. Those with abnormal findings could be selected for specific testing for *Chlamydia.* Asymptomatic male partners of women with mucopurulent cervicitis, pelvic inflammatory disease, or asymptomatic chlamydial infection should also be screened and then given empirical therapy. In homosexual men with suspected proctitis, *C. trachomatis* testing should be done to confirm the suspected diagnosis. Tables 4-3 and 4-4 summarize diagnostic criteria for various *C. trachomatis* infections in men and women, respectively.

Selection of the Appropriate Test

Selection of the most appropriate laboratory test for detection of *C. trachomatis* depends on local availability and expertise, the prevalence of infection in the test population, and the purpose of the test. Isolation in cell culture remains the most sensitive and specific test and thus should be used when it is available and when transport conditions, cost, and other logistic factors permit its use. Because of their high specificity, cell cultures may be of greatest value in screening low-risk populations. The difficulty of culture and other factors, however, have limited the culturing of *C. trachomatis* to larger centers.

Noncultural methods for detection of *C. trachomatis* antigen in infected secretions are also available. Two general approaches to antigen detection have been taken: (1) direct immunofluorescence staining of smears using monoclonal antibodies and (2) detection of chlamydial antigen eluted from swabs and measured by enzyme-linked immunosorbent assay (ELISA) with polyclonal or monoclonal antibodies. DNA probe (Gen Probe) is also widely used. Polymerase chain reaction (PCR) tests are being evaluated.

Serologic tests are not routinely used for diagnosis of chlamydial genital tract infections other than LGV because the baseline prevalence of antibody in populations that are sexually active and likely to be at risk for *C. trachomatis* infection is high, presumably because of past infection and/or persistent, chronic asymptomatic infection. In addition, because of the absence of abrupt onset of symptoms, many patients are seen during periods when IgM

TABLE 4-3. Diagnosis of *C. trachomatis* Infections in Men*

Associated findings	Clinical criteria	Laboratory criteria	
		Presumptive	Diagnostic
NGU	Dysuria, urethral discharge	Urethral GS with 5 or more PMNs/high-power (×1000) field; pyuria on FVU	Positive culture or direct antigen test (urethra)
Acute epididymitis	Fever, epididymal or testicular pain, evidence of NGU, epididymal tenderness or mass	Same as for NGU	Same as for NGU; positive culture on epididymal aspirate
Acute proctitis (non-LGV strain)	Rectal pain, discharge, bleeding; abnormal anoscopy (mucopurulent discharge, pain, spontaneous or induced bleeding)	Rectal GS with 1 or more PMN/high-power (×1000) field	Positive culture or direct FA (rectal)
Acute proctocolitis (LGV strain)	Severe rectal pain, discharge, hematochezia; markedly abnormal anoscopy (as above) with lesions extending into colon; fever, lymphadenopathy	Rectal GS with 1 or more PMN/high-power (×1000) field	Positive culture or direct FA (rectal); complement fixation antibody titer

*GS = Gram stain; PMN = polymorphonuclear leukocyte; NGU = nongonococcal urethritis; FA = fluorescent antibody; FVU = first-void urine; LGV = lymphogranuloma venereum. Reproduced with permission from the *Annals of Internal Medicine.*

51

TABLE 4-4. Diagnosis of *C. trachomatis* Infections in Women*

Associated findings	Clinical criteria	Laboratory criteria	
		Presumptive	Diagnostic
Mucopurulent cervicitis	Mucopurulent cervical discharge, cervical ectopy and edema, spontaneous or easily induced cervical bleeding	Cervical GS with greater than 30 PMNs/high-power (×1000) field in nonmenstruating women	Positive culture or direct antigen test (cervix)
Acute urethral syndrome	Dysuria-frequency syndrome in young sexually active women; recent new sexual partner; often more than 7 days of symptoms	Pyuria, no bacteriuria	Positive culture or direct antigen test (cervix or urethra)
PID	Lower abdominal pain; adnexal tenderness on pelvic exam; evidence of MPC often present	Same as for MPC; cervical GS positive for gonorrhea; endometritis on endometrial biopsy	Positive culture or direct antigen test (cervix, endometrium, tubal)
Perihepatitis	Right upper quadrant pain, nausea, vomiting, fever; young sexually active women; evidence of PID	Same as for MPC and PID	High-titer IgM or IgG antibody to *C. trachomatis*

*GS = Gram stain; PMN = polymorphonuclear leukocyte; PID = pelvic inflammatory disease; MPC = mucopurulent cervicitis. Reproduced with permission from the *Annals of Internal Medicine.*

antibody or rising or falling titers of IgG antibody cannot be demonstrated. Hence, these serologic parameters of recently acquired infection are often absent.

THERAPY

The treatment of choice for *C. trachomatis* infection is tetracycline or doxycycline. The recommended length of therapy ranges from 7 to 21 days. However, there is as yet no evidence that prolongation of tetracycline therapy beyond 1 week is necessary, provided that sex partners can be treated concurrently.

Uncomplicated Urethral, Endocervical, or Rectal *C. trachomatis* Infections

Recommended Regimen
Doxycycline 100 mg orally 2 times a day for 7 days *or* **azithromycin 1g orally, once.**
Alternative Regimens
Ofloxacin 300 mg orally 2 times a day for 7 days *or* **erythromycin base 500 mg orally 4 times a day or equivalent salt for 7 days** *or* **erythromycin ethylsuccinate 800 mg orally 4 times a day for 7 days.**
If erythromycin is not tolerated due to side effects, the following regimen may be effective: **sulfisoxazole 500 mg orally 4 times a day for ten days or equivalent.**
Other drugs that have demonstrated activity against *C. trachomatis* in tissue culture are rifampin, sulfonamides, clindamycin, and some fluoroquinolones. Ofloxacin has greater activity than ciprofloxacin. Ciprofloxacin has been associated with high relapse rates among men with NGU. Penicillin, ampicillin, cephalosporins, and spectinomycin in single-dose regimens given for treatment of gonorrhea usually do not eradicate concomitant chlamydial infection, while 7 or more days of treatment with tetracycline or erythromycin eradicates *C. trachomatis* from nearly all men, at least as determined by short-term follow-up. However, chlamydial infection recurs 3 to 6 weeks after treatment with tetracycline or erythromycin in 5 to 10 percent of men with chlamydial urethritis and cannot be clearly designated as reinfection or relapse. In addition, despite apparent elimination of *C. trachomatis,* 10 to 15 percent of men develop persistent or relapsing symptoms, perhaps due to simultaneous infection with another agent.
Regimen for Pregnant Women
Erythromycin base 500 mg orally 4 times a day for 7 days.

Test of Cure

Because antimicrobial resistance of *C. trachomatis* to recommended regimens seldom has been observed, test-of-cure evaluation is not necessary when treatment has been completed.

Sex Partners of Patients with *C. trachomatis* Infections

Sex partners of patients with *C. trachomatis* infection within the past 30 days should be tested for *C. trachomatis.* If testing is not available, they should be treated with the appropriate antimicrobial regimen.

PREVENTION

A major hindrance to effective prevention of chlamydial genital tract infection is the absence of specific diagnostic testing in most STD clinics or physicians' offices. At least 40 percent of all chlamydial infections seen in STD clinics are asymptomatic, and an even greater proportion of chlamydial infections in sexually active populations not seeking health care are probably asymptomatic. Establishment of diagnostic screening procedures for *C. trachomatis* in high-risk populations seen in STD clinics, family planning clinics, prenatal clinics, juvenile detention centers, adolescent medicine clinics, and gynecology clinics seems critical to identify and treat asymptomatically infected individuals who constitute the major reservoir for *C. trachomatis.*

Prevention of genital chlamydial infection may be a readily achievable goal with appropriate use of screening to identify unrecognized cases.

ADDITIONAL READING

Faro S et al: Effectiveness of ofloxacin in the treatment of *Chlamydia trachomatis* and *Neisseria gonorrhoeae* cervical infection. *Am J Obstet Gynecol* 164:1380, 1991

Hooton TM et al: Erythromycin for persistent or recurrent nongonococcal urethritis. A randomized, placebo-controlled trial. *Ann Intern Med* 113:21, 1990

Iwen PC et al: Comparison of the Gen-Probe PACE 2 system, direct fluorescent-antibody, and cell culture for detecting *Chlamydia trachomatis* in cervical specimens. *Am J Clin Pathol* 95:578, 1991

Johnson RB: The role of azalide antibiotics in the treatment of *Chlamydia. Am J Obstet Gynecol* 164:1794, 1991

Jones RB: New treatments for *Chlamydia trachomatis. Am J Obstet Gynecol* 164:1789, 1991

Jones RB et al: Partial characterization of *Chlamydia trachomatis* isolates resistant to multiple antibiotics. *J Infect Dis* 162:1309, 1990

Katz BP et al: A randomized trial to compare 7- and 21-day tetracycline regimens in the prevention of recurrence of infection with *Chlamydia trachomatis. Sex Transm Dis* 18:36, 1991

McGagny SE et al: Urinary leukocyte esterase test: A screening method for the detection of asymptomatic chlamydia and gonococcal infections in men. *J Infect Dis* 165:573, 1992

Palmer HM et al: Detection of *Chlamydia trachomatis* by the polymerase chain reaction in swabs and urine from men with non-gonococcal urethritis. *J Clin Pathol* 44:321, 1991

Ramstedt K et al: Contact tracing in the control of genital *Chlamydia trachomatis* infection. *Int J STD AIDS* 2:116, 1991

Ratti G et al: Detection of *Chlamydia trachomatis* DNA in patients with non-gonococcal urethritis using the polymerase chain reaction. *J Clin Pathol* 44:564, 1991

Rietmeijer CA et al: Unsuspected *Chlamydia trachomatis* infection in hetero-sexual men attending a sexually transmitted diseases clinic: Evaluation of risk factors and screening methods. *Sex Transm Dis* 18:28, 1991

Sellors JW et al: Comparison of cervical, urethral, and urine specimens for the detection of *Chlamydia trachomatis* in women. *J Infect Dis* 164:205, 1991

Weinstock HS et al: *Chlamydia trachomatis* infection in women: A need for universal screening in high prevalence populations? *Am J Epidemiol* 135:41, 1992

For a more detailed discussion, see Schachter J: Biology of *Chlamydia trachomatis,* Chap. 15, p. 161; Stamm WE, Holmes KK: *Chlamydia trachomatis* Infections of the Adult, Chap. 16, p. 181; and Stamm WE, Mårdh P-A: *Chlamydia trachomatis,* Chap. 74, p. 917, in STD-2.

Lymphogranuloma venereum (LGV) is a sexually transmitted disease usually caused by one of three serovars of *Chlamydia trachomatis:* L1, L2, or L3. These serovars can be distinguished from those usually associated with trachoma and other genital tract infections by use of appropriate monoclonal or polyclonal antibodies, but these tests are not routinely available.

LGV is a chronic disease that has a variety of acute and late manifestations. Three stages of infection are recognized. The primary lesion is a small, inconspicuous genital papule or herpetiform ulcer of short duration and few symptoms. The secondary stage is characterized by suppurative regional lymphadenopathy with fever and other constitutional symptoms caused by systemic spread of infection. The vast majority of patients recover clinically from LGV after the secondary stage, but in untreated patients the infection may persist and progress to a late stage characterized by fibrosis and abnormal lymphatic drainage. The proportion of patients whose illness progresses to late stage is uncertain, since the early stages are poorly diagnosed and reported.

EPIDEMIOLOGY

LGV is a sporadic disease throughout North America, Europe, and Australia. It is endemic in east and west Africa, India, parts of southeastern Asia, South America, and the Caribbean. Like other sexually transmitted diseases, LGV is more common in urban than in rural areas, among those with many sexual contacts, and among members of lower socioeconomic classes.

Acute LGV occurs most frequently during the third decade. It is reported much more frequently in men than in women, with the ratio often exceeding 5:1. This is because symptomatic infection is less common in women, who usually are diagnosed during early infection only if they develop acute proctocolitis or, less commonly, inguinal buboes. Late complications such as hyperplasia, ulceration and hypertrophy of the genitalia (esthiomene), and rectal strictures are reported to be more frequent in women than in men. Homosexual men who are recipients of anal intercourse may also present with acute proctocolitis rather than inguinal buboes and may develop rectal strictures.

PATHOGENESIS

Chlamydia probably gain entry through minute lacerations and abrasions. Laboratory-acquired infections following inhalation of highly concentrated virulent cultures have been reported.

LGV is predominantly a disease of lymphatic tissue. The primary pathologic process is thrombolymphangitis and perilymphangitis with spread of the inflammatory process from infected lymph nodes into the surrounding tissue. Inflammation mats the adjacent lymph nodes together by periadenitis with evidence of "stellate abscesses" on histologic examination. As inflammation progresses, the abscesses coalesce and rupture the node, forming loculated abscesses, fistulas, or sinus tracts.

The inflammatory process lasts several weeks or months before subsiding. Healing occurs by fibrosis, which destroys the normal structure of lymph nodes and obstructs subcutaneous and submucous lymph vessels. The resulting chronic edema and sclerosing fibrosis causes induration and enlargement of the affected parts. Fibrosis also compromises the blood supply to the overlying skin or mucous membrane, and ulceration occurs.

Although the primary pathologic process in LGV may be localized to one or two groups of lymph nodes, the organisms spread systematically in the bloodstream and can enter the central nervous system. Dissemination and local extension of disease is limited by host immunity. Host immunity ultimately limits chlamydial multiplication but may not eliminate organisms from the body, and a state of latency ensues.

CLINICAL MANIFESTATIONS

Table 5-1 outlines the lesions of LGV.

TABLE 5-1. Lesions of Lymphogranuloma Venereum

Early	Late
Inguinal syndrome:	
Primary genital lesion(s)	Genital elephantiasis
Inguinal buboes	Genital ulcers and fistulas
Bubonulus	
Anorectal syndrome:	
Proctitis	
	Rectal stricture
	Lymphorrhoids
	Perirectal abscesses
	Anal fistula
Other:	
Urethritis	
Cervicitis	
Salpingitis	Frozen pelvis
Parametritis	Infertility
Conjunctivitis	
Regional lymphadenitis	Scarring
Meningitis	

Primary Lesion

The primary lesion of LGV may take one of four forms: a papule, a shallow ulcer or erosion, a small herpetiform lesion, or nonspecific urethritis. The most common of these is the herpetiform ulcer, which appears at the site of infection after an incubation period of 3 to 12 days or longer. The primary lesion, although occasionally erosive, is usually asymptomatic and inconspicuous. It heals rapidly and leaves no scar and is therefore often not recognized. The lesions are sometimes noted on the penis or scrotum of infected men or the labia, fourchette, or posterior vagina of women.

Primary LGV lesions in men may be associated with a cordlike lymphangitis of the dorsal penis and formation of a large, tender lymphangial nodule, or "bubonulus." Bubonuli may rupture and form draining sinuses and fistulas of the urethra as well as fibrotic, deforming scars at the base of the penis. Lymphangitis is often accompanied by local and regional edema, which may produce varying degrees of phimosis in men and genital swelling in women.

Inguinal Syndrome

Inflammation and swelling of the inguinal lymph nodes is the most common manifestation of the secondary stage of LGV in men and is the reason most patients seek medical attention. Other lymph nodes may be involved; the likelihood of such involvement depends on the location of the primary lesion (Table 5-2). The incubation period for this manifestation is 10 to 30 days, but it may be delayed for as long as 4 to 6 months after infection.

The inguinal bubo is unilateral in two-thirds of cases. It begins as a firm, slightly painful mass which enlarges over 1 to 2 weeks. Constitutional symptoms are often seen in this stage and may be associated with systemic spread of chlamydia. During this stage of infection, LGV organisms have been recovered from the blood and the cerebrospinal fluid of patients both with and without symptoms of meningoencephalitis and abnormal cerebrospinal fluid. Other

TABLE 5-2. Site of Primary LGV Infection Determining Subsequent Lymphatic Involvement

Site of primary infection	Affected lymph nodes
Penis, anterior urethra	Superficial and deep inguinal
Posterior urethra	Deep iliac, perirectal
Vulva	Inguinal
Vagina, cervix	Deep iliac, perirectal, retrocrural, lumbosacral
Anus	Inguinal
Rectum	Perirectal, deep iliac

manifestations of systemic spread are hepatitis, pneumonitis, and possibly arthritis. Leukocytosis, abnormal liver function tests, and elevated erythrocyte sedimentation rates are common.

Within 1 to 2 weeks the bubo becomes fluctuant and the overlying skin takes on a characteristically livid color ("blue balls") that predicts rupture of the bubo. Rupture through the skin usually relieves pain and fever. Numerous sinus tracts are formed which drain thick, tenacious, yellowish pus for several weeks or months with little or no discomfort. Healing occurs slowly, leaving contracted scars in the inguinal region. The disappearance of the inguinal bubo usually marks the end of the disease in men, and the majority suffer no serious sequelae. Bubonic relapse occurs in about 20 percent of untreated cases, however.

Only about one-third of inguinal buboes become fluctuant and rupture; the others slowly involute and form firm inguinal masses without undergoing suppuration. In about 20 percent of cases the femoral lymph nodes are also affected and may be separated from the enlarged inguinal lymph nodes by Poupart's ligament; this process creates a groove that is said to be pathognomonic for LGV (Fig. 5-1).

Only 20 to 30 percent of women with LGV present with the

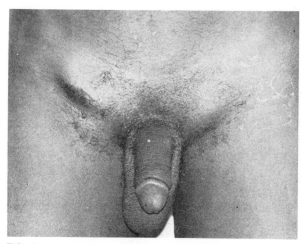

FIG. 5-1. Early inguinal syndrome of LGV showing a small vesicular primary lesion and bilateral inguinal lymphadenitis with cleavage of the enlarged right inguinal and femoral lymph nodes by the inguinal ligament, the characteristic "groove" sign.

inguinal syndrome. About one-third of female cases without proctitis, however, complain of lower abdominal and back pain, especially when supine. This symptom is characteristic of involvement of the deep pelvic and lumbar lymph nodes and may be mistaken for acute appendicitis or a tuboovarian abscess.

Differential diagnosis includes genital herpes, syphilis, chancroid, and Hodgkin's disease. Other infectious diseases which cause inguinal lymphadenitis and bubo formation are plague, tularemia, and tuberculosis.

ANOGENITORECTAL SYNDROME

Proctocolitis is an early subacute manifestation of this syndrome. Chronic or late manifestations include perirectal abscesses, ischiorectal and rectovaginal fistulas, anal fistulas, and rectal stricture or stenosis.

In men, the rectal mucosa can be directly inoculated with chlamydia during receptive anal intercourse or by lymphatic spread from the male posterior urethra. In women, the rectal mucosa can also be directly inoculated with chlamydia during anal intercourse, or it can be contaminated by migration of infectious vaginal secretions or by lymphatic spread from the cervix and posterior vaginal wall.

The early symptoms of rectal infection are anal pruritis and a mucous rectal discharge. The mucosa becomes hyperemic and friable after several weeks. Multiple superficial ulcerations appear and are gradually replaced by granulation tissue. With secondary bacterial infection of the rectal mucosa, the discharge becomes mucopurulent. If left untreated, the granulomatous process progressively involves all layers of the bowel wall. The muscle layers are replaced by fibrous tissue which may eventually cause rectal strictures or stenosis. Rectovaginal fistulas may form in women.

Symptoms of proctocolitis include fever, rectal pain, and tenesmus. The left lower quadrant of the abdomen is tender, and the pelvic colon may be palpably thickened. The rectal mucosa feels granular on digital examination, and movable, enlarged lymph nodes may be palpated immediately under the bowel wall. Additional symptoms that occur with rectal stricture include varying degrees of constipation, passage of "pencil" stools, attacks of ileus with colic and abdominal distension, and weight loss. Perirectal abscesses and anal fissures may form in the rectal mucosa below the stricture and skin around the anus. Obstruction of the lymphatic and venous drainage of the lower rectum may produce perianal outgrowths of lymphatic tissue which grossly resemble hemorrhoids but are called lymphorrhoids or perianal condylomas.

Differential diagnosis of anogenitorectal syndrome in homosexual men includes the infectious causes of proctitis (gonorrhea, herpes, syphilis, and non-LGV serovars of *C. trachomatis*), infectious causes of anal ulcers (herpes, syphilis, and chancroid); and infectious causes of proctocolitis (*Shigella, Campylobacter,* and *Entamoeba histolytica*), and noninfectious causes of proctitis and proctocolitis, such as ulcerative colitis and Crohn's disease. Rectal strictures of LGV may resemble those caused by trauma, actinomycosis, tuberculosis, schistosomiasis, and malignancy.

Other Manifestations

Less common manifestations include genital elephantiasis, chronic vulvar ulcerations (esthiomene), and follicular conjunctivitis, which may develop as a result of autoinoculation of infectious discharge.

DIAGNOSIS

The diagnosis of LGV is usually based on positive serologic tests or isolation of LGV chlamydia from infected tissue and secretions.

The complement fixation (CF) test is one of the more commonly used serologic tests. The CF test is more sensitive and is positive earlier than the previously used Frei antigen test. The CF test gives cross-reactions in infections caused by other chlamydial infections, and the antibody may persist in high or low titer for many years. In general, active LGV infections have CF titers of 1:64 or greater, but high CF titers are occasionally found in asymptomatic patients and those with other chlamydial infections. The microimmunofluorescent (micro-IF) test is considerably more sensitive than the CF test but is used primarily in a few specialized laboratories and is not routinely available.

Isolation of chlamydia from infected tissue by inoculation of mouse brain, yolk sac, or tissue culture is the definitive means of diagnosis, but the yield is frequently low. Bubo pus is the most practical clinical material, but the recovery rate is often less than 30 percent.

TREATMENT

A variety of different drugs have been used to treat LGV, but there is no singularly effective drug that will assure bacteriological cure.

Recommended Regimen
Doxycycline 100 mg orally 2 times a day for 21 days.
Alternative Regimen
Erythromycin 500 mg orally 4 times a day for 21 days *or* **Sulfisoxazole 500 mg orally 4 times a day for 21 days** *or* **equivalent sulfonamide course.**

Pregnant and nursing women should be treated with the erythromycin regimen.

Constitutional symptoms generally improve 1 to 2 days after antibiotic therapy is started. Chemotherapy appears to have only a minimal effect in shortening the duration of the bubonic lesions, although antibiotics reduce the frequency of complications. Fluctuant buboes may require frequent aspiration to prevent rupture. Surgery may be necessary to repair strictures, fistulas, and elephantiasis.

PREVENTION

Prevention of LGV requires identification and treatment of sexual contacts of proved or suspected cases. These contacts should receive prophylactic antibiotics if recently exposed to infection, in order to prevent reinfection as well as to eliminate a potential reservoir.

ADDITIONAL READING

Buntin DM et al: Sexually transmitted diseases: Bacterial infections. *J Am Acad Dermatol* 25:287, 1991
Burgoyne RA: Lymphogranuloma venereum. *Primary Care* 17:153, 1990
Martin DH: Chlamydial infections. *Med Clin North Am* 74:1367, 1990

For a more detailed discussion, see Perine PL, Osoba AO: Lymphogranuloma Venereum, Chap. 17 in STD-2, p. 195.

MICROBIOLOGY

Treponema pallidum, the causative organism of syphilis, is one of a small group of treponemes, members of the order Spirochaetales, that are virulent for human beings. *T. pallidum* is indistinguishable by known morphologic, chemical, or immunologic methods from treponemes which cause yaws, pinta, or endemic syphilis. Studies of *T. pallidum* are severely restricted by the inability to readily grow this organism in vitro. In vivo replication time, slow relative to most bacteria, is about 30 h.

The organism has a length of 6 to 15 μ (usually 10 to 13 μ) and a width of only 0.15 μ, which renders it below the level of resolution and, therefore, not visible by light microscopy—hence, the reliance on the dark-field microscope in clinical practice or electron microscopy in special clinical and investigational situations. *T. pallidum* has regular, tight spirals; when fixed, it appears wavelike with a wavelength of 1.1 μ and an amplitude of 0.2 to 0.3 μ. Dark-field microscopic examination of a wet preparation reveals a characteristic rotatory movement with flexion and back-and-forth motion.

Animal models for studying syphilis have been problematic. Experimental primary and secondary infection can be produced in rabbits. However, there is no known parallel in the rabbit, or in any other animal, including subhuman primates, for tertiary syphilis.

EPIDEMIOLOGY

The incidence of syphilis has risen dramatically in the United States during the past few years. From 1965 through 1980, overall rates of primary and secondary syphilis changed very little, although the ratio of male/female cases increased steadily, probably due to the increasing numbers of men reporting homosexual activity who acquired disease during this period. During the late 1980s the proportion of men with primary and secondary syphilis who named other men as sex partners drastically declined, probably due to altered sexual behavior in this group as a result of the AIDS epidemic. However, during 1987, the incidence of early infectious syphilis increased sharply in both men and women, particularly among black heterosexuals. Increased use of anonymous sexual partners and exchange of sex for drugs (cocaine) have contributed to this situation. Congenital syphilis also has increased dramatically since 1987, reflecting increased syphilis rates in young women. In recent years many sporadic, local syphilis outbreaks have emerged and contribute substantially to the national increase. Interestingly, these outbreaks have occurred in New York, in Los Angeles, in some areas in Texas, and in south Florida, areas where recent outbreaks of chancroid have occurred and where heterosexual HIV seropositivity rates are highest.

TRANSMISSION

Syphilis is usually acquired by sexual contact. The rate of acquisition from an infected sexual partner has been estimated at about 30 percent. Transmission by sexual contact requires exposure to moist mucosal or cutaneous lesions, and therefore a person ordinarily is able to transmit syphilis only during the first few years of infection, during the time of susceptibility to spontaneous mucocutaneous secondary relapses.

Infants acquire congenital infection by transplacental transmission of *T. pallidum*. Women may transmit infection to their fetus in utero shortly after onset of infection. Fetal transmission has been documented as early as the ninth week of pregnancy. Women may remain potentially infectious for the fetus for many years, although the risk of infecting a fetus declines gradually during the course of untreated illness.

STAGES OF SYPHILIS

Both congenital and acquired syphilis are divided into early and late stages. Early acquired syphilis is further subdivided into an incubation period, primary, secondary, and early latent stages. The U.S. Public Health Service uses 1 year as the dividing point between early and late latent disease.

EARLY SYPHILIS IN THE ADULT

Pathogenesis

T. pallidum probably requires a break in squamous or columnar epithelium to enter the body; macroscopic and microscopic trauma readily occur during sexual contact. Some organisms lodge at the site of entry; others escape via the lymphatic system to the regional lymph nodes and disseminate throughout the body. Wherever they lodge they may proliferate and stimulate an immune response. Many clinical manifestations of the disease are probably due to the immune response to infection.

The incubation period has a mean of 21 days with extremes of 10 to 90 days. Experimentally, large inocula are associated with short incubation periods and small inocula with longer intervals, but the reason for incubation periods over 5 weeks is unclear.

The immunobiology and pathogenesis of syphilis in humans and the immune response are still not completely understood. Untreated disease runs a roughly predictable but variable course; reasons for the clinical variability are obscure. In part, variations in expression of disease reflect differences in the immune status of the hosts.

Clinical Manifestations

Primary syphilis

The first clinical manifestation is usually a local lesion at the site of entry. This is usually a site of genital trauma, such as the coronal sulcus, glans, frenum, prepuce, and shaft of the penis, and near the anus, in the anal canal, or in the rectum in the homosexual or bisexual male. In the female the lesion is found on the fourchette or elsewhere on the vulva and on the cervix. Unilateral edema may accompany labial lesions, but rectal and cervical lesions are often asymptomatic.

The lesion starts as a dull red macule which rapidly becomes papular and then ulcerates. The classical ulcer, the chancre, is rounded with a well-defined margin, and a rubbery, thickened, indurated base; it is painless and nontender and produces more serum and less blood than ulcers due to other causes (Fig. 6-1). The early chancre has a clear red base, but later this becomes covered with a gray slough.

Classical chancres are becoming less common, at least in the

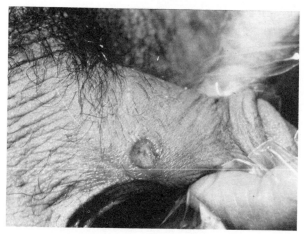

FIG. 6-1. Primary chancre of the shaft of the penis; typical clear-based lesion with indurated margin. *(Courtesy of E Stolz.)*

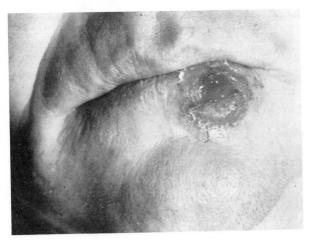

FIG. 6-2. Primary syphilitic chancre of the lip. *(Courtesy of E Stolz.)*

western parts of the world, and all genital and anorectal ulcers in
at-risk persons should be regarded as suspect. Chancres have been
reported at other sites including lips, tongue, breasts, and fingers
(Fig. 6-2). Lesions at extragenital sites may be atypical, and a high
index of suspicion is necessary to make this diagnosis.

Untreated, a chancre will persist for 3 to 6 weeks and then heal.
Relapse of the primary chancre is rare.

In most cases regional lymphadenopathy develops within a week
of the appearance of the chancre. Nodes are painless, nontender,
small to moderate in size, rubbery, and nonsuppurative. With
genital and anal chancres, nodes are often bilateral, but with
chancres elsewhere, they are unilateral.

If an ulcer becomes secondarily infected with pyogenic bacteria,
it may be painful and tender, and the nodes may develop the same
features.

Secondary syphilis

T. pallidum disseminate widely throughout the body. About 3 to 6
weeks after the appearance of the chancre the symptoms and signs
of secondary syphilis appear. It is at this stage that the disease is
seen to be systemic. The more common symptoms include sore
throat, malaise, headaches, weight loss, variable fever, and musculoskeletal pains. A rash occurs in 75 to 100 percent, lymphadenopathy in 50 to 86 percent, and mucosal ulceration in 6 to 30

percent of persons. The chancre may, rarely, persist into the secondary stage.

The rash starts as a faint macular eruption of rose pink rounded lesions 0.5 to 1.0 cm in diameter on the trunk and flexor surfaces of the upper limbs. It gradually becomes dull red and papular and spreads to involve the whole body, characteristically including the palms and soles, where the papules gradually become squamous (Fig. 6-3). Once the papular stage is reached, the rash is polymorphic and is usually nonirritant.

Variations of the rash include follicular lesions, annular lesions which are more common in blacks than in whites, and corymbose lesions with one central papule surrounded by a ring of smaller ones. Papules affecting intertriginous areas may become eroded and fissured. In warm, moist areas papules may become large and raised and may resemble viral warts, but they are characteristically broad and flat—so-called condylomata lata. These may develop around

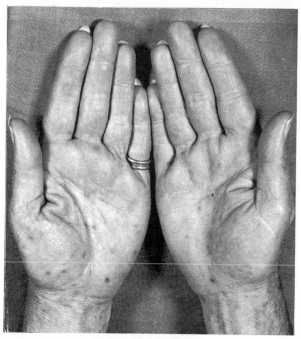

FIG. 6-3. Secondary syphilis: rash on palms.

the anus, on the scrotum, on the vulva, and sometimes in the axillae, under the breasts, and in other areas.

Less common manifestations include pustules, patchy alopecia, and diffuse thinning of the hair. Mucosal ulcers ("mucous patches") may affect any mucous membrane, the mouth, pharynx, larynx, and genitals being the most commonly involved.

With or without treatment all manifestations of secondary syphilis resolve. Pustules may heal with hypo- or hyperpigmentation.

A number of other manifestations may also accompany secondary syphilis. Generalized lymphadenopathy is common, with involvement of inguinal, suboccipital, posterior cervical, axillary, and epitrochlear nodes. Nodes are usually only moderately enlarged, rubbery, discrete, and nontender.

Involvement of other systems occurs in 10 percent of cases or less. Arthritis, bursitis, and osteitis have all been described. Hepatitis, nephrotic syndrome due to syphilitic glomerulonephritis, anterior uveitis, and acute choroiditis are sometimes seen.

Neurologic involvement occurs in a small proportion of patients. Meningitis, cranial nerve palsies, transverse myelitis, thrombosis of cerebral arteries, and syphilitic nerve deafness have all been described. Examination of the cerebrospinal fluid (CSF) shows abnormalities in about one-third of patients (increased cell count, increased protein), but most patients with abnormal CSF do not exhibit clinical symptoms or signs of neurologic disease.

Laboratory Tests

Dark field microscopy

Dark field microscopy is sensitive and specific for the diagnosis of primary syphilis. Dark field examinations should also be performed on papules, condylomata lata, or mucous patches of secondary syphilis, although saprophytic treponemes on mucosal surfaces may cause confusion. Lesions should be cleaned with 0.9% sterile saline and gently abraded to provoke oozing. Presence of red blood cells impedes recognition of *T. pallidum.* The organism is recognized by its morphology and characteristic movement. It may be necessary to examine several slides before treponemes are found.

Direct fluorescent antibody tests

The direct fluorescent antibody test for syphilis (DFA-TP) is a practical alternative to direct dark field examination when smears cannot be examined immediately and when examining oral lesions. The lesion material fixed to the slide is stained with fluorescein-labeled anti–*T. pallidum* globulin. The test offers the advantage of specifically detecting *T. pallidum,* thereby eliminating confusion with other spiral organisms, especially in oral lesions. In addition, motile organisms are not required for diagnosis.

The demonstration of treponemes with characteristic morphology and motility for *T. pallidum* by dark field microscopy or reactive DFA-TP results constitutes a positive diagnosis of syphilis in primary, secondary, early congenital, and infectious relapse stages. However, failure to find the organism does not exclude a diagnosis of syphilis. Failure to demonstrate *T. pallidum* from typical lesions may be due to the age or condition of the lesion, treatment of the patient either locally or systemically before the specimen was taken, and most commonly, poor technique in collecting and reading the specimen.

Serologic tests

Serologic tests for syphilis measure two different types of antibodies: nonspecific nontreponemal antibody and specific treponemal antibody.

Nontreponemal tests Nontreponemal tests are useful as a screen for disease and disease activity. All nontreponemal tests measure antilipid IgG and IgM antibodies formed by the host in response to lipid from the treponemes' cell surfaces. Commonly used tests in clinical practice include the Venereal Disease Research Laboratory (VDRL) test, rapid plasma reagin (RPR) test, automated reagin screen test (ART), unheated serum reagin (USR) test, and the reagin screen test (RST).

False-positive results occur in the general population at a rate of 1 to 2 percent regardless of the nontreponemal test used. In populations of intravenous drug users, more than 10 percent of the sera may give false-positive results. In general, 90 percent of the false-positive titers are less than 1:8, but low titers are also seen in latent and late syphilis. In low-risk populations, all reactive test results should be confirmed by a treponemal test since over 50 percent of the reactive nontreponemal tests may be false-positive in such populations.

Treponemal tests Specific treponemal antibody tests confirm the high probability of past or present treponemal infection. Tests in use today include the fluorescent antibody absorption (FTA-ABS) test, FTA-ABS double staining (DS), microhemagglutination assay for antibodies to *T. pallidum* (MHA-TP), and the hemagglutination treponemal test for syphilis (HATTS). All the treponemal tests use *T. pallidum* as the antigen, are based on the detection of antibodies against treponemal cellular components, and are designed as confirmatory tests.

About 1 percent of the general population have false-positive results in the treponemal tests. While the FTA-ABS is the most sensitive of all these tests, it also has the greatest possibility for laboratory error.

Diagnosis

Primary syphilis

Clinical suspicion   The prerequisite in diagnosis is clinical suspicion. Age, sexual behavior, and contact history are important clinical clues. A single painless, indurated, nontender ulcer suggests a high probability of primary syphilis.

Microscopy   Dark field microscopy is the investigation of first choice for diagnosis of primary syphilis, as the VDRL test gives negative results at the time of diagnosis in 30 to 50 percent of patients with primary infection. If the initial examination is negative in a suspect case, the procedure should be repeated on at least 2 successive days.

Serologic tests   Serologic tests can be a useful adjunct in diagnosis, especially when antimicrobial use has rendered dark-field microscopy negative, or in situations in which this technique is unavailable. The VDRL test gives positive results approximately 14 days after the appearance of the chancre and in 50 to 70 percent of patients at the time of diagnosis. The FTA-ABS and MHA-TP tests give positive results around the time of the appearance of the chancre and in 70 to 90 percent of patients at the time of diagnosis. A presumptive diagnosis of primary syphilis can be made in patients in whom the dark field examination is negative if they have suggestive clinical features supported by a history of contact and have reactive serologic tests, provided these include reactive FTA-ABS or MHA-TP results. If there is doubt in the interpretation of the initial investigations, the serologic tests should be repeated. A rising VDRL titer indicates a high probability of primary syphilis.

Secondary syphilis

Clinical suspicion   As with primary syphilis, a high index of suspicion is important. Features which suggest secondary syphilis include a papular rash affecting the palms and soles, condylomata lata, and mucous patches, especially if there is lymphadenopathy and malaise.

Dark field microscopy   Dark field examination should be performed on papules, condylomata lata, or mucous patches of secondary syphilis; saprophytic treponemes on mucosal surfaces may cause confusion. The preferred lesion is a papule at a distance from an orifice.

Serologic tests Serologic tests are almost always reactive in secondary syphilis, the VDRL test often reaching a high titer (reactive at a serum dilution of 1:16 or higher). Excessive amounts of antibody can interfere with the test, leading to a nonreactive, weakly reactive or atypical reaction (the prozone phenomenon). This effect can be prevented by diluting the serum. Typical clinical features, repeated reactive results to the VDRL test in a titer of 1:16 or higher, and a reactive FTA-ABS or MHA-TP result lead to a presumptive diagnosis of secondary syphilis. Skin biopsy may be quite helpful.

Latent infection

In latent infection there are, by definition, no positive clinical features. Diagnosis depends on positive results of serologic tests which must include a VDRL or similar test and either an FTA-ABS or an MHA-TP test. At least two samples taken at an interval of a week must be examined. If there are conflicting results, further samples are necessary. The CSF should be examined to exclude CNS involvement. A chest radiograph may be indicated to look for calcification in the ascending aorta. Further investigation such as computerized tomography (CT) may be considered if CSF or chest radiograph show suspicious abnormalities.

Differential Diagnosis

Primary syphilis

All genital ulcers and all anorectal lesions in at-risk persons should be regarded as possible primary syphilis. Differential diagnosis of a primary chancre principally includes genital herpes simplex and chancroid. The ulcers of recurrent genital herpes may be single and thus mimic a syphilitic chancre. Ulcers of chancroid typically are more necrotic and painful than the syphilitic chancre. Other considerations include secondary syphilis, erosive balanitis, trauma with or without secondary pyogenic infection, scabies, furuncle, herpes zoster, carcinoma, fixed drug eruption, Vincent's ulcers, and orogenital ulceration including Reiter's syndrome, Stevens-Johnson syndrome, and Behçet's syndrome. If there has been exposure in a tropical climate, one should consider granuloma inguinale, lymphogranuloma venereum, tuberculosis, and amoebic ulceration.

Secondary syphilis

The differential diagnosis of secondary syphilis is wide. The macular rash may resemble a drug eruption, measles, rubella, pityriasis rosea, tinea versicolor, seborrheic dermatitis, erythema multiforme, and leprosy. The papular rash may resemble drug eruption, lichen planus, acne vulgaris, and scabies. Squamous eruption may be confused with psoriasis or seborrheic dermatitis. Annular lesions may resemble fungal infection, impetigo, erythema multiforme, and more rarely the annular form of lichen planus and granuloma annulare. Mucosal ulcerations may be confused with those seen in herpes simplex and the orogenital ulceration syndromes mentioned above. Condylomata lata may be confused with human papillomavirus warts. The alopecia due to secondary syphilis must be distinguished from alopecia areata.

The lymphadenopathy of secondary syphilis can resemble that of Epstein-Barr virus and cytomegalovirus mononucleosis, HIV infection, Hodgkin's disease, and lymphomas.

Treatment of Early Syphilis (Primary, Secondary, Early Latent)

Penicillin is the preferred drug for treatment of syphilis. For patients with penicillin allergy, tetracyclines are useful but less effective than penicillin. In HIV-infected persons, penicillin is needed, and skin testing, with desensitization if necessary, should be done.

Jarisch-Herxheimer reaction

The Jarisch-Herxheimer reaction is an acute febrile reaction, often accompanied by headache, myalgia, and other symptoms, that may occur after any therapy for syphilis, and patients should be so warned. Jarisch-Herxheimer reactions are more common in patients with early syphilis. Antipyretics may be recommended, but there are no proven methods for preventing this reaction. Pregnant patients, in particular, should be warned that early labor may occur.

HIV-negative patients

Recommended Regimen
Benzathine penicillin G, 2.4 million units IM, in one dose.
Alternative Regimen for Penicillin-Allergic Patients
Doxycycline, 100 mg orally 2 times daily for 2 weeks, *or* **tetracycline, 500 mg orally 4 times daily for 2 weeks.** Doxycycline and tetracycline are equivalent therapies. There is less clinical experience with doxycycline, but compliance is better. In patients with penicillin allergy who cannot tolerate doxycycline or tetracycline, three options exist:

1. If follow-up or compliance cannot be ensured, the patient should have skin testing for penicillin allergy and be desensitized if necessary.

2. If compliance and follow-up are ensured, **erythromycin, 500 mg
orally 4 times a day for 2 weeks,** can be used.

Follow-up

Treatment failures can occur with any regimen. Patients should be
reexamined clinically and serologically at 3 and 6 months. If
nontreponemal antibody titers have not declined fourfold by 6
months (by 3 months with primary or secondary syphilis), or if signs
or symptoms persist and reinfection has been ruled out, patients
should have a CSF examination and be re-treated appropriately.

Lumbar puncture in early syphilis

CSF abnormalities are common in adults with early syphilis. Despite
the frequency of these CSF findings, very few HIV-negative patients
develop neurosyphilis with the treatment regimens described above.
Therefore, unless clinical signs and symptoms of neurologic involvement exist, such as optic, auditory, cranial nerve, or meningeal
symptoms, lumbar puncture is not recommended for routine evaluation of early syphilis.

HIV-infected patients

All syphilis patients should be encouraged to be counseled and tested
for HIV infection. HIV-positive patients should be treated with
penicillin, using desensitization if penicillin-allergic. Anecdotal evidence suggests that HIV-positive patients are more likely to relapse
after any syphilis therapy. However, no treatment regimens have
been shown more effective in preventing neurosyphilis than those
recommended for persons without HIV infection. HIV-positive
patients should have careful follow-up serologic testing at 1, 2, 3,
6, 9, and 12 months.

Persons exposed to syphilis (epidemiologic treatment)

Sexual partners of patients diagnosed with infectious syphilis within
the last 90 days should be evaluated clinically and serologically for
evidence of syphilis. Even if no indication of infection exists, they
should be treated with a regimen recommended for early syphilis.
Patients who have other STDs may also have been exposed to
syphilis and should have a serologic test for syphilis. The dual
therapy regimen currently recommended for gonorrhea (ceftriaxone
and doxycycline) probably effectively treats incubating syphilis. If
a different nonpenicillin antibiotic regimen is used, the patient
should have a repeat serologic test for syphilis in 3 months.

TABLE 6-1. Classification of Neurosyphilis

Asymptomatic neurosyphilis
Early
Late
Meningeal neurosyphilis
Acute syphilitic meningitis
Spinal syphilitic pachymeningitis
Meningovascular neurosyphilis
Cerebral form
Spinal form
Parenchymatous neurosyphilis
General paresis
Tabes dorsalis
Optic atrophy
Gummatous neurosyphilis
Cerebral form
Spinal form

SOURCE: After Merritt et al.[3]

NEUROSYPHILIS

Pathogenesis

T. pallidum often invades the meninges early during the course of systemic dissemination of syphilitic infection. After the initial spirochetal invasion of the CNS has occurred, untreated or inadequately treated infection may take one of several courses: spontaneous resolution, asymptomatic syphilitic meningitis, or symptomatic acute syphilitic meningitis. Progression of meningeal infection eventually causes either continuing asymptomatic neurosyphilis, meningovascular syphilis, tabes, or paresis.

Classification of neurosyphilis is complex because of the multitude of histopathologic reactions induced, anatomic sites involved, and clinical syndromes produced. Table 6-1 provides one traditional schema. Although distinctive individual forms of disease exist, features of several of the entities commonly coexist to create overlapping presentations, such as combinations of meningitis and vasculitis, or tabes and paresis.

Asymptomatic Neurosyphilis

Asymptomatic neurosyphilis is defined by the presence of abnormalities in the CSF in the absence of neurologic symptoms or findings. Thus examination of the CSF is essential for diagnosis.

Laboratory findings

Serologic examination of the blood is positive in almost every case of asymptomatic neurosyphilis. The CSF usually reveals a cell count of fewer than 100 lymphocytes per cubic millimeter, a normal or slightly elevated (<100 mg/dl) protein concentration, and a positive nontreponemal serologic test. It is relatively common, unfortunately, to encounter patients with positive blood serologic test results and an elevated level of CSF protein, with or without slight pleocytosis, but negative CSF serologic test results. Diagnosis is ambiguous in such patients, and alternative diagnoses should be considered. A positive CSF VDRL test is nearly always proof of neurosyphilis in the absence of CSF contamination by peripheral blood.

Meningeal Syphilis

Acute syphilitic meningitis

Symptoms and signs Syphilitic meningitis is most common in young adults. The incubation period in the majority of patients is less than 1 year. Fewer than 10 percent of patients have a secondary rash at the time of the meningitis; in about one-quarter of patients, meningitis is the first clinical manifestation of syphilis.

Patients may present with the constellation of headache, fever, photophobia, and stiff neck combined with CSF findings of a mild lymphocytic pleocytosis that suggests a viral aseptic meningitis. A positive nontreponemal serologic test (e.g., VDRL test) provides the important clue to diagnosis. Response to penicillin is prompt, and fever and other clinical findings clear within several days.

One-third of patients present with acute syphilitic hydrocephalus. Principal symptoms (headache, nausea, and vomiting) are those of increased intracranial pressure. Fever is only low-grade or may be absent. Neck stiffness, Kernig's sign, and papilledema are the principal findings.

Syphilitic meningitis with cerebral changes accounts for one-quarter of the cases. Symptoms (seizures, aphasia, and hemiplegia) are a combination of those of increased intracranial pressure and those of focal cerebral involvement. Clinical findings usually include stiff neck, confusion or delirium, and papilledema. Occasionally, cranial nerve palsies are present and most commonly involve the third and sixth cranial nerves.

Syphilitic meningitis with prominent cranial nerve palsies occurs in a substantial proportion of cases of syphilitic meningitis. The principal neurologic manifestations are cranial nerve palsies (especially the third, sixth, seventh, and eighth) and, less commonly, increased intracranial pressure. Early acquired syphilis is a cause of potentially reversible sudden sensorineural deafness in a young adult that must be considered in diagnosis even in the absence of clinical findings of secondary syphilis or of overt lymphocytic meningitis. Response to penicillin therapy is usually good.

Laboratory findings Serum treponemal and nontreponemal tests are usually positive. CSF changes include elevated pressure, mononuclear pleocytosis of 10 to 500 cells per cubic millimeter (occasionally as high as 1000 to 2000 cells per cubic millimeter), elevated protein concentration (45 to 200 mg/dl), and hypoglycorrhachia (less than or equal to 40 mg/dl) in 45 percent of cases. The CSF VDRL test is almost uniformly positive.

Diagnosis and differential diagnosis Diagnosis of acute syphilitic meningitis is based on the clinical picture of aseptic meningitis, lymphocytic CSF response (with or without mild hypoglycorrhachia), and positive nontreponemal blood and CSF serologic test results.

Differential diagnosis includes the various causes of a lymphocytic meningitis, including enteroviruses, leptospirosis, tuberculous meningitis, cryptococcal meningitis, and the meningitis of Lyme disease.

When Lyme disease occurs in the absence of extrameningeal findings, the distinction between the two processes becomes more difficult. Serum and CSF of patients with the neurologic involvement of Lyme disease are nonreactive in nontreponemal tests. However, the sera of 11 percent of patients with Lyme disease show reactivity on the FTA-ABS test. Moreover, some patients with syphilis show serologic reactivity with *Borrellia burgdorferi*. Distinction between the meningeal syndromes of the two spirochetal diseases can be readily made, however, by the clinical and epidemiologic features of the two diseases as well as VDRL reactivity and *B. burgdorferi* antibody testing of serum and CSF.

Meningovascular Syphilis

Cerebrovascular syphilis

Vascular neurosyphilis involves all parts (cerebrum, brain stem, and spinal cord) of the CNS. The underlying processes include chronic meningitis and production of areas of infarction secondary to syphilitic endarteritis. Most patients are 30 to 50 years of age. Cases generally occur 5 to 12 years after initial infection, which is earlier than the occurrence of paresis or tabes, but cases have occurred after a latent period of less than 2 years. If untreated, a patient with cerebrovascular syphilis may ultimately develop either tabes or paresis.

Symptoms and signs The possibility of meningovascular syphilis should be considered when cerebrovascular accidents occur in a young adult. Among the most common manifestations are hemiparesis or hemiplegia, aphasia, and seizures. The most common site of involvement is the middle cerebral artery, but other arteries are occasionally occluded. Neurologic syndromes produced are comparable to those caused by arteriosclerotic thrombotic lesions, but in neurosyphilis the site of thrombosis more often involves smaller branches and produces less extensive infarcts.

Laboratory findings Serum treponemal and nontreponemal antibody tests are positive in meningovascular syphilis. The CSF cell count is usually between 10 and 100 cells per cubic millimeter (virtually all lymphocytes). The CSF protein level is elevated (40 to 250 mg/dl), and the CSF VDRL test is usually positive. Angiographic changes may include diffuse irregularity and "beading" of anterior and middle cerebral arteries and segmental (sausagelike) dilatation of the pericallosal artery. CT shows low-density areas with variable degrees of contrast enhancement, consistent with multifocal infarctions. Magnetic resonance imaging shows focal regions of high signal intensity on T_2-weighted sequences, compatible with foci of ischemia.

Diagnosis and differential diagnosis The diagnosis is suggested when an acute cerebrovascular accident occurs in a young adult without a history of hypertension or findings suggestive of embolic cardiac disease (infective endocarditis, atrial thrombus, or myxoma) and when there is a positive serum VDRL test or a history of previously untreated or inadequately treated early syphilis. Differential diagnosis includes other causes of stroke syndromes such as hypertension, atherosclerotic vascular disease, cerebral emboli, or various types of cerebral vasculitis. A positive CSF serologic test is important in establishing the diagnosis.

Meningovascular syphilis of the spinal cord

Spinal syphilis represents only about 3 percent of neurosyphilis cases. Spinal cord involvement consists principally of syphilitic meningomyelitis (the most common form) and spinal vascular syphilis (acute syphilitic transverse myelitis). The basic underlying process is chronic spinal meningitis, which may result in degeneration of the cord, atrophy of peripheral myelinated fibers, cord infarction, and/or myelomalacia.

Parenchymatous Neurosyphilis

General paresis

General paresis, now a rare disease, is a meningoencephalitis associated with direct invasion of the cerebrum by *T. pallidum.* The clinical illness is a chronic process that evolves over many years and declares itself in middle to late adult life, 15 to 20 years after initial infection. Untreated, the course is progressively downhill, terminating in death.

TABLE 6-2. Symptoms of General Paresis

Early	Late
Irritability	Defective judgment
Memory loss	Emotional lability
Personality changes	(depression, agitation, euphoria)
Impaired capacity to concentrate	Lack of insight
and learn	Confusion and disorientation
Carelessness in appearance	Delusions of grandeur
Headache	Paranoia
Insomnia	Seizures

Symptoms and signs The clinical picture is that of a combination of psychiatric manifestations and neurologic findings. It may mimic almost any type of psychiatric or neurologic disorder. The illness is commonly insidious in onset but may occasionally become suddenly evident. Early features are usually of a psychiatric nature, and the course of illness is that of a dementing process. Early symptoms include gradual memory loss, impairment of intellectual function, and personality changes (Table 6-2). As the disease progresses other symptoms appear: defects in judgment, emotional lability, delusions, and inappropriate behavior. Adult-onset seizures may be the initial manifestation of paresis.

The most common neurologic findings (Table 6-3) in general paresis are pupillary abnormalities; lack of facial expression; tremors of the lips, tongue, facial muscles, and fingers; and impaired handwriting and speech. A true Argyll Robertson pupil is not frequent in early paresis; at this stage the pupils may be large, unequal, and sluggishly reactive to light and accommodation. Over the course of months, normal pupils may change to the Argyll Robertson type defined by the following characteristics: (1) the retina is sensitive (i.e., eye is not blind); (2) pupils are small, fixed, and do not react to strong light; (3) pupils react normally to convergence-accommodation; (4) mydriatics (atropine) fail to dilate pupils fully; and (5) pupils do not dilate on painful stimuli.

As the untreated paretic process advances, apathy, hypotonia, unsteadiness, dementia, and physical deterioration dominate the clinical picture. The duration of untreated paresis, from the onset of detectable mental symptoms until death, has ranged from a few months, in cases of sudden onset, to 4 or 5 years.

Laboratory findings Serum nontreponemal serologic tests are positive in 95 to 100 percent of cases of paresis. The serum FTA-ABS test is uniformly reactive. Characteristic CSF findings include: (1) normal or, occasionally, slightly increased pressure; (2) lymphocytic pleocytosis (usually 8 to 100 lymphocytes per cubic millimeter); (3) increased

TABLE 6-3. Neurologic Signs of
General Paresis*

Sign	Percent
Common	
Pupillary abnormalities	57
Argyll Robertson pupils	26
Slurred speech	28
Expressionless facies	—
Tremors (tongue, face, hands)	18
Impaired handwriting	—
Reflex abnormalities (↑ or ↓)	52
Uncommon	
Focal signs	1–2
Eye muscle palsies	—
Optic atrophy	2
Extensor plantar responses	—

*Where percentages are noted they are
derived from compilation of 134 cases
from two series studies dealing with
patients observed in the period 1950–
1969.[1,2]

SOURCE: After Dewhurst;[1] Dawson-
Butterworth and Heathcote.[2]

protein concentration (usually 50 to 100 mg/dl); (4) increased globulin
concentration; (5) normal or, occasionally, mildly reduced glucose
levels; and (6) a reactive nontreponemal test. False-positive VDRL
test results are extremely unusual. Thus, a positive CSF VDRL test
is very strong evidence for a diagnosis of neurosyphilis. However, a
negative result does not completely exclude the diagnosis, as the
sensitivity of the test may be less than 100 percent.

Diagnosis and differential diagnosis The diagnosis is based on the
clinical picture, which is readily recognizable in its full-blown form
but is more difficult to define when atypical or incomplete, plus
characteristic spinal fluid abnormalities. Differential diagnosis includes cerebral tumor, subdural hematoma, cerebral arteriosclerosis,
Alzheimer's disease, multiple sclerosis, senile dementia, and chronic
alcoholism.

Tabes dorsalis

Tabes dorsalis, now an uncommon form of syphilis, occurs in
untreated patients in the fifth and sixth decades of life after an
average latent period of 20 to 25 years.

Symptoms and signs The early clinical features of tabes are light-ning pains, paresthesias, decreased deep tendon reflexes (manifes-tations of posterior root and posterior column dysfunction), and poor pupillary responses to light. In more advanced stages of the disease, other symptoms and signs become prominent (Table 6-4). Lightning pains are sudden paroxysms of severe stabbing pains that usually occur in the lower extremities but may be felt anywhere on the body. Visceral crises are related to lightning pains, tending to recur in attacks of marked severity that may mimic acute surgical emergencies. The most common form is a gastric crisis consisting of intense epigastric pain, nausea, and vomiting. In some patients, impotence and urinary retention or dribbling may be early symp-toms of sacral root dysfunction. Other symptoms that become evident with more advanced tabes include broad-based, stamping gait and Charcot's joint (unstable, painless, markedly enlarged joint).

Diminished or absent knee and ankle reflexes are almost essential

TABLE 6-4. Symptoms and Signs
of Tabes Dorsalis*

	Percent
Symptoms	
Lightning pains	75
Ataxia	42
Bladder disturbances	33
Paresthesias	24
Visceral crises	18
Visual loss (optic atrophy)	16
Rectal incontinence	14
Signs	
Pupillary abnormalities	94
Argyll Robertson pupils	48
Absent ankle jerks	94
Absent knee jerks	81
Romberg's sign	55
Impaired vibratory sense	52
Impaired position sense	45
Impaired touch and pain sense	13
Ocular palsies	10
Charcot's joints	7

*Data from 150 cases.
SOURCE: After Merritt et al.[3]

diagnostic findings in tabes. Muscular power is usually well maintained until the late stages. Ataxia is evident on testing.

Involvement of cranial nerves (particularly the second, third, and sixth) is often overlooked. Primary optic atrophy may result in blindness if untreated. Oculomotor weakness and eighth nerve involvement with resultant hearing loss are also seen. Antibiotic treatment cannot reverse the extensive changes of advanced disease.

Laboratory findings Laboratory findings may be quite variable, depending on the stage of tabes, whether partial or full treatment has been administered in the past, and whether the process has spontaneously burned out. Ten percent of patients have negative serum VDRL titers. CSF findings may be normal or may include (1) lymphocytic pleocytosis (5 to 160 lymphocytes per cubic millimeter), (2) moderately elevated protein levels (45 to 100 mg/dl), and (3) increased globulin concentration. Normal CSF can be found in the late stages of treated or burned out tabes in a patient who continues to have lightning pains and Charcot's joints; this finding reflects the irreversible damage already produced in the spinal cord and dorsal roots.

Diagnosis and differential diagnosis A clinical diagnosis of tabes is most likely in a patient with lightning pains and ataxia who exhibits findings of absent deep tendon reflexes, Argyll Robertson pupils, and a positive Romberg sign. Differential diagnosis includes a variety of neurologic disorders, such as Adie's syndrome (absent deep tendon reflexes and myotonic pupil) and diabetic neuropathy.

Other now uncommon manifestations of neurosyphilis include isolated optic atrophy with resultant blindness and mass lesions of the brain and spinal cord due to syphilitic gummas.

Treatment of Neurosyphilis

CNS disease may occur during any stage of syphilis. Clinical evidence of neurologic involvement (optic and auditory symptoms, cranial nerve palsies, etc.) warrants CSF examination.

Recommended Regimen

Aqueous crystalline penicillin G, 12 to 24 million units daily (2 to 4 million units every 4 hours IV), for 10 to 14 days.

Alternative Regimen (if outpatient compliance can be ensured)

Procaine penicillin IM, 2.4 million units IM daily, and probenecid, 500 mg orally 4 times daily, both for 10 to 14 days.

Many authorities recommend addition of benzathine penicillin, 2.4 million units IM weekly for three doses after completion of these neurosyphilis treatment regimens. No systematically collected data have evaluated therapeutic alternatives to penicillin. Patients who cannot tolerate penicillin should be skin-tested, and desensitized if necessary, or managed in consultation with an expert.

Follow-Up

If an initial CSF pleocytosis was present, CSF examination should be repeated every 6 months until the cell count is normal. If it has not decreased at 6 months, or is not normal by 2 years, retreatment should be strongly considered.

HIV Infection and Neurosyphilis

Although there is only anecdotal evidence that HIV infection alters extra-CNS features of syphilis, mounting evidence suggests that conventional syphilis treatment fails more often in HIV-infected patients. Moreover, persons with HIV demonstrate accelerated progression to early neurosyphilis, often after conventional therapy for early syphilis. HIV infection itself can cause aseptic meningitis. At least partly as a result of the AIDS epidemic, neurosyphilis (particularly early neurosyphilis) has become much more common among young adults in the past few years than in preceding decades. Other infections (e.g., CMV, toxoplasmosis), of course, can mimic neurosyphilis and are common in HIV-infected patients.

Early neurosyphilis has been demonstrated in a substantial number of AIDS patients. Early manifestations include optic neuritis or neuroretinitis which may present with blurred vision or blindness, cranial nerve palsies, polyradiculopathy, or cerebrovascular accident. Most patients have positive CSF VDRL tests, but CSF abnormalities are not otherwise distinctive. Varying levels of derangement have been found in CSF cell count and protein and glucose levels.

Treatment of HIV-infected patients

Although critical data are lacking, most experts treat neurosyphilis in HIV-infected patients with intravenous penicillin for at least 10 days followed by benzathine penicillin weekly for three doses (see "Treatment of Neurosyphilis" above). Careful follow-up is necessary to ensure adequacy of therapy.

Patients should be followed clinically and with quantitative nontreponemal serologic tests (VDRL, RPR) at 1, 2, 3, 6, 9, and 12 months after treatment. Patients with early syphilis whose titers fail to decrease fourfold within 6 months should undergo CSF examination and be re-treated.

CARDIOVASCULAR SYPHILIS

At the turn of this century tertiary syphilis was a major cause of cardiovascular disease, but syphilitic heart disease is now relatively uncommon. Regardless of its incidence, syphilitic heart disease may present unpredictably after a long latent period and should be considered in the evaluation of diseases of the aorta and aortic valve.

Pathology and Pathophysiology

The cardiovascular system is not clinically affected in the early stages of syphilis, but it is involved morphologically in up to 80 percent of occurrences of the tertiary stage of the disease. Clinical manifestations of cardiovascular syphilis, however, may occur in only about 10 percent of such occurrences.

T. pallidum presumably spreads to the heart during the early stages of syphilis, possibly via the lymphatics, and the organisms lodge in the aortic wall, where they remain dormant for years. The spirochetes appear to have a predilection for the vasa vasorum of the aorta; they produce transmural inflammatory lesions which result in endarteritis of these vessels. Ultimately, all layers of the aortic wall are affected; varying degrees of thickening, scarring, and destruction of the intima, media, and adventitia occur with development of atherosclerotic plaques and calcification.

Clinical Manifestations

Because cardiovascular syphilis is manifested only in the tertiary stage of the disease, which is preceded by a latent period of 15 to 30 years, most patients with clinical evidence of cardiovascular syphilis are between 40 and 55 years of age. Men are affected three times as often as women. The major clinical cardiac problems posed by syphilis are thoracic aneurysm, aortic valve incompetence, and coronary ostial stenosis. Antibiotic therapy is not helpful because dysfunction at this late stage is due to degenerative changes and not active infection.

Aneurysm almost always involves the thoracic aorta, particularly the proximal ascending aorta immediately at and above the sinuses of Valsalva. Dissecting aneurysms do not occur, probably because of the medial scarring and wall thickening of the chronic inflammatory process. Typical presentations include persistent chest pain or symptoms of a mass lesion compressing adjacent structures.

Coronary artery involvement is usually restricted to the ostia or the most proximal few millimeters of the coronary arteries. When syphilitic endarteritis significantly narrows the coronary ostia, it may lead to ischemic heart disease, including angina pectoris or sudden death.

Aortic regurgitation without stenosis is a common cardiovascular manifestation of syphilis. Regurgitation appears to be due to aortic root dilatation with stretching of the aortic valve. If aortic stenosis is also present, the cause is unlikely to be syphilis. The differential diagnosis of chronic pure aortic insufficiency (i.e., without a component of stenosis) includes healed infective endocarditis, Marfan's syndrome, ankylosing spondylitis, Reiter's syndrome, and congenitally malformed valves.

LATE BENIGN SYPHILIS

Late benign syphilis is now rare. It represents an inflammatory process [either proliferative or destructive (gummatous)] that involves structures generally not essential to the maintenance of life. This process may occur in both acquired and prenatal infection. Most of these manifestations occur in the skin and the bones, with a lower frequency in the mucosae and certain of the viscera, muscles, and ocular structures. Resulting scar tissue may impair function of the structures involved.

Pathogenesis and Pathophysiology

In late benign syphilis the inflammatory response to a few *T. pallidum* organisms results in formation of a gumma. Syphilitic inflammation is generally relatively mild but chronic, and slow destruction of tissue eventually leads to fibrosis. The early inflammatory nodule has a granulomatous character which closely resembles the lesion of tuberculosis. Grossly, gummas are nodules which may be found in any tissue or organ and may vary from microscopic size to many centimeters in diameter. The necrotic material in the larger nodules is of a gummy consistency, hence the term *gumma*. The lesion is encapsulated by proliferating connective tissue. When the skin or mucous membrane is involved, an ulcer develops. Deep scarring accompanies the healing of gummas.

Ulcerative, nodular, noduloulcerative, and gummatous lesions may invade the skin, skeleton, oral cavity, upper and lower respiratory tracts, and digestive system. Because of the rarity of this manifestation, there are few data concerning the response of late benign syphilis to penicillin therapy. Available information suggests that penicillin is highly efficacious.

TREATMENT OF LATE LATENT SYPHILIS (GREATER THAN 1 YEAR'S DURATION), GUMMAS, AND CARDIOVASCULAR SYPHILIS

All patients should have a thorough clinical examination. Ideally, all patients with syphilis of greater than 1 year's duration should have CSF examination; however, performance of lumbar puncture can be individualized. In older (>50 years) asymptomatic individuals, the yield of lumbar puncture is relatively low; however, CSF examination is clearly indicated in specific situations [neurologic signs or symptoms, treatment failure, serum nontreponemal titer $\geq$ 1:32, other evidence of active syphilis (e.g., aortitis), non-penicillin therapy planned, positive HIV antibody test].

Recommended Regimen

Benzathine penicillin G, 7.2 million units total, administered as 3 doses of 2.4 million units IM, given 1 week apart for 3 consecutive weeks.

If patients are allergic to penicillin, alternative drugs should be used only after CSF examination has excluded neurosyphilis. Penicillin allergy is best determined at present by careful history taking, but skin testing may be used if the major and minor determinants are available.

Alternative Regimen

Doxycycline, 100 mg orally 2 times a day for 4 weeks *or* **tetracycline, 500 mg orally 4 times a day for 4 weeks.**

Note: If CSF examination is performed and reveals findings consistent with neurosyphilis, patients should be treated for neurosyphilis

Follow-Up

Quantitative nontreponemal serologic tests should be repeated at 6 and 12 months. If titers increase fourfold, or if an initially high titer (greater than or equal to 1:32) fails to decrease, or if the patient develops signs or symptoms attributable to syphilis, the patient should be evaluated for neurosyphilis and retreated appropriately.

REFERENCES

1. Dewhurst K: The neurosyphilitic psychoses today: A survey of 91 cases. *Br J. Psychiatry* 115:31, 1969
2. Dawson-Butterworth K, Heathcote PEM: Review of hospitalized cases of general paralysis of the insane. *Br J. Vener Dis* 46:295, 1970
3. Merritt HH et al: *Neurosyphilis.* New York, Oxford, 1946

ADDITIONAL READING

Grey MR: Syphilis and AIDS in Belle Glade, Florida, 1942 and 1992. *Ann Intern Med* 116:329, 1992

Hook EW III, Marra CM: Acquired syphilis in adults. *N Engl J Med* 326:1060, 1992

Hutchinson CM et al: Characteristics of patients with syphilis attending Baltimore STD clinics. Multiple high-risk subgroups and interactions with human immunodeficiency virus infection. *Arch Intern Med* 151:511, 1991

Lukehart SA et al: Invasion of the central nervous system by *Treponema pallidum:* Implications for diagnosis and treatment. *Ann Intern Med* 109:855, 1988

Matlow GA, Rachlis A: Syphilis serology in human immunodeficiency virus-infected patients with symptomatic neurosyphilis: Case report and review. *J Infect Dis* 12:703, 1990

Musher D: Syphilis, neurosyphilis, penicillin, and AIDS. *J Infect Dis* 163:1201, 1991

Musher DM et al: Effect of human immunodeficiency virus (HIV) infection on the course of syphilis and on the response to treatment. *Ann Intern Med* 113:872, 1990

Romanowski B et al: Serologic response to treatment of infectious syphilis. *Ann Intern Med* 114:1005, 1991

Zenilman JM et al: Effect of HIV posttest counseling on STD incidence. *JAMA* 267:843, 1992

For a more detailed discussion, see Musher DM: Biology of *Treponema pallidum,* Chap. 18, p. 205; Sparling PF: Natural History of Syphilis, Chap. 19, p. 213; Thin RN: Early Syphilis in the Adult, Chap. 20, p. 221; Swartz MN: Neurosyphilis, Chap. 21, p. 231; Healy BP: Cardiovascular Syphilis, Chap. 22, p. 247; Larsen SA, Hunter EF, Creighton ET: Syphilis, Chap. 75, p. 927; Jaffe HW, Musher DM: Management of the Reactive Syphilis Serology, Chap. 76, p. 935, in STD-2.

DEFINITION

Chancroid is a sexually transmitted ulcerative disease which is often associated with an inguinal bubo. Its cause is *Haemophilus ducreyi,* a gram-negative bacillus.

EPIDEMIOLOGY

Chancroid occurs throughout the world but has a particularly high incidence in developing countries. The number of reported cases in the United States, however, has increased markedly since 1985, with the majority of cases occurring in New York City, Dallas, Boston, and several communities in Florida. The disease is more prevalent in persons from lower socioeconomic groups who frequent prostitutes.

H. ducreyi appears to spread from person to person only by sexual contact with no known alternate routes. Autoinoculation of fingers or other sites is reported occasionally. Men have a much higher incidence of chancroid than women do; lack of circumcision further increases susceptibility of males to infection. There is no evidence for a continuing reservoir of *H. ducreyi* in the absence of clinical cases of chancroid. It is presumed that individuals capable of transmitting the infection to others have ulcers. In women, ulcers may often be subclinical, and sexual activity continues. Thus, women with multiple sexual contacts, ulcers, and few if any symptoms may be an efficient reservoir for continued dissemination of *H. ducreyi* throughout a community.

EPIDEMIOLOGIC ASSOCIATION WITH HIV-1

Studies in Africa provide substantial evidence that chancroid, like other genital ulcer diseases, is a risk factor for the heterosexual spread of HIV-1. In Africa and probably in many other developing regions, most genital ulcers are due to chancroid. It has recently been observed that both men and women with chancroid and asymptomatic HIV-1 infection are much more likely to have treatment fail. This observation has major implications for treatment protocols in countries in which HIV-1 is prevalent. If both pathogens are present, chancroid and HIV-1 presumably act synergistically with increased infectivity, susceptibility, and, for *H. ducreyi,* failure to respond to treatment. Chancroid may be one of the major reasons for the rapid heterosexual spread of HIV-1 in eastern and southern Africa.

MICROBIOLOGY

H. ducreyi is a small, pleomorphic, gram-negative, facultative anaerobic bacillus. All strains are oxidase-positive and catalase-negative and reduce nitrate. Like several other members of the genus *Haemophilus, H. ducreyi* requires hemin (X factor) for growth. The organism grows well on nutritionally enriched media such as chocolate blood agar or hemoglobin agar with complex supplements (IsoVitaleX or CVA).

Ampicillin-resistance (β-lactamase producing) plasmids have been identified in *H. ducreyi.* These plasmids are similar to those found in *H. influenzae, H. parainfluenzae,* and *Neisseria gonorrhoeae.* Studies have shown that *H. ducreyi* is able to accept and donate plasmids during conjugation with other species of *Haemophilus.* This suggests that widespread dissemination of antibiotic-resistance determinants and other genes is possible in this species.

PATHOGENESIS

The pathogenesis of genital ulcers due to *H. ducreyi* has not been extensively investigated. Trauma or abrasion is thought to be necessary for organisms to penetrate the epidermis. The inoculum size required for infection is not known, and no toxins or extracellular enzymes of the organism have been discovered.

Some strains of *H. ducreyi* are virulent, whereas others are apparently avirulent. Virulent strains are relatively resistant to phagocytosis and killing by human polymorphonuclear leukocytes and are resistant to complement-mediated killing by normal human and rabbit sera.

CLINICAL MANIFESTATIONS

The incubation period ranges between 3 and 10 days with a median of 4 to 7 days. There are no prodromal symptoms.

Men usually present because of ulcerative lesions or inguinal tenderness. Depending on the site of the ulcer, women often present with less obvious symptoms including pain on voiding, pain on defecation, rectal bleeding, dyspareunia, or vaginal discharge.

The chancre begins as a tender papule surrounded by erythema. Over the course of 24 to 48 h it becomes pustular, eroded, and ulcerated. Vesicles are not seen at any stage of the disease. The ulcer is usually quite painful in males, but it frequently is not painful in females. Most women with ulcers are unaware of their infection. The ulcer has ragged undermined edges, is sharply demarcated, and is without induration. Its base may be covered by a gray or yellow necrotic purulent exudate, and its friable granulomatous base may bleed on scraping. There is little inflam-

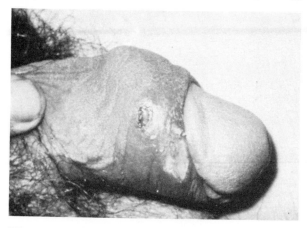

FIG. 7-1. Typical chancroidal ulcer in a male.

mation of the surrounding skin. Several lesions may merge to form giant ulcers (greater than 2 cm) or serpiginous ulcers. Occasionally, lesions may remain pustular, the so-called dwarf chancroid, and resemble a folliculitis or pyogenic infection. One-half of men have a single ulcer, but women often have multiple lesions.

Most lesions in males are on either the external or internal surface of the prepuce, on the frenulum, or in the coronal sulcus. The glans meatus and the shaft of the penis can also be involved but are involved less frequently (Fig. 7-1).

In females most lesions are at the entrance to the vagina and include lesions on the fourchette, labia, vestibule, and clitoris. Longitudinal ulcers are often present at the posterior fourchette; large periurethral ulcers are not uncommon. Rectovaginal fistulas have been reported as a complication of chancroid. Extragenital lesions are less common but have been described on the breasts, fingers, and thighs, and within the mouth.

Differential diagnosis of chancroid includes other causes of genital ulcers such as syphilis, genital herpes, lymphogranuloma venereum, and donovanosis (see Chap. 26).

Painful inguinal adenitis, a characteristic feature of chancroid, may be present in up to 50 percent of patients. The adenitis is unilateral in most patients, and erythema of the overlying skin is usually present. Buboes form and can become fluctuant and rupture spontaneously (Fig. 7-2). Bubo pus is usually thick, creamy, and

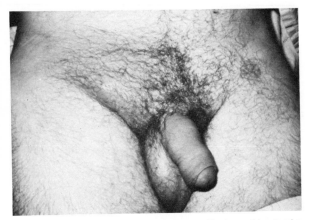

FIG. 7-2. Ruptured inguinal bubo in a patient with chancroid; extensive destruction of soft tissues and skin is evident.

viscous. Both lymphadenitis and bubo formation are less common in females.

Mild constitutional symptoms can accompany the illness. However, *H. ducreyi* has not been shown to cause systemic infection or to spread to distant sites. Occasionally, superinfection with anaerobes such as *Fusobacterium* spp. or *Bacteroides* spp. leads to gangrenous phagedenic ulceration and extensive destruction of genital tissue.

H. ducreyi has not been noted to cause opportunistic infection or to become more invasive in immunocompromised hosts. However, among HIV-infected persons, ulcers due to chancroid are larger, persist for longer periods of time, and are associated with less extensive lymphadenoapathy than is noted among normal hosts.

Chancroid has not been reported to cause disease in infants born to women with active chancroid at delivery.

LABORATORY DIAGNOSIS

Diagnosis of chancroid depends on the isolation of *H. ducreyi* from a genital ulcer or bubo and the exclusion of other diseases associated with similar clinical findings, especially ulcers due to herpes simplex, syphilis, and lymphogranuloma venereum.

Specimens should be taken from the purulent ulcer base with either cotton or calcium alginate swabs. The organism will only survive for 2 to 4 h on a swab unless refrigerated. Numbers of *H. ducreyi* in ulcer exudates are substantial and probably in the range of 10^7 to 10^8 per milliliter of pus. On the other hand, no organisms are seen in bubo pus, and culture from the bubo is always sterile unless it has ruptured and an inguinal abscess is present.

Direct examination of clinical material by a Gram stain sometimes reveals pleomorphic gram-negative organisms in a "school of fish" pattern, but these smears may be difficult to interpret because of the polymicrobial flora of most genital ulcers.

It is best to confirm the diagnosis by culture, but recovery rates are variable—probably because of the fastidious growth requirements of the organism. The best single media have been prepared from a nutritionally rich agar base supplemented with hemoglobin and serum, such as gonococcal agar supplemented with hemoglobin and fetal calf serum. Other media have also been used successfully. Growth usually occurs in 2 to 4 days but may take as long as 7. Alternatives to culture diagnosis are not yet widely available.

TREATMENT

Clinically significant antimicrobial resistance has become common. Plasmid-mediated antibiotic resistance has been described for ampicillin, sulfonamides, chloramphenicol, tetracycline, streptomycin, and kanamycin.

Recommended Regimen
Azithromycin 1g orally, once, *or* ceftriaxone 250 mg IM in a single dose *or* erythromycin base 500 mg orally 4 times a day for 7 days.

Alternative Regimens
Amoxicillin 500 mg plus clavulanic acid 125 mg orally 3 times a day for 7 days *or* ciprofloxacin 500 mg orally 2 times a day for 3 days.

We do not recommend single-dose therapy for HIV-infected persons, as higher failure rates have been noted with one-dose regimens in this population.

Relapse after complete healing occurs at the site of the original ulcer in about 5 percent of patients. Retreatment with the original regimen is usually successful. Persons who have been sexual partners within the 10 days preceding onset of symptoms in an infected patient should be examined and treated, whether symptomatic or not. This presumptive treatment helps avoid reinfection of the index patient and prevent further dissemination of the disease.

ADDITIONAL READING

Farris JR et al: Chancroid in Dallas: New lessons from an old disease. *Tex Med* 87:78, 1991

Schmid GP: Treatment of chancroid, 1989. *Rev Infect Dis* 12:S580, 1990

For a more detailed discussion, see Ronald AR, Albritton W: Chancroid and *Haemophilus ducreyi,* Chap. 24, p. 263 in STD-2.

Donovanosis is a chronic, progressively destructive bacterial infection of the genital region which is believed to be sexually transmitted. The disease has been known by many names, including granuloma inguinale and granuloma venereum.

MICROBIOLOGY

The etiology of donovanosis is *Calymmatobacterium granulomatis,* a gram-negative bacterium measuring 1.5 by 0.7 µm. In tissue smears the bacteria appear enclosed in vacuolar compartments in large histiocytic cells or occasionally in polymorphonuclear leukocytes or plasma cells. The bacteria reproduce in multiple foci within these cells until the vacuole contains 20 to 30 organisms, which mature and are then liberated when the infected cell ruptures.

The organisms have a surrounding cell membrane and overlying cell wall and possess a sharply defined capsule when mature. Small filamentous projections, of the size of bacterial fimbriae or pili, extend from the cell wall. Culture in the chick embryonic yolk sac has been reported, but the organism is difficult to grow on artificial media. Its biochemical and bacteriological characteristics have not been well defined.

PATHOGENESIS

The primary lesion begins as an indurated nodule which erodes to form a beefy, exuberant, granulomatous, heaped ulcer. This process usually progresses slowly, often coalescing with adjacent lesions or forming new lesions by autoinoculation, particularly in the perineal region. Little is known about microbial toxins or other virulence factors or the role of the immune system in the pathogenesis of donovanosis. The infecting organisms invade mononuclear endothelial cells, and when mature, feature metachromatic bars that stain blue or black with Wright's stain. The pathognomonic feature of donovanosis is the large infected mononuclear cell, 15 to 90 µm in diameter, containing many intracytoplasmic cysts filled with deeply staining Donovan bodies (Figs. 8-1 and 8-2).

EPIDEMIOLOGY

Although rarely reported in the United States or other developed countries, donovanosis is among the most prevalent sexually transmitted diseases in some developing communities. The disease is endemic among aborigines living in the central deserts of Australia

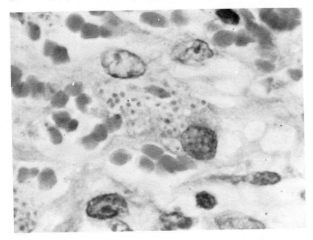

FIG. 8-1. Donovanosis. H&E stain of biopsy specimen, showing intracytoplasmic Donovan bodies.

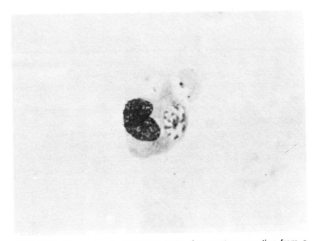

FIG. 8-2. Donovanosis. Giemsa's stain of a crust preparation from a biopsy specimen, showing a single cell with many intracytoplasmic Donovan bodies.

and is common in India, the Caribbean, Africa, and many other tropical or subtropical environments. A recent epidemic of 20 cases was reported in Texas.

The role of sexual transmission is controversial. In most cases, lesions cannot be detected in sexual contacts, but a number of studies have detected infection in 12 to 52 percent of steady sexual partners. The disease is only mildly contagious, and repeated exposure is apparently necessary for the development of most clinical cases. The long incubation period or inconspicuous location of lesions (such as rectum or vagina) favors low detection rates in sexual partners.

CLINICAL MANIFESTATIONS AND SEQUELAE

The incubation period has been ill defined but is probably 8 to 80 days. The disease begins as single or multiple subcutaneous nodules which erode through the skin to produce clean, granulomatous, sharply defined lesions which are usually painless (Fig. 8-3). These lesions, which bleed readily on contact, slowly enlarge; there may be abundant, beefy-red granulation tissue. Secondary infection of an ulcer or its margin may occur, but surrounding cellulitis is rarely

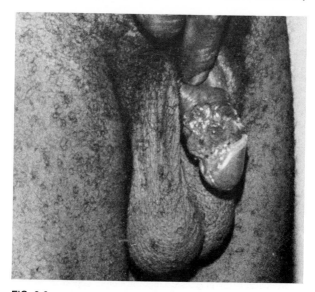

FIG. 8-3. Donovanosis. Typical beefy granuloma of the penis.

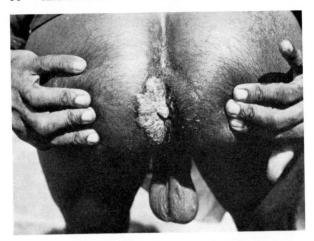

FIG. 8-4. Perianal donovanosis. *(Courtesy of CN Sowmini.)*

seen. Fibrosis occurs concurrently with extension of the primary lesion, and phimosis or lymphedema of distal tissues is common in the active phase of the disease. Inguinal involvement may mimic the buboes of other genital infections (pseudobuboes).

The genitalia are involved in 90 percent of cases, the inguinal region in 10 percent, the anal region in 5 to 10 percent, and distant sites in 1 to 5 percent. A verrucous form of disease is likely to occur in the perianal area (Fig. 8-4). Lesions are limited to the genitalia in approximately 80 percent of cases and to the inguinal region in less than 5 percent. Cervical or intravaginal lesions may be an uncommon cause of vaginal bleeding but may account for the predominance of females among patients who suffer hematogenous spread of the organism.

In the male, lesions usually occur on the prepuce or glans; in the female, lesions on the labia are the most common. The most frequently involved distant sites are on the head (mouth, lips, throat, face), but involvement of the liver, thorax, and bones has also been reported.

DIAGNOSIS

Clinical manifestations are highly suggestive of the diagnosis in most cases. Wright's or Giemsa's stain of crush preparations from the lesion confirms the diagnosis. Donovan bodies appear as clusters of blue- or black-staining organisms with a safety pin appearance (from bipolar chromatin condensation) in the cytoplasm of large mononuclear cells.

Light microscopic examination of biopsy specimens which have been formalin-fixed and wax-embedded is a less reliable diagnostic procedure since the pathognomonic Donovan bodies are infrequently seen. However, the organisms may be identified by electron microscopy or by light microscopy of sections prepared for electron microscopy by glutaraldehyde fixation and plastic embedding.

Investigation for other sexually transmitted disease is warranted in patients in whom donovanosis is suspected. Coexisting diseases such as syphilis are common.

DIFFERENTIAL DIAGNOSIS

Penile donovanosis is frequently misdiagnosed as carcinoma. This confusion may occur relatively early in the disease process, and in advanced cases of donovanosis or when unusual sites are affected, the simulation of carcinoma may be even more convincing. With external lesions histologic examination definitively resolves diagnostic confusion, but where this is not readily available, therapeutic trial with chloramphenicol or another appropriate antibiotic can resolve the diagnostic dilemma within a few weeks.

Perianal donovanosis lesions are frequently diagnosed as condylomata lata of secondary syphilis. Patients may be referred because of persisting condylomata lata following penicillin therapy—a history that is virtually diagnostic of donovanosis in areas where the disease is common. Syphilis serologic examination may add to the confusion because it may be positive due to past or concomitant treponemal infection, although the reagin titer is usually low, which makes secondary syphilis unlikely.

Amebiasis and donovanosis may be confused because both may produce necrotic ulceration of the penis following anal intercourse, and the two diseases may coexist. If all findings are consistent with donovanosis and the diagnosis cannot be resolved by histologic examination, a therapeutic trial with chloramphenicol is warranted.

TREATMENT

Tetracycline (500 mg orally 4 times daily) is probably the most widely used drug for treating donovanosis and, although resistance has been encountered, is recommended as first-line therapy in developed communities where there are high compliance and follow-up rates. Chloramphenciol or gentamicin is reserved for resistant cases. **Chloramphenicol (500 mg 4 times daily),** which is cheap, highly effective, and associated with higher compliance rates than tetracycline (possibly because of gastrointestinal side effects of the latter drug), may be the most appropriate therapy in developing communities. **Erythromycin (500 mg 4 times daily)** may be considered in pregnancy, but the results are often disappointing unless it is combined with another antibiotic. No data are available concerning the efficacy of azithromycin or the fluoroquinolones for treatment of donovanosis.

Medication should be continued until lesions have completely healed and until a minimum of 3 weeks of therapy has been given. When drugs are stopped before this time, healing usually continues, but the recurrence rate is greater.

If an antibiotic is effective, clinical response should be evident in 7 days. Within a few days of the start of treatment, the lesions become paler, less exuberant, and less friable. Total healing, except in severe cases, usually occurs within 3 to 5 weeks. Relapse occurs frequently, especially if an antibiotic is discontinued before the primary lesion has completely subsided. An area of depigmentation may occur at the border of the healed lesion.

PREVENTION

No method of prophylaxis has been assessed. Disastrous sequelae such as complete genital erosion or urethral occlusion are caused solely by delay in seeking treatment. When treated at the time of appearance of the initial subcutaneous nodule, donovanosis is a benign disease. Control strategies should therefore focus on encouraging people to seek treatment as soon as they are aware of genital or inguinal lesions.

ADDITIONAL READING

O'Farrell N et al: Genital ulcer disease in women in Durban, South Africa. *Genitourin Med* 67:322, 1991

O'Farrell N et al: Genital ulcer disease in men in Durban, South Africa. *Genitourin Med* 67:327, 1991

O'Farrell, N, Hammond M: HLA antigens in donovanosis (granuloma inguinale). *Genitourin Med* 67:400, 1991

For a more detailed discussion, see Hart G: Donovanosis, Chap. 25, p. 273, in STD-2.

Clinical Manifestations of HIV Infection in Adults in Industrialized Countries

The clinical spectrum of illnesses associated with the human immunodeficiency virus (HIV) is wide. Complications of HIV infection involve almost every organ system. This chapter will review the clinical features of HIV disease and its complications in adults in industrialized countries.

VIROLOGY

The etiologic agent of acquired immunodeficiency syndrome (AIDS) is HIV, a member of a subfamily of retroviruses called lentiviruses because they characteristically cause slow infections in which months or years separate invasion of the host from the appearance of symptoms. All retroviruses have RNA genomes which are replicated through a DNA intermediate in the cell. The name *retrovirus* refers to this reversed flow of genetic information catalyzed by an RNA-directed DNA polymerase, or reverse transcriptase, of the virus.

Structure of the Virus

Figure 9-1 is a structural model of the distinctive features of HIV. Mature virions are roughly spherical and about 100 nm in diameter (Fig. 9-2), but the range in sizes and shapes is extensive. Seventy to 80 knoblike projections protrude above the surface of the virion, and these envelope structures have two component glycoproteins, gp120 and gp41. The major structural protein of the virus core is p24; other polypeptides derived from a common precursor form a shell around the core (p17), or complex with virion RNA (p7).

Some genes are common to all retroviruses. *Gag* and *env* code for retroviral structural proteins. *Pol* encodes for reverse transcriptase, a protease, and integrase. Long terminal repeats (LTRs) have also been identified in all retroviruses. However, HIV also has at least six additional genes—designated *vif, vpr, vpu, tat, rev,* and *nef*—which play a role in viral replication.

Viral Replication

The life cycle of HIV (Fig. 9-3) begins with the attachment of virus to T-helper lymphocytes and other cells with the CD4 cell surface antigen. Attachment is followed by fusion of the viral envelope and entry of virions. The reverse transcriptase then synthesizes a double-stranded DNA copy of the RNA genome, and viral DNA (proviral genome) then integrates itself into the host cell's chromo-

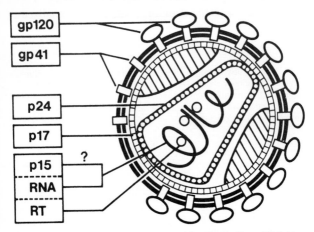

FIG. 9-1. Structural model of the organization of HIV. *(From HR Gelder-blom et al, Virology 156: 171, 1987, with permission.)*

somal DNA. Viral DNA is subsequently transcribed by host cell RNA polymerase II, and the resulting viral mRNAs are translated into the structural proteins. The viral proteins and two copies of the genomic RNA assemble at the cell membrane, and virions are released from the cell by a budding process.

The rate and extent of virus production in tissue culture is governed by the products of the previously described regulatory genes *tat*, *rev*, and *nef*, and by the products of a number of cellular genes. Coinfection by viruses in the herpes and papovavirus families may also reactivate transcription of latent HIV.

DIAGNOSIS

Diagnosis is discussed in Chap. 34.

PATHOGENESIS

In the first step of infection, invasion of the host, HIV is introduced into the bloodstream, either directly or from other sites through intimate contact with infected secretions. Virus attaches and penetrates T-helper lymphocytes, monocytes, macrophages, and possibly epithelial cells, to initiate the multiplication stage of infection. Within the first week or two, individuals become viremic, and circulation of cell-free virus spreads the infection to secondary sites, where a variety of cell types may participate in replication.

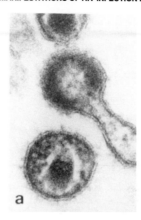

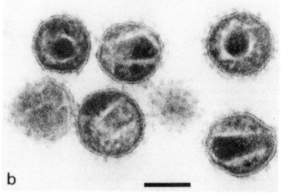

FIG. 9-2. Electron micrographs of thin sections of HIV. *(A)* The most completely budded particle contains an open, electron-dense ribonucleoprotein shell apposed to the viral membrane. Virus surface projections are visible on the left half of the bud. *(B)* "Mature" particles showing different core orientations, lateral bodies, and a continuous dense layer adjacent to the inner membrane. Bar represents 100 nm. *(From HR Gelderblom et al, Virology 156: 171, 1987, with permission.)*

During the period of viral dissemination, the infected individual mounts both a humoral and a cell-mediated response (Fig. 9-4). Seroconversion is often complete by the second to seventh weeks (occasionally much longer). These first antibodies are directed against gp160 and p24, but, in time, antibodies to all other structural

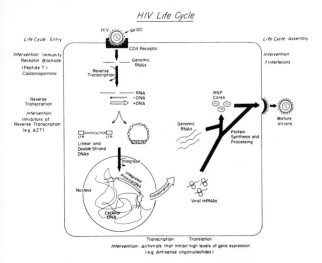

Intervention: Antivirals that inhibit high levels of gene expression
(e.g. Antisense oligonucleotides)

FIG. 9-3. HIV life cycle with points of potential intervention. HIV binds to the CD4 cell surface antigen and enters the cell, where the released viral RNA genomes are copied into DNA. Synthesis is initiated at the 5′ end of the viral RNA using the bound tRNA as primer. Ribonuclease H activity of the reverse transcriptase degrades the RNA in the RNA-DNA hybrid to free sequences complementary to the repeated sequences at the 5′ and 3′ end of the RNA. Base pairing of the (−) strand DNA to the 3′ end of a second viral RNA accomplishes the first transcriptional jump and provides one of the LTRs. As the (−) strand DNA is elongated, ribonuclease H cleavage of RNA at a polypurine tract provides the primer for (+) strand DNA synthesis. In a second transcriptional jump this species is transferred to the end of (−) strand DNA to form the second LTR. A viral integrase facilitates the integration of viral DNA into the host genome. In a productive life cycle, viral DNA is transcribed and translated to generate the RNA cores and viral subcomponents which are assembled into viral particles at the cell surface.

proteins and nonstructural proteins are demonstrable and IgM is replaced by other immunoglobulin classes.

Despite the immune response, HIV persists in its hosts. Its perplexing ability to elude immune surveillance has been attributed to restricted gene expression in the majority of infected cells. Most infected cells harbor the viral genome in an immunologically silent state in which viral antigens are not produced or are not presented in sufficient quantities for efficient detection and destruction by host defenses.

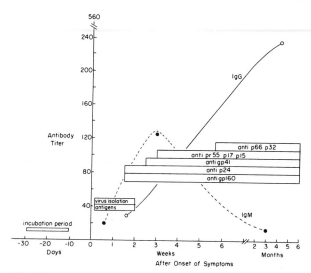

FIG. 9-4. Hypothetical time course of relation of viral isolation and antigenemia to the humoral immune response. Virus may be isolated from peripheral blood lymphocytes throughout the course of the infection, while cell-free viremia again becomes common late in disease.

HIV fuses infected and uninfected cells to form giant cells and syncytia which degenerate as the characteristic cytopathic effect of in vitro infections. Fusion is mediated by interactions between CD4 on the cell's surface and gp41 on the viral envelope. Cell fusion, however, is not the only mechanism of cell death in culture, as HIV kills T cells without fusion, and there are viral mutants which fuse without killing.

In moving from the pathogenesis of cell injury in vitro to pathologic lesions at the organismal level, the mechanisms may be expected to be more complex. First, although the dysfunction and depletion of CD4+ helper cells are central to the immunocompromised state in AIDS, only a relatively small fraction of the lymphocyte population contains evidence of viral infection. This discrepancy between the profound general effects of infection and the limited number of infected cells implies an amplification mechanism set in motion by viral replication. Current speculations include (1) destruction of progenitor cells or other immune cell subsets which affect T cell proliferation and function, (2) elimination of uninfected cells through syncytium formation with infected cells, (3) shedding of the viral glycoprotein which is directly or indirectly immunosuppressive, and (4) an autoimmune state with a target antigen of cellular origin induced by HIV which stimulates production of antilymphocyte antibodies.

EPIDEMIOLOGY

The World Health Organization estimates that by the end of 1990, the AIDS pandemic resulted in approximately 1.3 million AIDS cases worldwide. By the end of that year 156 countries had reported at least one case. As of February 1992, 209,693 cases had been reported in the United States alone since the start of the epidemic.

HIV can be transmitted in three ways: sexually; perinatally; and through exposure to contaminated blood, body fluid, or needles.

Sexual Transmission

Homosexual men have remained the most affected group in almost all developed countries. Approximately 57 percent of the AIDS cases reported to Centers for Disease Control (CDC) are homosexual or bisexual men [including homosexual and bisexual men who are also injecting drug users (IDUs)]. However, HIV infection rates in selected cohorts of homosexual men in major U.S. cities have clearly declined since the early years of the epidemic. This has been attributed to adoption of protective sex practices such as condom use. Objective evidence of such changes can also be found in the falling incidence of other STDs, such as gonorrhea, in homosexual men since 1982. Declines in HIV infection and other STDs in homosexual men have also been noted in Europe, where heterosexual IDUs account for an ever-increasing proportion of AIDS cases.

However, decreases in HIV infection rates in homosexual and bisexual men obscure the fact that in cities such as San Francisco, where half or more of homosexual men have HIV infection, exposure to relatively few partners may lead to infection. Also, it is expected that the number of AIDS cases in homosexual men will continue to increase as persons infected years ago become ill. It will probably be several more years before the incidence of AIDS in homosexual men substantially decreases.

Worldwide, heterosexual contact is the most common means of HIV infection. Although most AIDS cases in the United States are due to homosexual transmission, an increasing proportion are attributed to heterosexual acquisition. Of the second 100,000 AIDS cases reported to the CDC, 7 percent were acquired through heterosexual contact.

Although HIV appears to be transmitted more efficiently from men to women, transmission from women to men is well documented and occurs frequently in the developing world.

Injection Drug Use

After homosexual and bisexual men, IDUs are the next largest category of AIDS patients in the industrialized world. Of the second 100,000 reported AIDS cases in the United States, 24 percent occurred among persons with a history of injection drug use. The extent of drug use since 1978, needle-sharing frequency, and time spent in "shooting galleries" all increase one's risk of HIV infection. Conversely, use of sterile needles and length of time in treatment (methadone) programs are associated with lower rates of infection. Seroprevalence among IDUs in New York City has been estimated to be about 50 percent, and seroprevalence in Europe reportedly varies from 17 to 70 percent.

IDUs are an important link between the reservoir of HIV in the infected population and the uninfected heterosexual population. Women who acquire HIV infection from sexual contact more frequently report sexual contact with IDUs than with bisexual men, transfusion-infected men, or hemophilic men. Conversely, female-to-male spread of HIV may result from contact with prostitutes, who are often IDUs or sex partners of IDUs. Finally, about 80 percent of U.S. pediatric AIDS cases occur in infants born to HIV-infected mothers; most of these infected mothers are IDUs or the sex partners of IDUs. Thus, the current high prevalence and continued incidence of HIV infection in IDUs is not a problem limited to themselves.

Blood and Clotting Factor Transfusion

With the availability and widespread use of an enzyme immunoassay for screening blood for HIV antibodies, HIV infections from blood transfusion have been almost completely eliminated. Such screening began by April 1985 in almost all U.S. blood collection centers and shortly thereafter in most European countries. However, before the widespread screening, an estimated 12,000 U.S. residents may have been infected by transfused blood and survived the illness or procedure for which they received blood.

Persons with hemophilia receive clotting factors harvested from plasma of thousands of blood donors. About 80 percent of men with hemophilia in the United States became infected with HIV through transfusion of infected clotting factor in the early 1980s. Heat treatment has since been widely adopted, making infection of previously uninfected persons with hemophilia exceedingly rare in industrialized countries.

Perinatal Transmission

Children may acquire HIV infection through any of the mechanisms listed above, such as by transfusion of blood or antihemophilic clotting factors and, rarely, through sexual exposures. However, in most countries, most HIV transmission to children is perinatal; in the United States, about 80 percent of children under 13 years old who have AIDS have a parent with or at risk for AIDS. As noted earlier, perinatal transmission is closely linked to HIV infection in IDUs and their sex partners.

The actual risk of HIV infection in the perinatal period has varied widely from report to report, but pooled data and larger studies suggest that infants born to infected mothers have about a 30 percent risk of acquiring infection from their mothers.

Risk Factors for Acquisition and Transmission of HIV

Large cohort studies of homosexual men in developed countries have yielded important data about behavioral risk factors for HIV infection. These studies have uniformly shown that large numbers of sexual partners and receptive anal intercourse, unprotected by condoms, both substantially increase a homosexual man's likelihood of becoming infected by HIV. The data regarding risk of HIV infection from insertive anal intercourse and from receptive or insertive oral intercourse have been much less clear, mainly because it is almost impossible to find a sufficient number of persons who engage in just one of these practices to the exclusion of other sexual activities. However, because these behaviors involve the exchange of semen or mucosal–mucosal (and perhaps blood-to-blood) contact, they should not generally be regarded as safe sex practices in regard to HIV transmission.

Other risk factors that have emerged from several recent studies are either a previous history of genital ulcer disease, such as chancroid, syphilis, or herpes simplex virus type 2 (HSV-2), or lack of circumcision. It seems biologically plausible that genital ulcers could predispose to HIV infection because mucosal lesions (even when they are not apparent) might facilitate entry of HIV to the bloodstream. Similarly, other sexually transmitted diseases which cause microulcerations, such as gonorrhea and chlamydia, also appear to increase the risk of HIV transmission. Lack of circumcision provides a larger mucosal surface for virus entry in men and probably predisposes to various causes of genital ulcer disease as well.

Biological host factors that might enhance transmissibility from an HIV-infected to an uninfected person are hard to evaluate. Available evidence suggests that persons with advanced HIV disease have higher levels of viremia and may be more infectious than those with early disease.

CLINICAL MANIFESTATIONS

Several classification systems for HIV-related illnesses have been proposed. Tables 9-1 and 9-2 respectively outline the 1986 CDC and Walter Reed classification systems. The CDC's 1992 revised AIDS case definition and HIV classification system are discussed later in this chapter. The CDC classification offers the advantage of simplicity, whereas the Walter Reed system utilizes laboratory abnormalities, for example, T-helper cell numbers and cutaneous delayed hypersensitivity reactivity, to help with staging. Although categorization is somewhat artificial and often misleading to patients, it is useful for surveillance, epidemiologic studies, and studies of therapeutic intervention. This chapter will use the CDC classification system.

Acute Primary Infection Syndromes

Many HIV seroconversions are asymptomatic or subclinical. However, some seroconverters develop a self-limited mononucleosis or influenza-like syndrome characterized by various combinations of fever, rigors, arthralgias, myalgias, malaise, lethargy, anorexia, nausea, diarrhea, sore throat, and a truncal maculopapular, urticarial, or vesicular rash. Neurologic signs and symptoms may predominate, including headaches, stiff neck, retroorbital pain, neuritis, myelopathy, photophobia, irritability, depression, or frank encephalopathy. The illness may last 2 to 3 weeks but usually results in clinical recovery.

Laboratory abnormalities may include transient leukopenia, lym-

TABLE 9-1. CDC Classification for HIV Infections (1986)

Group I	Acute infection
Group II	Asymptomatic infection*
Group III	Persistent generalized lymphadenopathy*
Group IV	Other disease:
Subgroup A	Constitutional disease
Subgroup B	Neurologic disease
Subgroup C	Secondary infectious diseases
Category C-1	Specified secondary infectious diseases listed in the CDC surveillance definition for AIDS†
Category C-2	Other specified secondary infectious diseases
Subgroup D	Secondary cancers
Subgroup E	Other conditions

*Patients in groups II and III may be subclassified on the basis of a laboratory evaluation.
†Includes those patients whose clinical presentation fulfills the definition of AIDS used by CDC for national reporting.
This classification system has been replaced by the 1992 system.

TABLE 9-2. The Walter Reed Staging Classification for HIV Infection

WR stage	HIV antibody or virus detection	Chronic lymphadenopathy	T-helper cells/mm³	Delayed hypersensitivity	Thrush	Opportunistic infections
0	−	−	>400	+	−	−
1	+	−	>400	+	−	−
2	+	+	>400	+	−	−
3	+	±	<400	+	−	−
4	+	±	<400	Partial anergy	−	−
5	+	±	<400	Complete and/or	+	−
6	+	±	<400	Partial or complete anergy	±	+

108

phopenia, relative monocytosis, thrombocytopenia, and elevated erythrocyte sedimentation rate. The T4/T8 ratios in peripheral blood may become inverted, largely as a result of increased numbers of T8 cells, and atypical lymphocytes may be seen on blood smears.

Incubation periods range from a few days up to 3 months, and seroconversion usually occurs 2 to 10 weeks after onset of acute illness. HIV can be isolated from blood, and HIV p24 antigen can often be detected in plasma during the acute illness. HIV has been isolated from CSF during episodes of acute meningitis.

Immunofluorescent antibody (IFA) techniques reveal IgM antibodies to HIV in serum which peak at 24 ± 17 days after onset of acute illness and disappear by 81 ± 27 days. IgG IFA titers are detectable somewhat later, peak at 133 ± 63 days, and persist. Detection of seroconversion by enzyme immunosorbent assay (ELISA) varies in time from day 31 ± 14 to 58 ± 32, depending on the kit used.

Asymptomatic Infection and Persistent Generalized Lymphadenopathy

The duration of an asymptomatic carrier state is unpredictable but may be prolonged. In adults, mean asymptomatic incubation periods before development of AIDS have been estimated at 10 years.

It is not clear what viral, host, or environmental factors are responsible for the variable disease progression among HIV-infected individuals. In a Multicenter AIDS Cohort Study of homosexual and bisexual HIV seropositive men, decreased numbers of CD4 cells, increased numbers of CD8 cells, high titers of cytomegalovirus (CMV) antibodies, low levels of HIV antibodies, and history of sex with someone in whom AIDS developed were independently associated with subsequent progression to AIDS. It is not clear whether these are determinants or merely markers of disease progression.

Asymptomatic HIV carriers often have persistent generalized lymphadenopathy (PGL), defined as palpable lymphadenopathy (nodes ≥ 1 cm) at two or more extrainguinal sites for more than 3 months in the absence of an identifiable cause other than HIV infection. Nodal histologic examination demonstrates pronounced follicular hyperplasia with prominent capillary endothelial cell proliferation. As patients develop clinical symptoms, lymph node histologic findings change to reflect atrophy of germinal centers, progressing to lymphocyte depletion and fibrosis. Thus, lymph node regression may, paradoxically, herald disease progression.

Symptomatic HIV Infection

After a variable period of asymptomatic HIV seropositivity, a variety of signs or symptoms may herald clinical deterioration.

Chronic fevers, night sweats, diarrhea, weight loss, herpes zoster, oral thrush, or hairy leukoplakia may occur individually, simultaneously, or sequentially. The term *AIDS-related complex* (ARC) is often used to characterize the presence of two or more symptoms and two or more laboratory findings indicative of immune dysfunction.

AIDS represents the most advanced stage of HIV disease and is characterized by the development of opportunistic infections, malignancies (e.g., Kaposi's sarcoma), wasting syndrome, and/or HIV encephalopathy. Table 9-3 outlines the 1987 CDC case definition of AIDS.

In December 1992, the CDC further revised the classification system for HIV infection and expanded the case definition for AIDS among adolescents and adults. Category A includes documented HIV infection with no symptoms, persistent generalized lymphadenopathy, or acute (primary) HIV infection with accompanying illness or history of acute HIV infection. Category B includes conditions such as oropharyngeal candidiasis and oral hairy leukoplakia in the presence of HIV infection. Category C includes all clinical conditions in the 1987 AIDS surveillance case definition, recurrent pneumonia, invasive cervical cancer, and pulmonary TB. The expanded AIDS case definition now includes documentation of a $CD4^+$ count less than 200 cells/mm^3 in an HIV-infected person, or any of the clinical conditions listed in Category C.

MANIFESTATIONS OF HIV INFECTION BY BODY SYSTEM

Skin

As immune deficiency develops later in the course of HIV infection, a variety of mucocutaneous manifestations develop. These may be of infectious, neoplastic, allergic, or undefined cause. Table 9-4 lists some of the conditions observed in HIV-infected patients.

Generalized pruritus is one of the most common manifestations of early HIV infection. Pruritus often develops as the patient's CD4 count falls to 500/mm^3. A substantial proportion of HIV-infected patients with pruritus have scabies or positive scrapings for *Demodex* mites; treatment with an antiscabetic agent often relieves their symptoms. Some patients with generalized pruritus have folliculitis and growth of *Staphylococcus* from cultures; these patients sometimes improve with antibiotic therapy.

Seborrheic dermatitis develops in up to 83 percent of patients with AIDS. It is frequently severe and may resemble psoriasis in its appearance, with papular and scaling lesions involving scalp (sometimes with alopecia), face, trunk, groin, and extremities. Diffuse erythroderma may be seen as well. Although the pathogenesis of HIV-associated hyperkeratotic disorders is unclear,

TABLE 9-3. CDC Case Definition of AIDS (1987)

I. *Without laboratory evidence regarding HIV infection.* If laboratory tests for HIV were not performed or gave inconclusive results and the patient had no other cause of immunodeficiency listed in section I.A below, then any disease listed in section I.B indicates AIDS if it was diagnosed by a definitive method.

A. Causes of immunodeficiency that disqualify diseases as indicators of AIDS in the absence of laboratory evidence for HIV infection

1. High-dose or long-term systemic corticosteroid therapy or other immunosuppressive or cytotoxic therapy ≤3 months before the onset of the indicator disease

2. Any of the following diseases diagnosed ≤3 months after diagnosis of the indicator disease: Hodgkin's disease, non-Hodgkin's lymphoma (other than primary brain lymphoma), lymphocytic leukemia, multiple myeloma, any other cancer of lymphoreticular or histiocytic tissue, or angioimmunoblastic lymphadenopathy

3. A genetic (congenital) immunodeficiency syndrome or an acquired immunodeficiency syndrome atypical of HIV infection, such as one involving hypogammaglobulinemia

B. Indicator diseases diagnosed definitively

1. Candidiasis of the esophagus, trachea, bronchi, or lungs
2. Cryptococcosis, extrapulmonary
3. Cryptosporidiosis with diarrhea persisting >1 month
4. Cytomegalovirus disease of an organ other than liver, spleen, or lymph nodes in a patient >1 month of age
5. Herpes simplex virus infection causing a mucocutaneous ulcer that persists longer than 1 month; or bronchitis, pneumonitis, or esophagitis for any duration affecting a patient >1 month of age
6. Kaposi's sarcoma affecting a patient <60 years of age
7. Lymphoma of the brain (primary) affecting a patient <60 years of age
8. Lymphoid interstitial pneumonia and/or pulmonary lymphoid hyperplasia (LIP/PLH complex) affecting a child <13 years of age
9. *Mycobacterium avium* complex or *M. kansasii* disease, disseminated (at a site other than or in addition to lungs, skin, or cervical or hilar lymph nodes)
10. *Pneumocystis carinii* pneumonia
11. Progressive multifocal leukoencephalopathy
12. Toxoplasmosis of the brain affecting a patient >1 month of age

111

TABLE 9-3. CDC Case Definition of AIDS (1987) (Continued)

II. With laboratory evidence for HIV infection. Regardless of the presence of other causes of immunodeficiency (I.A), in the presence of laboratory evidence for HIV infection, any disease listed above (I.B) or below (II.A or II.B) indicates a diagnosis of AIDS.
  A. Indicator diseases diagnosed definitively
    1. Bacterial infections, multiple or recurrent (any combination of at least two within a 2-year period), of the following types affecting a child <13 years of age: septicemia, pneumonia, meningitis, bone or joint infection, or abscess of an internal organ or body cavity (excluding otitis media or superficial skin or mucosal abscesses), caused by Haemophilus, Streptococcus (including pneumococcus), or other pyogenic bacteria
    2. Coccidioidomycosis, disseminated (at a site other than or in addition to lungs or cervical or hilar lymph nodes)
    3. HIV encephalopathy (also called "HIV dementia," "AIDS dementia," or "subacute encephalitis due to HIV")
    4. Histoplasmosis, disseminated (at a site other than or in addition to lungs or cervical or hilar lymph nodes)
    5. Isosporiasis with diarrhea persisting >1 month
    6. Kaposi's sarcoma at any age
    7. Lymphoma of the brain (primary) at any age
    8. Other non-Hodgkin's lymphoma of B-cell or unknown immunologic phenotype and the following histologic types:
       a. Small noncleaved lymphoma (either Burkitt or non-Burkitt type)
       b. Immunoblastic sarcoma (equivalent to any of the following, although not necessarily all in combination: immunoblastic lymphoma, large-cell lymphoma, diffuse histiocytic lymphoma, diffuse undifferentiated lymphoma, or high-grade lymphoma)
       Note: Lymphomas are not included here if they are of T-cell immunologic phenotype or their histologic type is not described or is described as "lymphocytic," "lymphoblastic," "small cleaved," or "plasmacytoid lymphocytic"
    9. Any mycobacterial disease caused by mycobacteria other than M. tuberculosis, disseminated (at a site other than or in addition to lungs, skin, or cervical or hilar lymph nodes)
    10. Disease caused by M. tuberculosis, extrapulmonary (involving at least one site outside the lungs, regardless of whether there is concurrent pulmonary involvement)
    11. Salmonella (nontyphoid) septicemia, recurrent
    12. HIV wasting syndrome (emaciation, "slim disease")

B. Indicator diseases diagnosed presumptively

Note: Given the seriousness of diseases indicative of AIDS, it is generally important to diagnose them definitively, especially when therapy that would be used may have serious side effects or when definitive diagnosis is needed for eligibility for antiretroviral therapy. Nonetheless, in some situations, a patient's condition will not permit the performance of definitive tests. In other situations, accepted clinical practice may be to diagnose presumptively based on the presence of characteristic clinical and laboratory abnormalities.

1. Candidiasis of the esophagus
2. Cytomegalovirus retinitis with loss of vision
3. Kaposi's sarcoma
4. Lymphoid interstitial pneumonia and/or pulmonary lymphoid hyperplasia (LIP/PLH complex) affecting a child <13 years of age
5. Mycobacterial disease (acid-fast bacilli with species not identified by culture), disseminated (involving at least one site other than or in addition to lungs, skin, or cervical or hilar lymph nodes)
6. *Pneumocystis carinii* pneumonia
7. Toxoplasmosis of the brain affecting a patient >1 month of age

III. *With laboratory evidence against HIV infection*. With laboratory test results negative for HIV infection, a diagnosis of AIDS for surveillance purposes is ruled out unless:

A. All the other causes of immunodeficiency listed above in section I.A are excluded; *and*

B. The patient has had either:

1. *Pneumocystis carinii* pneumonia diagnosed by a definitive method; *or*
2. *a.* Any of the other diseases indicative of AIDS listed above in section I.B diagnosed by a definitive method; *and*
   b. A T-helper/inducer (CD4) lymphocyte count <400/mm^3

113

TABLE 9-4. Mucocutaneous Manifestations of HIV Infection

Infections
  Viruses:
    Herpes simplex
    Varicella zoster
    Molluscum contagiosum
    Human papilloma virus
    Hairy leukoplakia (EBV)
  Bacteria:
    Mycobacterium avium or *M. marinum*
    Treponema pallidum (syphilis)
    Staphylococcus aureus
  Fungi:
    Candida albicans
    Cryptococcus neoformans
    Histoplasma capsulatum
  Mites:
    Scabies
Neoplasms
  Kaposi's sarcoma
  Squamous cell carcinomas
  Basal cell carcinomas
  Cutaneous lymphomas (?)
Miscellaneous
  Seborrheic dermatitis
  Telangiectasis
  Ichthyosis
  Erythroderma
  Papules
  Drug reactions

both ketoconazole and topical steroids are sometimes useful in their management.

Papular eruptions with noncoalescing 2- to 5-mm skin-colored papules, often pruritic, have been described in over 20 percent of patients with AIDS. These papules, histologically characterized by a nonspecific perivascular mononuclear cell infiltration, often persist for prolonged periods.

Allergic skin reactions occur in over 50 percent of AIDS patients treated with trimethoprim-sulfamethoxazole. An erythematous, maculopapular rash is often associated with fever, neutropenia, thrombocytopenia, and transaminase level elevation. The mechanisms underlying HIV-associated drug hypersensitivity are unclear.

Infections with HSV are often quite severe and chronic. If untreated, they can become erosive and secondarily infected. Varicella zoster can disseminate or become chronic. Moreover, the appearance of varicella zoster in a previously asymptomatic HIV carrier may herald progression to AIDS. Molluscum contagiosum, induced by a poorly defined pox virus, occurs commonly in genital or facial areas and may require surgery or cryosurgery for eradication. Therapeutic options include liquid nitrogen, cryosurgery, electrocoagulation, and curettage. Treatment yields variable results. A number of other opportunistic pathogens, including *Candida albicans, Mycobacterium avium* complex, *Cryptococcus neoformans, Histoplasma capsulatum,* and papilloma viruses, may also cause skin lesions in HIV-infected patients.

Lungs

Pulmonary complications are common in patients with HIV disease. Pyogenic bacterial infections (due to organisms such as *Haemophilus influenzae* and *Streptococcus pneumoniae*) and tuberculosis are more common than opportunistic infections (OIs) early in the course of HIV disease, but the incidence of opportunistic infections markedly increases as immunodeficiency progresses. Table 9-5 outlines the relative frequency of pulmonary pathogens in AIDS patients with respiratory symptoms.

Pulmonary OIs in HIV-infected patients typically have an insidious onset, often preceded by prolonged periods of constitutional

TABLE 9-5. Relative Frequency of Pulmonary Disease in 441 Patients with AIDS

Pathogen or disorder	Number of patients, %
Pneumocystis carinii	85
Without other pathogen	58
With other pathogen	27
Cytomegalovirus	11
Mycobacterium avium complex	8
M. tuberculosis	3
Legionella	2
Cryptococcus	2
Other	1
Other Infections	21
M. avium complex	8
Cytomegalovirus	5
Pyogenic bacteria	2
Legionella	2
Fungi	2
Other	2
Kaposi's sarcoma	8

SOURCE: JF Murray et al, N Engl J Med 310:1682, 1984.

symptoms such as fevers, night sweats, and weight loss. Most patients note the progressive onset of chest tightness, exertional dyspnea, dry cough, and fatigue, in addition to worsening constitutional symptoms. Sputum production, pleuritic chest pain, and rapid progression of symptoms are common when infection is caused by pyogenic organisms.

Physical examination usually reveals fever (38 to 40.5°C) and tachypnea; oral candidiasis or hairy leukoplakia may be present. Chest examination often reveals only diffuse fine rales, or may be unremarkable. The remainder of the examination is often normal. The white blood cell count is frequently low with an absolute lymphopenia ($<1000/mm^3$) but may be normal or elevated in patients with bacterial pneumonia. A mild anemia may be present, and the erythrocyte sedimentation rate and the serum lactate dehydrogenase levels are usually elevated.

The AIDS patient with respiratory complaints may have one or more OIs or malignancies. The most frequent pulmonary OI, by far, is *Pneumocystis carinii* pneumonia (PCP). PCP characteristically presents with a history of prodromal constitutional symptoms for several weeks with increasing respiratory symptoms and spiking fevers over several days. Occasionally PCP may present with an abrupt onset followed by rapid deterioration. In contrast, HIV-infected patients with a community-acquired pyogenic infection are most likely to have the acute onset of fever, productive cough, pleuritic chest pain, dyspnea, and focal radiographic infiltrates. Tuberculosis is more common in persons with an increased risk of prior infection with *Mycobacterium tuberculosis* (e.g., IDUs and persons from developing countries and areas of high *Mycobacterium tuberculosis* endemicity in the United States), and extrapulmonary disease sites are frequently noted. *Mycobacterium avium* complex (MAC) is often isolated from the sputum of patients with PCP, but whether MAC causes pulmonary disease in AIDS patients is unclear. Likewise, CMV is isolated in the respiratory specimens of approximately 40 percent of patients with PCP, but the contribution that CMV makes to pulmonary disease is unknown. Pulmonary cryptococcal infection may present with nonspecific respiratory symptoms and a focal nodule or cavity on chest x-ray films. Pulmonary Kaposi's sarcoma should be suspected in patients with other sites of tumor who have pleural effusions on the chest radiograph, or who have lesions seen during bronchoscopy.

Initial evaluation should include chest radiographs and sputum induction by administration of hypertonic saline with an ultrasonic nebulizer. Samples should be stained for bacteria (Gram stain), acid-fast bacilli, and PCP and cultured for bacteria, mycobacteria, fungi, and viruses. Bronchoscopy may be necessary if these studies do not yield a diagnosis.

Central Nervous System

Infections of the central nervous system (CNS) are common in patients with advanced HIV infection and for clinical purposes can be divided into two groups, those that affect the brain or spinal cord (encephalitis and abscesses) and those of the cerebrospinal fluid (meningitis).

Encephalitis or Abscesses

When patients with advanced HIV infection present with headache, a change in mental status, or focal neurologic symptoms, a diagnosis of CNS toxoplasmosis should immediately be considered. The presentation is often vague and nonspecific. Headaches are usually present and described as dull and constant, but they may be severe and unresponsive to analgesics; fever is present in less than 50 percent of patients. Two-thirds of patients have altered mental status; focal neurologic abnormalities occur in one-third. Generalized abnormalities such as weakness, myoclonus, and ataxia are also common.

While *Toxoplasma gondii* is by far the most frequent cause of encephalitis in the AIDS patient, other infectious and noninfectious causes may occur. Primary CNS lymphoma is the most common of these. Focal tuberculoma is seen in patients with prior tubercular anergy and evidence of disseminated disease. Rarely, fungi may cause focal abscesses, and viral infections due to papovavirus or HSV may occasionally present with focal disease.

Routine laboratory tests are of little value in establishing the diagnosis of toxoplasmic encephalitis. However, this disease is undoubtedly due to reactivation of latent infection, and thus the serologic tests for toxoplasma IgG antibody are usually positive. Absence of toxoplasma IgG antibody is strong (but not absolute) evidence against the diagnosis. Computerized axial tomography (CT) scanning or magnetic resonance imaging (MRI) are the most important diagnostic tests. Imaging typically reveals multiple, hypodense, ring-enhancing discrete lesions, often involving the basal ganglia, brainstem, or posterior fossa. Lymphomas, tuberculomas, and mycetomas caused by fungi are more likely to be seen on CT scans as single lesions that involve the cerebral cortex. Occasionally the CT scan is normal, but lesions may still be demonstrated by MRI. In patients with AIDS who have positive IgG serologic findings for toxoplasmal antibodies, focal neurologic findings, and multiple ring-enhancing lesions visualized by CT or MRI scanning techniques, a presumptive diagnosis of toxoplasmosis can be made and medical therapy initiated. However, if the patient is atypical in presentation, has negative serologic findings, is in a high-risk group for other causes of focal CNS disease, or fails to respond to antitoxoplasmal therapy in 2 to 3 weeks, a brain biopsy should be performed.

Meningitis

The most common cause of meningitis in AIDS patients is *Cryptococcus neoformans.* Cryptococcal meningitis occurs in 5 to 10 percent of all patients with advanced HIV infection and is the presenting condition in 2 to 3 percent of patients. Its presentation may be acute, subacute, or chronic and indolent. Fever and persistent headache occur in 80 to 90 percent of cases, and when present in AIDS patients should always suggest the disease. Other signs that are typical of meningitis in the non-AIDS population are unusual: nausea and vomiting occur in less than 50 percent, meningismus in 30 percent, alteration in mental status or photophobia in 20 to 25 percent, and seizures or other focal neurologic findings in 10 percent.

Although *C. neoformans* is the most common cause of meningitis in patients with advanced HIV infection, other pathogens, such as *Treponema pallidum, S. pneumoniae, H. influenzae,* and *M. tuberculosis,* may also infect the CSF and the meninges. Involvement of the meninges with aggressive B-cell lymphoma may also produce an illness indistinguishable from meningitis. HIV infection itself also causes an aseptic meningitis syndrome.

Ideally, any patient with HIV infection and central neurologic dysfunction should first undergo CT or MRI because of the possibility of a space-occupying lesion.

Cryptococcal antigen in the blood can be detected in more than 95 percent of patients with cryptococcal meningitis, and elevated antigen titers may provide evidence of CNS infection. Fungal cultures of blood, sputum, or urine sometimes yield *C. neoformans.* However, CSF examination most quickly establishes the diagnosis. Ninety-five percent of patients with cryptococcal meningitis have positive CSF cryptococcal antigen tests, and 99 percent have positive CSF cultures for the organism. When the cryptococcal antigen test is negative, tuberculosis becomes a more likely diagnosis, but acid fast bacillus (AFB) smears of the CSF are rarely positive. If cryptococcal antigen is not present and examination of the CSF reveals a more intense inflammatory response with a predominance of polymorphonuclear leukocytes or a reduction in CSF glucose to levels less than 50 percent of simultaneous serum levels, a bacterial infection (e.g., *S. pneumoniae, H. influenzae*) should be seriously considered. Syphilis must always be included in the differential diagnosis of meningitis when lymphocytes predominate and the CSF glucose is normal.

Gastrointestinal Tract

Infections of the Oral Cavity

Painful white lesions in the oral mucosa are usually caused by *C. albicans* infection. Pseudomembranous candidiasis (thrush) is one of the earliest clinical signs of immunodeficiency and is nearly ubiquitous in patients with severe immune impairment. Oral candidiasis may also present as red lesions on the tongue and palate (atrophic candidiasis), angular cheilitis, and bilateral white and red lesions on the buccal mucosa (chronic hypertrophic candidiasis).

Candidiasis must be distinguished from hairy leukoplakia and other white lesions of the oral mucosa. The diagnosis can be made by scraping the surface of lesions with a tongue depressor and microscopically examining the material obtained in a wet mount prepared with 10% potassium hydroxide. The presence of hyphae distinguishes infection from colonization. Fungal cultures are rarely indicated or helpful.

Hairy leukoplakia is a newly described disorder observed commonly in HIV-infected individuals. Like oral candidiasis, it may be predictive of the development of AIDS. Raised white areas on the tongue or buccal mucosa appear, often with a corrugated or "hairy" surface. Epstein-Barr virus has been implicated as the cause of this lesion. Lesions resolve after treatment with oral acyclovir but tend to recur.

A variety of viruses produce mucosal lesions in HIV-infected patients. The lesions of recurrent HSV gingivostomatitis are often indistinguishable from those found in immunocompetent patients, although large ulcerations, secondary infections, and slow healing sometimes occur. Viral cultures inoculated with fluid from an ulcer or a fresh unroofed vesicle usually confirm the diagnosis.

Gingivitis is a common complication of HIV infection. In general, the severity of gingival inflammation parallels the severity of immunosuppression, although the exact microbial cause of the condition is unknown. Acute necrotizing ulcerative gingivitis is diagnosed clinically by the presence of severe gingival inflammation with ulcerations, bleeding, and halitosis.

Esophagitis

Patients with esophagitis usually complain of odynophagia or dysphagia. Invasive *C. albicans* is the most common cause; HSV and CMV infections are less common causes of esophagitis in persons with AIDS. An empirical trial of oral ketoconazole or fluconazole is a rational management strategy in patients with AIDS and mild to moderate symptoms, particularly when oral thrush is present. The diagnosis may be confirmed by endoscopic biopsy.

Proctitis

HSV causes most cases of ulcerative proctitis in HIV-infected patients and can usually be diagnosed by direct IFA or culture. Chlamydial and gonococcal cultures should also be performed in sexually active homosexual patients with symptoms of proctitis.

Enteritis

Diarrhea and weight loss occur in more than 50 percent of patients with AIDS and are also common in those with less severe clinical manifestations of immunodeficiency. The wide range of infections, neoplasms, and inflammatory processes which produce these symptoms presents a difficult problem for the clinician. However, as with other clinical syndromes in AIDS, the approach to the patient with diarrheal illness can be simplified by emphasizing the identification of treatable causes and avoiding unnecessary invasive procedures. Common pathogens include *Salmonella, Shigella, Campylobacter, Clostridium difficile, Giardia lamblia, Entamoeba histolytica, Cryptosporidium, Mycobacterium avium intracellulare*, CMV, Microsporidia, and *Isospora belli.* Noninfectious causes of diarrhea, such as Kaposi's sarcoma, lymphoma, and carcinoma, occur as well. Evaluation by stool culture, and examination of stool for ova and parasites often reveals an infectious cause. Sigmoidoscopy, however, is sometimes necessary for diagnosis.

Malignancy

The incidence of several cancers is markedly increased among persons with HIV infection. These include Kaposi's sarcoma (KS), primary CNS non-Hodgkin's lymphomas, and high-grade peripheral B-cell lymphoma. These malignancies in the presence of HIV infection are, in fact, diagnostic of AIDS.

Most patients with AIDS-related KS have subcutaneous, painless, palpable, nonpruritic tumor nodules, or lymphatic involvement. Typically, lesions are first noted on the face or in the oral cavity, although they may begin in any site. The lesions are pigmented red to blue and are nonblanching; in deeper lesions the pigmentation may not be apparent. With advanced disease, plaques of coalesced lesions are common, especially over the medial aspect of the thigh. Cutaneous KS is readily recognized, but biopsy must be performed to establish a histologic diagnosis.

Eyes

Fifty to 90 percent of AIDS patients have abnormal ocular findings. Ophthalmic manifestations may be grouped into two major categories: noninfectious lesions such as cotton wool spots and retinal hemorrhages, and infections such as CMV retinitis.

Cotton wool spots, the most common ophthalmic lesion described in AIDS patients, have been reported in about 40 to 70 percent of cases. These lesions are not specific for AIDS but occur in a number of systemic diseases including hypertension and diabetes. Cotton wool spots appear as single or multiple fluffy white opacities with indistinct borders located in the superficial retina (nerve fiber layer) along the vascular arcades (Fig. 9-5). They are asymptomatic and transient, lasting 4 to 6 weeks. The clinical significance of these lesions is not fully understood. They are thought to be a result of focal ischemia, a focal infarct in the nerve fiber layer.

Retinal hemorrhages, another noninfectious microvascular disorder associated with AIDS, are visible in about 10 to 40 percent of patients. Like cotton wool spots, retinal hemorrhages are a transient and nonspecific finding which may also occur in a number of systemic diseases, such as diabetes, hypertension, and renal failure. They are usually either superficial flame-shaped hemorrhages lying within the posterior pole or deeper intraretinal blot-type hemorrhages found more anteriorly. Their presence does not correlate with disease activity.

CMV chorioretinitis is the most common opportunistic ophthalmic manifestation of AIDS, its prevalence ranging from about 5 to

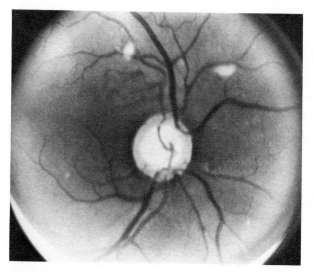

FIG. 9-5. Multiple cotton wool spots in a young homosexual man with HIV-1 infection.

50 percent. CMV retinitis is found more frequently in homosexuals with AIDS than in HIV-infected heterosexual IDUs.

The manifestations of CMV retinopathy are so characteristic that this diagnosis can be made clinically, even in the presence of negative CMV antibody titers. Characteristically, CMV retinopathy is a necrotizing infection which involves all layers of the retina as well as the retinal pigment epithelium. Involvement of the choroid, however, is minimal. The lesions appear initially as scattered white granular patches within the posterior pole. They are usually found along the vascular arcade and may be associated with sheathing of the retinal vessels. Superficial and deep hemorrhages are found adjacent to these lesions.

CMV retinitis is the major cause of visual loss in AIDS. With progression of CMV chorioretinitis, loss of retinal function occurs in 3 to 6 months. In addition, visual field defects with absolute scotomas may occur in areas corresponding to excessive retinal atrophy. Therapy of CMV retinitis is discussed in Chap. 12.

ADDITIONAL READING

Centers for Disease Control. *HIV/AIDS Surveillance Report.* Atlanta, CDC, 1992

Crowe SM et al: Predictive value of CD4 lymphocyte numbers for the development of opportunistic infections and malignancies in HIV-infected persons. *J Acquir Immune Defic Syndr* 4:770, 1991

Dover JS: Cutaneous manifestations of human immunodeficiency virus infection (part I). *Arch Dermatol* 127:1383, 1991

Dover JS: Cutaneous manifestations of human immunodeficiency virus infection (part II). *Arch Dermatol* 127:1549, 1991

Duvic M: Papulosquamous disorders associated with human immunodeficiency virus infection. *Dermatologic Clinics* 9:523, 1991

Farizio KM et al: Spectrum of disease in persons with human immunodeficiency virus infection in the United States. *JAMA* 267:1798, 1992

Holmes KK et al (eds): *AIDS DX/Rx.* New York, McGraw-Hill, 1990

Quinn TJ: Smith PD, moderator: Gastrointestinal infections in AIDS. *Ann Intern Med* 116:63, 1992

Saag MS et al: Comparison of amphotericin B with fluconazole in the treatment of acute AIDS-associated cryptococcal meningitis. The NIAID Mycoses Study Group and the AIDS Clinical Trials Group. *N Engl J Med* 326:83, 1992

Schuman JS et al: Ocular effects in the acquired immune deficiency syndrome. *Mt Sinai J Med* 50:443, 1983

World Health Organization. Global AIDS case surveillance, In *1990 World Health Statistics Annual.* Geneva, WHO, 1991

For a more detailed discussion, see Haase AT: Biology of Human Immunodeficiency Virus and Related Viruses, Chap. 28, p. 305;

Koenig S, Fauci AS: Immunology of HIV Infection, Chap. 29, p. 317; Hirsch MS: Clinical Manifestations of HIV Infection in Adults in Industrialized Countries, Chap. 30, p. 331; Holmberg SD, Curran JW: The Epidemiology of HIV Infection in Industrialized Countries, Chap. 31, p. 343; Quinn TC: Unique Aspects of Human Immunodeficiency Virus and Related Viruses in Developing Countries, Chap. 32, p. 355; Volberding PA: AIDS-Related Malignancies, Chap. 56, p. 685; and Chaisson RE, Gerberding JL, Sande MA: Opportunistic Infections in AIDS, Chap. 57, p. 691, in STD-2.

Since the early years of the AIDS epidemic, the primary care needs of HIV-infected people have been continuously evolving. Progression of HIV disease results in a variety of clinical syndromes, some of which have been outlined in Chap. 9. These conditions contribute to the morbidity and mortality of people with HIV infection and erode their quality of life. However, early intervention with antiretroviral agents and prophylactic therapy can decrease mortality and delay onset of some AIDS-related complications. Furthermore, many complications that once required hospitalization are now managed on an ambulatory basis. This chapter outlines some current concepts in the primary care of early HIV disease.

INITIAL CLINICAL EVALUATION

The goals of the initial clinical evaluation are to assess the stage of HIV infection, and the patient's prior exposures to potential opportunistic infections such as tuberculosis and toxoplasmosis, in order to determine the most appropriate intervention. In addition, necessary vaccinations can be provided, and strategies for health maintenance discussed.

History and Physical Examination

All patients should undergo a review of their full history and also a complete physical examination. The clinician should focus particular attention, however, on the presence or absence of constitutional symptoms such as fever, sweats, and weight loss; and localizing signs, such as skin changes, lymphadenopathy, oral findings (thrush, hairy leukoplakia, Kaposi's sarcoma), visual disturbances and funduscopic examination; and respiratory and genital symptoms and examination.

Certain aspects of the past medical and social histories are particularly important. History of travel and prior risk practices, including sexual practices, is obtained to assess potential exposures to infections and needs for counseling. Patients should be specifically queried concerning tuberculosis exposure and past diagnosis and treatment of sexually transmitted diseases—especially syphilis, herpes, hepatitis, and condyloma. Women should be asked about increases in symptoms of vaginal candidiasis and history of abnormal Papanicolaou (Pap) smears. HIV infection is associated with a more aggressive course of some of these conditions.

Laboratory Tests and Other Diagnostic Procedures

Of the tests currently available in clinical practice, enumeration of CD4+ lymphocytes has emerged as the most useful for staging HIV disease. Prognosis worsens when the absolute CD4+ count falls below 500/mm^3, and the risk of opportunistic infections markedly increases when the CD4+ count is less than 200/mm^3. This marker, however, is far from precise. Because infections other than HIV can lower the detected number of CD4+ cells, determination of lymphocyte markers should not be performed while patients have an intercurrent illness, if possible. Moreover, counts are subject to diurnal variation and sometimes vary from laboratory to laboratory. Therefore, CD4+ counts should be performed at the same time of day and by the same laboratory whenever possible.

All patients should receive skin testing for tuberculosis. Purified protein derivative (PPD) should be used for skin testing, and controls should be placed to help assess anergy. The presence of ≥ 5 mm of induration is considered a positive PPD test among HIV-infected persons. HIV infection results in an increased risk of tuberculosis reactivation, which can contribute substantially to morbidity and mortality of persons with HIV disease. Moreover, tuberculosis is one of the few infections which HIV-infected people can readily transmit to others.

Because of the high prevalence of syphilis and the aggressive course of this disease among persons with HIV infection, a quantitative nontreponemal test for syphilis (e.g., Venereal Disease Research Laboratory, VDRL) should be performed.

Serologic screening for antibodies to *Toxoplasma gondii* identifies those at risk for future toxoplasmosis. Conversely, serologic screening for absence of hepatitis B markers (HBsAg and anti-HBsAg) identifies those who remain at risk for hepatitis B and who may benefit from hepatitis B vaccination if they continue high-risk sexual or drug-using behaviors.

In addition to performing a complete pelvic examination, clinicians should obtain Pap smears in women at 6-month intervals, and colposcopy should be performed if a smear is abnormal. A high prevalence of cervical intraepithelial neoplasia (dysplasia) has been noted among women with HIV infection. Similarly, an increased prevalence of anal intraepithelial neoplasia (dysplasia) has been documented in homosexual men with HIV infection, particularly those who are immunosuppressed. Although not proven, it is possible that earlier detection and intervention may result in improved survival in patients with HIV disease and cervical or anal dysplasia.

INTERVENTIONS

All Patients

If the PPD is >5 mm, the clinician should obtain a chest radiograph, as well as sputum tuberculosis stains and culture, urine tuberculosis cultures, and other tests when clinically indicated to exclude active tuberculosis. If no evidence of active tuberculosis is found, the patient should receive isoniazid (INH) 300 mg orally per day for at least 12 months. When the patient is anergic and has a history of tuberculosis exposure or residence in a tuberculosis-endemic region, some clinicians prescribe INH after excluding active disease because of the high probability of prior infection and subsequent reactivation.

Evaluation and management of syphilis in this population is currently controversial. However, two issues remain virtually uncontested: (1) all patients with clinical evidence of neurologic involvement should receive a lumbar puncture with evaluation of cerebrospinal fluid and treatment for neurosyphilis if it is identified, and (2) regardless of the stage of syphilis, close follow-up of all HIV-infected patients is essential to ensure that therapy has been complete. See Chap. 6 for a more complete discussion.

Although there are as yet no substantive data to suggest that immunization per se may increase productive HIV replication in vaccine-stimulated CD4 cells, clinicians should be aware that this issue is still under investigation. Nonetheless, because of the high incidence of *Streptococcus pneumoniae* infection among HIV-infected persons, pneumococcal vaccine is commonly given to all patients as soon as HIV infection is diagnosed. Data concerning clinical efficacy of vaccine administration are limited. However, patients are more likely to mount an antibody response to the vaccine when immunized early during the course of HIV disease than when immunized late. Because HIV infection is associated with increased risk of *Haemophilus influenzae* infection, some clinicians immunize patients with *H. influenzae* B vaccine. However, since most *H. influenzae* pneumonias are not with *H. influenzae* type B, this practice is not universal. HIV-infected patients who are susceptible to hepatitis B should be immunized against this infection if they will remain at risk for acquiring it [e.g., active injecting-drug user (IDU), sexual partner of an IDU, some homosexual men]. The efficacy of hepatitis B vaccine is reduced in HIV infection, and the anti-HBsAg response should be checked after completion of the three-dose vaccine schedule. We also offer influenza vaccine during influenza season, although there are no data concerning increased virulence of influenza or efficacy of the vaccine in this population.

Patients with CD4+ Counts >500

CD4+ counts should be repeated at 3- to 6-month intervals for patients whose CD4+ counts are greater than 500/mm³. More frequent lymphocyte determinations should be considered when counts appear to be falling rapidly or when levels approach 500. There is no evidence at this time that antiretroviral therapy benefits patients in this category.

Patients with CD4+ Counts of 200 to 500

When CD4+ lymphocyte counts fall below 500, the clinician should recommend initiation of antiretroviral therapy with zidovudine and continue determination of CD4+ lymphocyte counts at 3- to 6-month intervals until counts fall to approximately 200/mm³. More frequent monitoring should be considered when levels are falling rapidly or approaching 200. Some clinicians continue to monitor even after counts fall below 200, because the rate and type of morbidity change with very low counts.

Patients with CD4+ Counts ≤200

When counts of CD4+ cells fall below 200/mm³, the clinician should recommend initiation of antiretroviral therapy with zidovudine if it has not already been given and begin prophylaxis against *Pneumocystis carinii* pneumonia, preferably with trimethoprim-sulfamethoxazole, alternatively with dapsone or aerosolized pentamidine, as discussed below.

ANTIRETROVIRAL THERAPY

As this book goes to press, three agents—zidovudine, didanosine, and zalcitabine—are licensed in the United States for treatment of HIV infection.

Zidovudine

Zidovudine (ZDV, formerly azidothymidine, or AZT) is a thymidine analogue which inhibits HIV reverse transcriptase and interrupts the growing DNA chain of the virus. ZDV decreases mortality and incidence of opportunistic infections when given to patients with AIDS and advanced HIV disease. ZDV also delays the onset of AIDS when given to asymptomatic HIV-infected persons with less than 500 CD4+ cells. A retrospective study showed that the drug increased survival of persons with early HIV disease and fewer than 350 CD4+ cells.

Current indications for ZDV therapy include AIDS, HIV infection with a CD4$^+$ count less than 500, and AIDS-related idiopathic thrombocytopenic purpura.

Recommended dose: Zidovudine 100 mg orally 5 times daily. Alternatively, 200 mg can be given 3 times daily to improve compliance. Total daily dose 500 to 600 mg. Higher doses may be required for HIV-related neurologic disease (for example, HIV cognitive-motor syndromes).

The major adverse effect of ZDV is hematologic toxicity, which is more common in patients with advanced disease than in those with early infection. Anemia and granulocytopenia are common, but in general, decreases in hemoglobin and neutrophil levels are reversible if the dose is decreased or the drug discontinued. Other reported side effects include headache, nausea, myopathy, and rarely, rashes or mania.

Hematologic parameters should be carefully monitored at least every 4 weeks. Several options exist for treatment of anemia. The drug can be temporarily discontinued, transfusion given if necessary, and therapy restarted at a lower dose (e.g., 300 or 400 mg daily) once the hemoglobin level has returned to an acceptable level. If toxicity recurs, permanent discontinuation of ZDV and substitution of didanosine (ddI) should be considered. Alternatively, ZDV may be continued with administration of erythropoietin if endogenous serum erythropoietin levels are less than 500 IU/l.

When neutrophil counts fall below 700/mm^3, ZDV should be temporarily discontinued and reinstituted at a lower dose when neutrophil counts rise above 800/mm^3. If granulocytopenia recurs repeatedly at lower ZDV doses, many clinicians discontinue the drug and recommend switching to ddI.

Didanosine

Like zidovudine, ddI is a nucleoside analogue which inhibits HIV reverse transcriptase. The drug is rapidly degraded by acid; the oral formulation contains buffering agents and should be taken on an empty stomach.

Substantially less clinical information is available for ddI than for ZDV. Didanosine is currently recommended for patients with advanced HIV disease who are unable to tolerate ZDV; who have demonstrated significant clinical or immunologic deterioration (for example, rapid fall in CD4$^+$ cell count) during ZDV therapy; or who have advanced disease and have received prolonged ZDV therapy, even when CD4$^+$ counts are stable below 250. The effect of ddI on patients with asymptomatic HIV infection is not yet known. Ongoing studies will address this issue as well as the drug's effect on survival of patients with advanced disease.

Recommended dose:
Weight >50 kg: ddI 200 mg orally twice a day.
Weight 35 to 49 kg: ddI 125 mg orally twice a day.

Didanosine has minimal hematologic toxicity but has been associated with a high incidence of dose-related peripheral neuropathy, and also with pancreatitis. Neuropathy is characterized by distal numbness, tingling, or pain in feet or hands and is often reversible if ddI is discontinued promptly after symptoms begin. Pancreatitis should be considered whenever patients taking ddI develop abdominal pain and nausea, vomiting, or biochemical evidence of pancreatitis. When these signs or symptoms occur, the drug should be discontinued until pancreatitis has been excluded.

Zalcitabine

Zalcitabine (ddC, formerly dideoxycytidine) is approved for use as combination therapy with ZDV for the treatment of HIV-infected adults with advanced HIV infection (CD4$^+$ lymphocyte counts <300) who have demonstrated clinical or immunologic deterioration. Like ZDV and ddI, ddC is a nucleoside analogue which inhibits HIV replication. The most common side effect is peripheral neuropathy, which usually resolves if ddC is discontinued soon after onset of symptoms. Pancreatitis occurs in less than 1 percent of patients.

Recommended dose: ddC 0.75 mg orally per day and ZDV 200 mg orally every 8 h.

Pneumocystis carinii PROPHYLAXIS

The risk of *P. carinii* pneumonia (PCP) rises markedly among HIV-infected patients when the CD4$^+$ lymphocyte count falls below 200/mm^3. Because appropriate antimicrobials decrease the risk of PCP, prophylaxis is recommended for patients with HIV who have CD4$^+$ counts less than 200/mm^3, or unexplained fever, or oral thrush (primary prophylaxis); or who have had an episode of PCP (secondary prophylaxis). The two most widely used agents are trimethoprim-sulfamethoxazole (TMP-SMX) and aerosolized pentamidine.

TMP-SMX has several advantages over pentamidine. TMP-SMX is inexpensive and convenient for patients to take, and its systemic absorption may protect against extrapulmonary pneumocystosis. Moreover, it appears to be more effective than aerosolized pentamidine for preventing or delaying recurrences of PCP. TMP-SMX appears to offer some protection against CNS toxoplasmosis, and perhaps against certain bacterial infections. However, TMP-SMX causes a high incidence of side effects in this population.

In contrast, pentamidine inhalation results in minimal systemic absorption, with minimal toxicity. However, pentamidine is considerably more expensive. Its administration is inconvenient for many patients and could contribute to the spread of tuberculosis if not given in an appropriately ventilated setting. Pulmonary tuberculosis should be excluded in patients before aerosolized pentamidine is given.

Recommended regimens:

TMP-SMX double strength, 1 tablet daily, or pentamidine 300 mg aerosolized monthly. Some patients require inhaled bronchodilators to alleviate bronchospasm precipitated by aerosolized pentamidine.

DERMATOLOGIC CONDITIONS

Skin disorders are among the earlier clinical manifestations in many persons with HIV infection. These conditions may be of infectious or neoplastic origin and often cause considerable distress. Common conditions include chronic generalized pruritus; severe seborrhea; generalized erythroderma; severe psoriasis; photosensitivity; and viral, bacterial, or fungal infections. Some common conditions, and therapy alternatives, are as follows:

Pruritus: Emollients, antihistamines (e.g., diphenhydramine), topical steroids, camphor menthol shake lotions (e.g., Sarna).

Seborrhea: Topical steroids, topical ketoconazole, or oral ketoconazole.

Staphylococcal folliculitis: Antistaphylococcal therapy (e.g., dicloxacillin 250 to 500 mg orally 4 times daily for 10 to 14 days).

Dermal candidiasis: Topical nystatin, clotrimazole, or oral ketoconazole.

Varicella zoster: Acyclovir (800 mg orally 5 times daily). If visceral or extensive cutaneous involvement is present, intravenous acyclovir (12 mg/kg every 8 h for 7 to 14 days) should be seriously considered.

Herpes simplex: Acyclovir (200 mg 5 times daily) for 7 to 10 days. Maintenance therapy should be considered for patients with recurrent episodes: Acyclovir (200 mg orally 4 times daily). HSV lesions that do not respond to acyclovir should be evaluated for the possibility of acyclovir resistance; foscarnet sometimes yields improvement.

ODYNOPHAGIA

Painful swallowing is a frequent presenting complaint of patients with HIV disease. The most common cause is esophagitis due to *Candida,* herpes simplex virus (HSV), or cytomegalovirus (CMV). Of these pathogens, *Candida* is the most common. Definitive diagnosis requires endoscopy with biopsy and/or brushings, but *Candida* is so common a cause of this condition that empirical therapy with ketoconazole or fluconazole is reasonable, especially if oral thrush is present. Endoscopy should be performed, however, if esophageal symptoms do not resolve with these regimens.

Recommended regimens:

Esophageal candidiasis: Ketoconazole (200 to 400 mg orally per day) or

Fluconazole (100 mg orally once a day). (Some clinicians initiate 200 mg orally per day and later decrease to 100 mg per day for maintenance therapy.)

HSV esophagitis: Acyclovir (200 mg orally 5 times daily for 10 to 14 days); severe disease may require parenteral therapy.

CMV esophagitis: Ganciclovir 5 mg/kg intravenously 2 times daily for 14 to 21 days.

SINUSITIS

Sinusitis is very common among persons with HIV disease and is frequently seen—even among persons who are otherwise asymptomatic. Fever, headache, or upper respiratory symptoms should arouse suspicion of sinusitis. Initial evaluation and treatment are the same as for patients without HIV disease and should include Gram stain and culture of nasal secretions, decongestants, empirical antibiotic therapy for coverage of *S. pneumoniae* and *H. influenzae* (e.g., amoxicillin–clavulanic acid) if signs of infection are noted. Sinus imaging, drainage, and culture are indicated for patients who worsen or do not rapidly improve despite appropriate medical therapy, or who display systemic toxicity or experience recurrent episodes of sinusitis.

BACTERIAL INFECTIONS

Bacterial infections are common in persons with HIV disease and in some patients represent an early manifestation of immune system compromise. IDUs and patients with indwelling catheters are at highest risk. Common presentations include bacteremia or endocarditis due to *Staphylococcus aureus* or pneumonia caused by *S. pneumoniae* or *H. influenzae*. Bacterial pneumonias are often more severe and accompanied by bacteremia and complications, such as empyema. Radiographic findings are often atypical. The incidence of bacteremia due to *Salmonella* species is also increased among HIV-infected patients. Disease tends to recur unless long-term suppressive therapy is given.

NEUROPSYCHIATRIC MANIFESTATIONS

Neuropsychiatric disease is extremely common among patients with HIV disease. Its presentation can range from depression or mild cognitive dysfunction to psychosis or dementia. Neuropsychiatric testing can be helpful in detecting cognitive impairment. Depression often responds to antidepressant medications.

A variety of peripheral neuropathies can complicate the course of HIV disease. Acute or chronic demyelinating neuropathy, for example, may occur during early infection. In patients with advanced disease, peripheral neuropathy is common and manifests itself as painful dysesthesias with symmetrical sensory loss and sparing of motor function. One of the tricyclic antidepressants, diphenylhydantoin, or carbamazepine, may ameliorate the severe neuropathic pain.

With the potential for drug interactions in patients receiving multiple medications, experienced neuropsychiatric consultation in managing these problems can be invaluable.

INITIAL EVALUATION OF PNEUMONIA

Initial evaluation should include chest radiographs and sputum induction by administration of hypertonic saline with an ultrasonic nebulizer. Focal pulmonary infiltrates in patients with relatively early HIV disease are often caused by pyogenic bacteria, such as *S. pneumoniae* or *H. influenzae,* while diffuse infiltrates in patients with CD4$^+$ lymphocytes <200/mm^3 suggest *P. carinii* or other opportunistic pathogens. However, aerosolized pentamidine prophylaxis may make radiographic diagnosis of PCP more difficult. Blood cultures should be obtained, and sputum samples should be stained for bacteria (Gram stain), acid-fast bacilli, and *P. carinii,* and cultured for bacteria, mycobacteria, fungi, and viruses. Although cryptococcal pneumonia is not common and is often cavitary, if initial stains and blood cultures do not identify a pathogen, serum cryptococcal antigen testing can be performed—especially if the patient's CD4$^+$ lymphocyte count is below 200/mm^3. Bronchoscopy may be necessary if these studies do not yield a diagnosis.

In the clinical setting, patients with pulmonary symptoms should wear respiratory masks until mycobacterial infection is excluded, to minimize nosocomial transmission of tuberculosis.

Treatment

Treatment should be directed by results of initial evaluation. However, for patients whose preliminary evaluation does not identify a pathogen, TMP-SMX is reasonable empirical therapy because of its broad antibacterial spectrum and activity against *P. carinii.*

PCP: TMP-SMX orally or intravenously at doses of 15 to 20 mg/kg per day TMP and 75 to 100 mg/kg per day SMX for 21 days in 4 divided doses or pentamidine isoethionate intravenously 4 mg/kg per day.

Alternate PCP therapy: Dapsone 100 mg orally per day (glucose 6-phosphate dehydrogenase deficiency must be excluded), plus TMP orally 20 mg/kg per day in divided doses or clindamycin 600 mg orally every 6 h plus primaquine 15 mg (base) per day orally.

Tuberculosis generally responds well to standard antituberculosis drugs, even in AIDS.

FEVER AND HEADACHE

Common causes of fever and headache or mental status changes in patients with HIV disease include cryptococcal meningitis, toxoplasmosis, aseptic meningitis, tuberculous meningitis, and lymphoma. Initial evaluation should include either head CT or MRI to exclude the presence of a space-occupying lesion or imminent herniation. Because *T. gondii* is the most common cause of multiple ring-enhancing lesions in patients with advanced HIV disease, patients with this finding should receive empirical treatment for cerebral toxoplasmosis, especially if serologic tests suggest past toxoplasmosis infection.

If imaging procedures do not reveal a contraindication to lumbar puncture, cerebrospinal fluid should be stained and cultured for bacteria, fungi, and mycobacteria and examined for cryptococcal antigen. Cerebrospinal fluid and serum nontreponemal serologic tests for syphilis should also be performed as well as blood cultures. Diagnoses of histoplasmosis and coccidioidomycosis should be pursued in patients with appropriate geographic exposure.

DIARRHEA

Diarrhea frequently contributes to the morbidity and mortality of patients with HIV disease. Routine enteric pathogens, such as *Salmonella, Shigella,* and *Campylobacter,* are the most common pathogens in early HIV infection, but as disease progresses the incidence of opportunistic pathogens, such as cytomegalovirus, *Mycobacterium avium* complex, *Cryptosporidium,* or *Microsporidia,* markedly increases. *Clostridium difficile* infection is not uncommon after hospitalization or antimicrobial therapy. Because clinical features seldom distinguish one cause of diarrhea from another, diagnosis can be exhausting for both patient and practitioner. Moreover, many causes of enteritis do not respond to treatment. Partly because of these issues, the evaluation and treatment of diarrhea in HIV-infected patients is controversial. Nonetheless, treatable causes should be sought, and symptoms should be alleviated to the extent possible.

The initial approach includes examination of stool for blood, leukocytes, bacteria, ova, and parasites. If no blood or leukocytes are identified, opiate constipating agents may be used. Patients with high fever or rigors should be treated empirically with antibiotics (e.g., ciprofloxacin) while awaiting results of stool and blood cultures or fecal *C. difficile* toxin assay. Fever or rigor in this setting can, of course, be due to causes unrelated to diarrhea. Therapy should be modified as results of preliminary evaluation dictate. If symptoms do not improve and the above evaluation yields no diagnosis, colonoscopy should be considered. This procedure can identify colitis due to cytomegalovirus or *M. avium* complex which sometimes improves with systemic therapy.

ADDITIONAL READINGS

Collier AC et al: Clinical manifestations and approach to management of HIV infection and AIDS, in *AIDS Dx/Rx,* Holmes KK et al (eds). New York, McGraw-Hill, 1990

Fischl M et al: Recombinant human erythropoietin for patients with AIDS treated with zidovudine. N Engl J Med 322:1488, 1990

Fischl MA et al: The efficacy of azidothymidine (AZT) in the treatment of patients with AIDS and AIDS-related complex: a double-blind, placebo-controlled trial. N Engl J Med 317:185, 1987

Glaser JP et al: Zidovudine improves response to pneumococcal vaccine among persons with AIDS and AIDS-related complex. Journal of Infectious Diseases 164:761, 1991

Graham NMH et al: The effects on survival of early treatment of human immunodeficiency virus infection. N Engl J Med 326:1037, 1992

Maiman M et al. HIV infection and cervical neoplasia. Gyneol-Oncol 38:377, 1990

Palefsky JM: HPV-associated anogenital neoplasms and other solid tumors in HIV-infected individuals. Current Opin Oncol 3:881, 1991

Phair J et al: The risk of *Pneumocystis carinii* pneumonia among men infected with human immunodeficiency virus type 1. N Engl J Med 322:161, 1990

Rubin JS, Honigberg R: Sinusitis in patients with the acquired immunodeficiency syndrome. *Ear Nose Throat J* 69:460, 1990

Sande MA, Volberding PA: *The Medical Management of AIDS,* 3d ed. Philadelphia, Saunders, 1992

Steinhoff MC et al: Antibody responses to *Haemophilus influenza* type B vaccine in men with HIV infection. N Engl J Med 325:1837, 1991

Volberding PA et al: Zidovudine in asymptomatic human immunodeficiency virus infection: a controlled trial in persons with fewer than 500 CD4$^+$-positive cells per cubic millimeter. N Engl J Med 322:941, 1990

For more detailed discussion, see Hirsch: "Clinical Manifestations of HIV Infection in Adults," Chapter 30, p. 331 and Chaisson RE, Gerberding JL, Sande MA: "Opportunistic Infections in AIDS," Chapter 57, p. 691, in STD-2.

Understanding of the natural history and epidemiology of genital herpes simplex virus (HSV) infection has advanced rapidly in the last two decades. The clinical morbidity, frequency of recurrences, characteristic complications, and relation to HIV infection concern patients and challenge health care providers.

VIROLOGY

Six different human herpesviruses have been recognized, including HSV types 1 and 2 (HSV-1 and HSV-2), varicella-zoster virus (VZV), Epstein-Barr virus (EBV), cytomegalovirus (CMV), and the recently discovered human herpesvirus 6 (HHV-6). HSV-2 and (less commonly) HSV-1 are the causes of genital herpes, while oral-labial lesions are more often associated with HSV-1 than HSV-2.

The herpesviruses contain a linear, double-stranded DNA core, an icosahedral capsid, and an outer lipid-containing membrane or envelope.

All herpesviruses produce latent infection, in which the viral genome is stably maintained by the cell, with only limited expression of certain viral genes, no production of infectious virus, and no evident virus-induced cytotoxicity. Latent infection can be converted to productive infection, with replication of infectious virus and cell death. Reactivation is more common with HSV than with VZV. Factors which stimulate reactivation remain poorly defined.

EPIDEMIOLOGY

Incidence Trends and Prevalence of Genital HSV Infections

How common is genital herpes? The annual number of office visits for first episodes of genital herpes increased from fewer than 18,000 in 1966 to more than 160,000 by 1988, remaining stable thereafter. This measure greatly underestimates the true incidence, as shown by recent seroepidemiologic studies. Older serologic methods, such as neutralizing or complement-fixing antibody assays, were unsatisfactory in differentiating HSV-1 and HSV-2 infection, even though these methods are still used. Newer methods, described below, accurately distinguish between antibody to HSV-1 and antibody to HSV-2. These antibodies persist after acute infection and reveal the true extent of HSV-1 and HSV-2 infection in the population.

In the United States, HSV-1 antibodies are found by age 30 in about 50 percent of adults of high socioeconomic status and 80 percent of those of low socioeconomic status. Antibodies to HSV-2 are not seen until puberty, but then increase rapidly in prevalence during teen and young-adult years. HSV-2 antibody prevalence rates subsequently reach about 20 percent in whites and 40 to 60 percent in blacks. Among blacks, rates are higher in women than in men. HSV-2 antibody has been found in nearly 50 percent of female STD clinic patients, and in up to 80 percent of homosexual male patients. Among sexually experienced female college students, about 20 percent have HSV-2 antibody; antibody prevalence rises with increasing numbers of sex partners, although the prevalence of antibody to HSV-2 is higher in female STD clinic patients than in female students even after controlling for number of partners. The lower risk of HSV-2 infection per partner among the students illustrates that the risk of acquiring an STD is a function not only of the number of sexual partners, but also of the ecological milieu and prevalence of infection in the pool of available partners.

The discrepancy between the number of office visits for symptomatic first episodes of genital herpes and the much greater prevalence of antibody to HSV-2—the most frequent cause of genital infection—is largely explained by the fact that only about one-quarter to one-third of HSV-2 infections are clinically apparent; of women with HSV-2 antibody, up to three-quarters have no prior history of symptomatic genital herpes.

PATHOGENESIS

Genital herpes is acquired through sexual contact with a person shedding virus from a mucosal or skin surface. Since HSV is inactivated at room temperature and by drying, aerosol and fomite spread are considered unusual means of transmission. Genital HSV-2 infection usually results from sexual intercourse, while genital HSV-1 infection can result from intercourse, fellatio, or cunnilingus.

Virus presumably enters susceptible mucosal epithelium (e.g., the oropharynx, cervix, conjunctivae) or through superficially eroded, abraded, or fissured keratinized epithelium. HSV infection causes focal necrosis and ballooning degeneration of cells, and eosinophilic intranuclear inclusions (Cowdry type A bodies). As viral replication is restricted, lesions reepithelialize.

With either symptomatic or asymptomatic initial infection, HSV ascends peripheral sensory nerves, enters sensory or autonomic nerve root ganglia, and establishes latent infection. The prevailing view of recrudescent episodes of genital herpes is that HSV is reactivated in the ganglion and travels peripherally down the nerve to the skin, producing viral shedding from lesions that range from trivial and subclinical to overt recurrent genital herpes lesions. The host-viral mechanisms responsible for latency and reactivation are poorly understood. Reinfection with different strains of virus occurs, but this is infrequent; recurrences are usually attributed to reactivation of virus from latently infected ganglia.

CLINICAL MANIFESTATIONS OF GENITAL HERPES

The clinical manifestations and recurrence rate of genital herpes are influenced by viral type and host factors such as site of infection, past exposure to HSV-1, previous episodes of genital herpes, and gender. The effects of other host factors, such as genetic background, or of viral inoculum size on the acquisition of infection or expression of disease are poorly understood.

The term *primary infection* refers to the first infection with HSV. As summarized in Table 11-1, patients with a first symptomatic episode of genital HSV-2 infection who have serologic evidence of prior HSV-1 infection have a milder illness than those experiencing true primary infection with either HSV-1 or HSV-2 and are said to have nonprimary initial infection. Most persons with nonprimary initial symptomatic episodes of genital herpes have HSV-2 isolates, with serologic evidence of past HSV-1 infection (presumably, prior oral HSV-1 infection in most cases). However, about 25 percent have genital HSV-2 isolates together with serologic evidence of past HSV-2 infection, a finding that suggests previous asymptomatic acquisition of genital HSV-2 infection.

Genital HSV-1 infections have been reported with increasing frequency, probably causing about 10 to 15 percent of all first episodes of genital herpes in the United States today. Most genital HSV-1 infections are true primary infections, as prior oral-labial HSV-1 infection or prior HSV-2 infection appear to protect against the acquisition of genital HSV-1 disease. In addition, prior HSV-1 infection ameliorates the severity of first episodes of genital (HSV-2) herpes.

Persons with first-episode nonprimary genital HSV-2 infection are less likely to have systemic symptoms and more likely to have

TABLE 11-1. Viral, Serologic, and Clinical Features of Primary and Nonprimary First Clinical Episodes of Genital Herpes

Infection	Viral isolate from genitalia	Serum HSV antibody	Comment
Primary genital HSV-2	HSV-2	None	Severe manifestations
Primary genital HSV-1	HSV-1	None	Severe
Nonprimary first episode of genital HSV-2	HSV-2	HSV-1	Less severe
Nonprimary first episode of genital HSV-1	HSV-1	HSV-2	Seldom documented

TABLE 11-2. Relation between Viral Type, Presence of HSV Antibody in Acute Sera, and Severity of Disease in Patients with First-Episode Genital Herpes*

	Primary HSV-1 infection	Primary HSV-2 infection	Nonprimary HSV-2 infection†
Number in study	20	189	76
Percentage with systemic symptoms	58	62	16
Mean duration local pain, days	12.5	11.8	8.7
Mean number of lesions	24.3	15.5	9.5
Percentage with bilateral lesions	100	82	55
Percentage forming new lesions during course of disease	68	75	45
Mean duration viral shedding from genital lesions, days	11.1	11.4	6.8
Mean duration lesions, days	22.7	18.6	15.5

*Only one patient with complement fixation and/or neutralizing antibody in acute-phase sera had HSV-1 isolated from the genital lesions.
†$p < 0.05$ for each comparison between nonprimary and primary HSV-2 infection (chi square or Student's t-test).

a shorter duration of symptoms and signs than persons with primary genital herpes due to either HSV-1 or HSV-2. The severity of local symptoms, duration of viral shedding from lesions, and duration of lesions appear similar in patients with primary HSV-1 and those with primary HSV-2 disease (Table 11-2). However, genital HSV-1 infection recurs much less frequently than genital HSV-2 infection. This is true for both symptomatic and asymptomatic recurrences.

Primary Genital Herpes

Signs and Symptoms

Systemic and local symptoms are often prominent in primary genital herpes. Of patients who do develop symptoms and seek consultation for primary genital HSV-2 infection (a biased sample of the sickest subset of patients), nearly 40 percent of men and 70 percent of women report fever, headache, malaise, and myalgias (Table 11-3). Systemic symptoms appear early, usually peak within the first 3 to 4 days after onset of lesions, and gradually recede over the subsequent 3 to 4 days (Fig. 11-1).

Pain, itching, dysuria, vaginal or urethral discharge, and tender

TABLE 11-3. Clinical Symptoms and Signs of Primary Genital HSV-2 Infection in Men and Women Followed at the University of Washington Genital HSV Clinic

	Men	Women
Percentage with constitutional symptoms	39*	68
Percentage with meningitis symptoms	11*	36
Percentage with local pain	95	99
Mean duration of local pain, days (range)	10.9 (1–40)	11.9 (1–37)
Percentage with dysuria	44*	83
Mean duration of dysuria, days (range)	7.2 (2–20)**	11.9 (1–26)
Percentage with urethral/vaginal discharge	27**	85
Mean duration discharge, days	5.6**	12.9
Percentage with tender adenopathy	80	81
Mean duration adenopathy, days	8.6**	14.2
Mean area of lesions, mm^2 (range)	427 (6–1671)	550 (8–3908)
Mean duration viral shedding from lesions, days	10.5	11.8
Percentage with HSV isolated from urethra	28*	76
Percentage with HSV isolated from cervix	—	88
Mean duration viral shedding from cervix, days	—	11.4
Mean duration lesions, days	16.5	19.7

*$p < 0.05$ by chi square.
**$p < 0.05$ by Student's t-test.

inguinal adenopathy are the predominant local symptoms. Dysuria, both external and internal, appears more frequently in women (83 percent) than in men (44 percent). About one-quarter of men with primary genital HSV-2 infection of the external genitalia have urethral discharge, which is usually clear and mucoid. Gram's stain of the discharge usually reveals between 5 and 15 polymorphonuclear leukocytes per oil-immersion field, although occasionally mononuclear cells predominate. HSV can be isolated from a urethral swab or from the first-voided urine. A small proportion of men presenting with nongonococcal urethritis have herpetic urethritis without external genital ulcers.

Pain and irritation from lesions gradually increase over the first 6 to 7 days of illness, reach their maximum intensity between days 7 and 11 of disease, and gradually recede over the second week of illness (Fig. 11-1). Tender inguinal adenopathy usually appears during the second and third week of disease and often is the last symptom to resolve. Inguinal and femoral lymph nodes are generally firm, nonfluctuant, and tender. Suppurative lymphadenopathy is very uncommon.

Widely spaced bilateral pustular or ulcerative lesions on the external genitalia are the most frequent presenting sign. Lesions

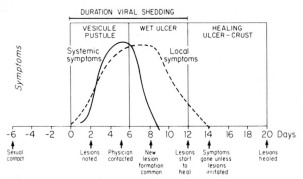

FIG. 11-1. Clinical course of primary genital herpes.

usually start as papules or vesicles which rapidly spread over the genital area. At the time of the first clinic visit, there may be multiple small pustular lesions which coalesce into large areas of ulcerations, although often patients have already passed into the ulcerative stage before seeking treatment. Ulcers persist from 4 to 15 days until crusting and/or reepithelialization occurs. Lesions of the penis and keratinized skin of the external genitalia of the female crust over before complete reepithelialization ensues. Crusting does not occur on mucosal surfaces. Secondary bacterial infection and residual scarring are uncommon.

The median duration of viral shedding as defined from the onset of lesions to the last positive culture is about 11 days (Table 11-3). The time from the onset of lesions to complete reepithelialization of all lesions is usually 2 to 3 weeks. Patients should be advised not to resume sexual activity until lesions have completely healed.

Herpes Cervicitis

HSV is isolated from the cervix of up to 90 percent of women with primary or nonprimary first-episode HSV-2 infection, compared with only 12 to 20 percent of women with recurrent external genital lesions. In primary genital herpes, cervicitis may produce purulent vaginal discharge or may be asymptomatic. In most cases of primary HSV cervicitis, inspection reveals areas of diffuse or focal ulcerative lesions of the exocervix, which may produce confluent epithelial necrosis. Bleeding is easily induced with a swab. Cervicitis can occur without external genital lesions in initial or recurrent episodes of genital herpes; sometimes symptoms of vaginal discharge, or signs of cervicitis are detected only on routine speculum exam.

Clinical differentiation between herpes cervicitis and chlamydial or gonococcal mucopurulent cervicitis may be difficult, although herpes can involve both the ectocervical squamous epithelium and any visible ectopic columnar epithelium, while chlamydia and gonorrhea spare the ectocervical squamous epithelium. Vaginal trichomoniasis produces ectocervical macular erythematous lesions ("strawberry cervix") best seen on colposcopy. In women with primary genital herpes, the mean duration of viral shedding from the cervix parallels that from lesions of the external genitalia.

Pharyngeal Infection

When the sexual exposure to an index case of herpes involves both intercourse and oral sex, then both pharyngeal and genital herpes often result, and pharyngeal symptoms are sometimes the chief complaint of individuals with primary infection of both sites. Either HSV-1 or HSV-2 can be transmitted to the pharynx with oral-genital exposure. Sore throat and pain on swallowing are often associated with constitutional symptoms such as fever, malaise, myalgia, and headache. Signs may include mild erythema, discrete or diffuse ulcers, or exudates involving the pharynx and posterior palate. Most patients with HSV pharyngitis have tender cervical nodes. Many are misdiagnosed as having streptococcal pharyngitis and/or infectious mononucleosis.

COMPLICATIONS OF GENITAL HERPES

Aseptic Meningitis

Symptoms compatible with aseptic meningitis have been reported in 36 percent of women and 11 percent of men with primary genital HSV-2 infection. HSV-1 and HSV-2 both have been isolated from CSF, although isolation of HSV-2 is much more common. Aseptic meningitis appears to be more frequently associated with genital than with oral-labial HSV infection. In contrast, HSV encephalitis in older children or adults is rarely due to HSV-2 infection.

Fever, headache, vomiting, photophobia, and nuchal rigidity are the predominant symptoms of HSV meningitis. Meningeal symptoms usually start from 3 to 12 days after onset of genital lesions. Symptoms generally increase in severity over 2 to 4 days and then gradually recede over 36 to 72 h. CSF is usually clear, and the opening pressures may be elevated. White blood cell counts in the CSF range from 10 to over 1000 cells per cubic millimeter (mean 550). The pleocytosis is predominantly lymphocytic in adults, although early in the course of disease and in neonates polymorphonuclear cells may predominate. The CSF glucose level is usually normal, although hypoglycorrhachia has been reported. The CSF protein level is slightly elevated.

The differential diagnosis of aseptic meningitis with genital ulcerations includes early syphilis, sacral herpes zoster, Behçet's syndrome, collagen vascular disease, and inflammatory bowel disease. In STD populations, the primary stage of human immunodeficiency virus (HIV-1) infection can be associated with meningitis and can be preceded by an episode of genital ulcer disease (e.g., syphilis, chancroid, or herpes).

Aseptic meningitis associated with genital herpes is a benign disease in immunocompetent persons. Signs and symptoms of encephalitis are unusual, and neurologic sequelae are rare. Early use of systemic antiviral chemotherapy for primary genital herpes decreases the subsequent development of aseptic meningitis. Although controlled trials of intravenous acyclovir for established HSV meningitis have not been conducted, it seems reasonable to give intravenous acyclovir 5 mg/kg every 8 h to hospitalized patients. Once symptoms have resolved, oral therapy can be continued to complete 10 to 14 days of therapy. For patients with HSV-1 encephalitis, higher doses of intravenous acyclovir should be given; oral therapy should not be attempted.

Other Neurologic Complications

Autonomic nervous system dysfunction, and rarely, transverse myelitis, have been described with genital HSV infection. Symptoms of autonomic nervous system dysfunction include hyperesthesia or anesthesia of the perineal, lower back, and sacral regions; difficulty urinating; constipation; and occasionally impotence. Physical examination reveals a large bladder, decreased sacral sensation, and poor rectal and perineal sphincter tone. CSF pleocytosis may be present. Electromyography usually reveals slowed nerve conduction velocities and fibrillation potentials in the affected area, and urinary cystometric examination shows a large atonic bladder. Most cases gradually resolve over 4 to 8 weeks. Whether autonomic nervous system dysfunction results from viral invasion of the central nervous system or an unusual immunologic response to infection is unknown.

Transverse myelitis is associated with decreased deep-tendon reflexes and muscle strength in the lower extremities, as well as with the autonomic nervous system signs and symptoms described above. Controlled clinical trials of antiviral or anti-inflammatory medications have not been performed for these neurologic complications.

Extragenital Lesions

Extragenital lesions frequently complicate the course of primary genital herpes but are uncommon in nonprimary first-episode or recurrent genital herpes. Such lesions usually involve the buttock, groin, or thigh area, and occasionally a finger or the conjunctivae. Characteristically, the extragenital lesions develop after the onset of genital lesions, often during the second week of disease. The majority probably result from autoinoculation of virus rather than from viremic spread.

Disseminated Infection

Blood-borne disseminated HSV infection can complicate primary mucocutaneous HSV infection during pregnancy or in immunosuppressed patients, especially those with impaired cellular immunity. Disseminated infection produces widespread cutaneous vesicles over the trunk and extremities, appears early in the disease, and is often associated with aseptic meningitis and severe visceral involvement, particularly hepatitis, as well as pneumonitis, or arthritis. This syndrome in immunosuppressed or pregnant adults resembles the manifestations of disseminated HSV infection of the neonate. Disseminated visceral infection is a disease of high mortality. Systemic antiviral chemotherapy should be given.

Superinfection

Bacterial superinfection of genital herpes lesions is uncommon in nonimmunosuppressed patients. However, vaginal yeast infection often develops during the second week of disease and is associated with a change in character of the vaginal discharge and reemergence of local symptoms such as vulvar itching and irritation.

SUMMARY OF THE CLINICAL COURSE OF FIRST EPISODES OF GENITAL HERPES

Primary first episodes of genital herpes lack serologic evidence of prior HSV-1 infection, whereas nonprimary episodes have antibody to HSV-1. Constitutional symptoms are more common with true primary episodes. Over one-half of patients with true primary genital herpes report constitutional complaints, and one-third of women complain of headache, stiff neck, and mild photophobia during the first week of disease. The duration of symptoms and frequency of complications are greater in women than in men.

Neutralizing antibody to HSV, present in those with prior HSV-1 infection, inactivates extracellular virus and interrupts the spread of HSV infection. In addition, a cellular immune response to HSV antigens appears earlier in persons with nonprimary first episodes of genital HSV than in persons with true primary infection. Both immune mechanisms may contribute to the clinical differences between primary and nonprimary first episodes of genital HSV-2 infection.

RECURRENT GENITAL HERPES: CLINICAL SIGNS AND SYMPTOMS

In contrast to the findings in first episodes of genital herpes, the symptoms, signs, and anatomic sites of infection in recurrent genital herpes are localized to the genitalia. Local symptoms such as pain and itching are milder with recurrent episodes, and the episodes usually last for about a week (Tables 11-4 and 11-5). Approximately 50 percent of attacks of recurrent genital herpes follow prodromal symptoms. The prodrome varies from a mild tingling sensation, occurring up to 48 h prior to the eruption, to "shooting pains" in the buttocks, legs, or hips 1 to 5 days prior to the episode.

As with first episodes of genital herpes, symptoms of recurrent genital herpes tend to be more severe in women than in men. Only about 10 to 30 percent of women with recurrent genital lesions experience concomitant cervical infection.

Recurrent lesions are usually confined to one side, with a much smaller area of involvement than that of first-episode genital infection. Tender, regional lymphadenopathy is also less common. The duration of viral shedding averages 4 days, and the mean time from the onset of lesions to crusting averages between 4 and 5 days. The mean time from onset of vesicles to complete reepithelialization of lesions is about 10 days. However, the severity and duration of

TABLE 11-4. Prevalence and Duration of Clinical Symptoms of Recurrent Genital Herpes in Patients Followed at the University of Washington Genital HSV Clinic

	Males	Females
Number in study	218	144
Percentage experiencing prodromal symptoms	53	43
Percentage with pain	67*	88
Mean duration pain, days (range)	3.9 (1–14)**	5.9 (1–13)
Percentage with itching	85	87
Mean duration itching, days (range)	4.6 (1–16)	5.2 (1–15)
Percentage with dysuria	9	27
Percentage with urethral/vaginal discharge	4	45
Mean duration discharge, days (range)	1.7 (1–5)**	5.3 (1–14)
Percentage with tender lymph nodes	23	31
Mean duration tender nodes, days (range)	9.2 (1–25)**	5.9 (1–15)

*$p < 0.01$ by chi square.
**$p < 0.01$ by Student's t-test.

TABLE 11-5. Clinical Signs of Recurrent Genital Herpes in Patients Followed at the University of Washington Genital HSV Clinic

	Males	Females
Number in study	218	144
Mean number of lesions at onset of episode, days (range)	7.5 (1–25)	4.8 (1–15)
Mean lesion area, mm^2 (range)	62.7 (2–270)	53.5 (4–208)
Percentage with bilateral lesions	15*	4
Percentage forming new lesions during episode	43*	28
Mean duration of new lesion formation, days (range)	5.2 (1–15)	5.4 (1–15)
Percentage with extragenital lesions	3	5
Mean time to crusting, days (range)	4.1 (1–15)	4.7 (2–13)
Mean time to healing, days (range)	10.6 (5–25)	9.3 (4–29)
Mean duration viral shedding from lesions, days (range)	4.4 (1–20)	4.1 (2–14)
Percentage shedding virus from cervix	—	12
Duration viral shedding from cervix, days (range)	—	3.2 (1–16)

*$p < 0.05$ by chi square.

recurrent episodes varies among patients, and from episode to episode in any one patient.

"Atypical" Genital HSV Infection

While the classic clinical findings of genital HSV are described above, recent studies illustrate a more diverse clinical spectrum of genital HSV. For example, among randomly selected women attending a Seattle STD clinic, in a setting in which chancroid, syphilis, and other genital ulcer diseases were uncommon, HSV was isolated from 30 percent of women with genital lesions not clinically suggestive of herpes; many of these lesions were small linear ulcerations, believed due to trauma. Serologic evidence of HSV-2 also was more common among women with HSV culture–negative atypical lesions than among those with no lesions, further suggesting that HSV-2 causes some of these lesions. Diagnostic tests for HSV-2 infection should be considered in evaluating any genital ulcerations or fissures.

OTHER CLINICAL SYNDROMES ASSOCIATED WITH GENITAL HSV INFECTION

Herpes Simplex Proctitis

First episodes of rectal herpes in men generally result from receptive anal intercourse among homosexually active men. In women, however, there is little association between anorectal HSV infection and rectal intercourse.

Patients with anorectal herpes usually present with acute onset of rectal pain, discharge, tenesmus, constipation, and bloody and/or mucoid rectal discharge, but not with true diarrhea. Fever, malaise, and myalgia are common, and urinary retention, perineal dysesthesia, and impotence may also be reported. About one-half of patients have external perianal lesions, and these cases may be accompanied by inguinal lymphadenopathy, since the anal lymphatic drainage goes to inguinal nodes, whereas lesions limited to the rectal mucosa drain to perirectal nodes.

Anoscopy generally reveals diffuse rectal mucosal inflammation, and sigmoidoscopy shows that this is limited to the distal 10 cm of the rectal mucosa with normal epithelium above this level. This establishes the diagnosis of proctitis (usually caused by HSV, *Chlamydia trachomatis, Neisseria gonorrhoeae,* or syphilis in homosexual men), as opposed to proctocolitis (where inflammation extends proximally, diarrhea is prominent, and other causes are involved). Herpes proctitis is manifested by ulceration, exudate, and easily induced mucosal petechiae or bleeding (positive wipe test). Discrete vesicular-pustular lesions are occasionally present and highly suggestive of herpetic proctitis. Histologic sections of the rectum demonstrate mucosal ulcerations with intranuclear inclusions in about 40 percent of cases. A controlled trial of systemic acyclovir showed clinical benefit. Recurrences of disease may be mild or asymptomatic in the absence of immunosuppression. However, chronic persistent anorectal herpes has become the most common form of proctitis in homosexual men with AIDS and clearly benefits from treatment with oral acyclovir, as discussed below.

Asymptomatic HSV Infection

As noted above, serosurveys show that the majority of people with HSV-2 antibody, presumed to reflect genital HSV-2 infection, are not aware of prior episodes of clinically apparent genital herpes. Among women presenting with an acute initial episode, routine frequent genital cultures obtained during follow-up showed that recurrent HSV-2 shedding was often detected in the absence of genital lesions, and the majority of recurrences were subclinical. Asymptomatic genital HSV shedding is an important source of transmission; source contacts of patients with initial episodes of genital herpes often are seropositive but unaware of their infection. Similarly, genital HSV-1 infection has been acquired by oral-genital sex with a partner experiencing asymptomatic oral excretion of virus.

Genital HSV Infection in the Immunocompromised Patient

Immunocompromised patients have more frequent and more prolonged mucocutaneous HSV infections. Such infections are usually associated with systemic complaints, prolonged local symptoms, and durations of viral shedding greater than 30 days.

Over 70 percent of renal and bone marrow transplant recipients who have serologic evidence of past HSV infection reactivate latent HSV infection within the first month after transplantation. Recurrent genital herpes in immunosuppressed patients often results in large numbers of vesicles which may coalesce into deep, necrotic, ulcerative lesions. Dissemination of virus may occur. Administration of prophylactic acyclovir prior to bone marrow transplantation has decreased the incidence of reactivated disease. In general, episodes of mucocutaneous herpes in the immunosuppressed patient should be treated with oral or intravenous acyclovir.

HSV Infection in the HIV-Infected Patient

Severe HSV infections are among the most common clinical manifestations of HIV infection. The severity and frequency of reactivation of HSV increase as the patient develops progressive immunodeficiency. Characteristically, HIV-infected patients with HSV reactivation present with chronic mucocutaneous ulcerations often involving large perianal, scrotal, penile, or vaginal areas. Pain and lesions may persist for months, and secondary infections with *Candida* are extremely common.

Lesions respond to oral acyclovir, and many patients benefit from chronic suppressive acyclovir therapy. Thymidine kinase–negative mutants resistant to acyclovir have been isolated with increasing frequency from HIV-infected patients who have persistent HSV infection unresponsive to systemic acyclovir. Alternative treatment with foscarnet may allow healing, although recurrences are common.

Role of HSV in Sexual Transmission of HIV

Several studies have implicated genital ulcerations, and specifically, the presence of HSV-2 antibodies, as risk factors for acquisition of HIV. As persons with HSV antibodies can develop genital ulcerations containing mononuclear cells, easier access of HIV to its cellular target may explain this phenomenon. Whether prevention and control of genital ulcer disease will decrease the rate of sexual transmission of HIV remains to be determined.

RATE OF RECURRENCE OF GENITAL HSV INFECTION

Following primary genital herpes, about 60 percent of patients with HSV-1 and 90 percent of those with HSV-2 infections develop symptomatic recurrences within the first 12 months of infection; the rate of asymptomatic viral shedding also is higher for HSV-2.

Rates of recurrence vary greatly between individuals. Over the first 2 years of follow-up after symptomatic primary HSV-2 infection, the median rate of clinical recurrence is five episodes per year. Asymptomatic viral shedding from the genitourinary tract occurs in 10 percent of women with HSV-1 and about 20 percent of women with HSV-2 infection during the first year after resolution of the initial episode of genital herpes. Viral and host determinants of the frequency of reactivation remain largely unknown.

GENITAL HSV INFECTION IN PREGNANCY

This topic is discussed in Chap. 28.

DIAGNOSIS OF GENITAL HERPES

Clinical Diagnosis

Differentiation between genital herpes and other infectious or noninfectious causes of genital ulceration may be difficult. In industrialized countries, the most common cause of genital ulcerations is HSV, but chancroid and primary syphilis have become resurgent since 1985 in the United States, especially in poor, inner city populations, and in association with crack cocaine use. In many developing countries, *Haemophilus ducreyi* and *Treponema pallidum* may be more prevalent, although there is some evidence from subsaharan Africa that genital ulcers are more likely to be due to HSV in HIV-infected persons than in those without HIV infection.

The differential diagnosis of ulcer adenopathy syndrome is discussed in detail in Chap. 26. Experienced clinicians realize it is usually not possible to differentiate various causes reliably without laboratory testing, especially now during the AIDS era. Briefly, however, with both genital herpes and chancroid, ulcers and nodes are painful and tender. Although vesicular lesions indicate herpes, and nodes may become fluctuant with chancroid, the two conditions are often indistinguishable at time of presentation. In contrast, primary syphilis usually produces firm, nonpainful, nontender ulcers and nodes. Donovanosis (rare in industrialized countries) produces painless, indolent, chronic genital ulcers without true adenopathy. Genital lymphogranuloma venereum generally causes only transient ulceration, with prominent inguinal adenopathy.

Noninfectious causes of genital ulcers, such as inflammatory bowel disease (Crohn's disease) or Behçet's syndrome, may also be confused with genital herpes. Ulcerative lesions due to noninfectious causes usually persist for much longer periods of time and appear larger and deeper than those typically seen in HSV infection. The genital lesions of Crohn's disease generally wax and wane with the symptoms of bowel disease. Persistent oral lesions, conjunctivitis, and/or central nervous system disease may help suggest Behçet's syndrome. Persistent lack of laboratory evidence of HSV or other infections supports the clinical diagnosis of these noninfectious entities.

Laboratory Diagnosis

Laboratory diagnosis is necessary to confirm genital herpes, unless characteristic vesiculopustular lesions are present. Syphilis should always be excluded by appropriate tests. Specific diagnosis is useful in (1) counseling regarding potential infectivity during current and future episodes of lesions, (2) identifying women at future risk for transmitting the infection to the neonate, and (3) selecting antiviral or other therapy.

Commonly used laboratory techniques for diagnosis of HSV include (1) isolation of virus in tissue culture; (2) demonstration of characteristic pathologic changes, such as giant cells or cells with typical "ground glass"–appearing intranuclear inclusions, in biopsies or lesion smears; these are stained by Giemsa or Pap smears and are less sensitive than other methods; (3) demonstration of viral antigen by immunologic methods, such as enzyme-linked immunosorbent assay (ELISA), immunofluorescence, or immunoperoxidase; or (4) demonstration of viral DNA in clinical specimens.

Viral culture is the most sensitive and specific method of confirming a diagnosis of genital herpes. In most clinical situations, the rapid appearance of HSV in tissue culture (1 to 4 days) makes viral isolation a simple method for laboratory confirmation when genital herpes is suspected. Alternatively, rapid detection methods which are fairly sensitive, such as solid-phase ELISA or immunofluorescence, are available.

Serology has limited utility in diagnosis of acute disease, although primary infection can be documented by demonstrating seroconversion. With new type-specific serologic methods, serology is of greater importance in determining if a person is an asymptomatic carrier of HSV-2. As most HSV-2 infections appear to be transmitted from persons who have undiagnosed disease or asymptomatic infection, more active identification of HSV-2 carriers has been advocated.

THERAPY

Acyclovir

The mainstay of therapy for genital HSV infection is the antiviral agent acyclovir (ACV), which has potent in vitro activity against both

HSV-1 and HSV-2. ACV is an acyclic nucleotide analogue that acts as a substrate for HSV-specific thymidine kinase (TK). HSV-infected cells selectively phosphorylate ACV to ACV-monophosphate (ACV-MP). Cellular enzymes then phosphorylate ACV-MP to ACV-triphosphate (ACV-TP), a competitive inhibitor of viral DNA polymerase. ACV-TP is incorporated into the growing DNA chain of the virus and causes chain termination. See Table 11-6 for current status of chemotherapy.

Recommended Regimen

First clinical episode of genital herpes: ACV 200 mg orally 5 times a day for 7 to 10 days or until clinical resolution occurs.

First clinical episode of herpes proctitis: ACV 400 mg orally 5 times a day for 10 days or until clinical resolution occurs.

Inpatient therapy is reserved for patients with severe disease or complications necessitating hospitalization: **ACV 5 mg/kg body weight IV every 8 h for 5 to 7 days or until clinical resolution occurs.**

When given during the first episode, ACV reduces fever and constitutional symptoms within 48 h of initiating therapy and rapidly relieves symptoms. While treatment of first episode infection markedly shortens the course of the episode, it unfortunately has no effect on the subsequent long-term natural history of recurrences.

Recurrent Episodes

Recurrent episodes of genital herpes in immunocompetent individuals are self-limited, and thus benefit little from therapy with ACV. If there is a pattern of recurrences, some patients who are able to start therapy at the beginning of the prodrome or very soon after onset of lesions may have significant benefit. Therapy, if given, should consist of: **ACV 200 mg orally 5 times a day for 5 days** *or* **ACV 800 mg orally 2 times a day for 5 days.**

Daily Suppressive ACV

Daily treatment reduces frequency of recurrences by at least 75 percent among patients with frequent (more than six per year) recurrences. Safety and efficacy have been clearly documented among persons receiving daily therapy for up to 3 years. ACV resistant strains of HSV have occasionally been isolated from immunocompetent persons receiving suppressive therapy but have not been associated with treatment failure or with documented sexual transmission. After 1 year of continuous daily suppressive therapy, ACV should be discontinued to reassess the patient's recurrence rate.

TABLE 11-6. Current Status of Antiviral Chemotherapy of Mucocutaneous HSV Infections

Type of infection	Treatment and benefits
Mucocutaneous HSV infections	
Immunosuppressed patients	
Acute symptomatic first or recurrent episodes	IV or oral ACV relieves pain and speeds healing; with localized external lesions, topical ACV may be beneficial.
Suppression of reactivation	IV or oral ACV taken daily prevents recurrences during high-risk periods (e.g., immediately after transplant); lesions will recur when therapy is discontinued.
Immunocompetent patients	
First episodes of genital herpes	Oral ACV is the treatment of choice. IV ACV may be used if severe disease or neurologic complications are present; topical ACV may be beneficial in patients without cervical, urethral, or pharyngeal involvement.
Symptomatic recurrent genital herpes	Oral ACV has some benefit in shortening lesions and viral excretion time; routine use for all episodes not recommended.
Suppression of recurrences	Daily oral ACV prevents reactivation of symptomatic recurrences. While licensure is at present limited to 6 months, recent studies suggest courses of up to 18 months are safe.
First episodes of oral-labial HSV	Oral ACV has not yet been formally studied but is likely to be effective.
Recurrent episodes of oral-labial HSV	Topical ACV is of no clinical benefit; oral ACV has minimal benefit.
Oral-labial UV-provoked HSV	One study indicates oral ACV will prevent UV-provoked lesions when started 24 h prior to exposure and continued through exposure period, usually 7–21 days.
Herpetic whitlow	Anecdotal reports suggest oral ACV is beneficial.
HSV proctitis	Oral ACV will shorten the course of disease.
Herpetic eye infections	Topical trifluorothymidine, vidarabine, idoxuridine, acyclovir, and interferon are all beneficial; debridement may be required; topical steroids may worsen disease.

TABLE 11-6. (continued)

Antiviral Dosages	
Immunosuppressed patients	IV ACV 5 mg/kg q 8 h for 7–14 days, depending on response. Oral ACV 200–400 mg p.o. 5 times a day for 7–14 days. Topical ACV 4–6 times a day for 7–10 days.
Immunocompetent patients	
First-episode genital herpes	Oral ACV 200 mg p.o. 5 times a day for 10 days.
Recurrent genital herpes	Oral ACV 200 mg p.o. 5 times a day for 5 days.
Meningitis	IV ACV 5 mg/kg q 8 h for 5 days
Encephalitis	IV ACV 10 mg/kg q 8 h for 10 days. Oral ACV not recommended.

Suppression of HSV Infection	
Immunosuppressed patients	400 mg p.o. tid (higher dosages can be utilized if clinically necessary).
Immunocompetent patients	ACV 200 mg tid or 400 mg p.o. bid (higher or lower dosages can be utilized depending on clinical response).

Recommended regimen: ACV 400 mg orally 2 times a day
Alternative regimen: ACV 200 mg orally 2 to 5 times a day.

Genital Herpes in HIV-Infected Patients

It has not yet been established whether higher-than-standard doses of oral ACV are needed for patients with early HIV infection who are otherwise immunocompetent. Immune status, not HIV infection per se, is the likely predictor of disease severity and response to therapy. Immunocompromised patients, as well as immunocompetent hosts in whom initial therapy fails, may benefit from an increased dose of ACV.

Emergence of Resistance

In vitro resistance to ACV can result from TK-deficient, TK-altered, or DNA-polymerase-resistant strains of HSV. TK deficiency is the most common mechanism of HSV resistance to ACV. Most of the resistant isolates have been recovered from immunocompromised patients undergoing multiple courses of therapy for established infection. Recently, increasing ACV resistance has been seen in

HIV-infected patients who have received long courses of intermittent and/or suppressive therapy. Persistent cutaneous lesions in this setting have cleared with the use of intravenous foscarnet.

At present, routine in vitro testing of HSV isolates for ACV sensitivity is not recommended. However, isolates from patients with mucocutaneous infections which persist on ACV therapy (especially among HIV-infected patients) should be tested for ACV resistance.

Acyclovir in Pregnancy

Although ACV is not teratogenic in animals, oral ACV in pregnancy generally cannot be advocated until studies of its efficacy and safety in pregnancy have been completed.

Foscarnet

Foscarnet is a viral DNA polymerase inhibitor with potent antiviral activity. It can be given only intravenously or topically. The drug causes renal toxicity and changes in calcium and phosphorous balance and has therefore been reserved for therapy of serious herpesvirus infection, especially CMV and HSV infection in immunosuppressed patients. Foscarnet is the preferred drug for treatment of disease due to ACV-resistant strains of HSV.

PREVENTION OF INFECTION

No proven effective means of prophylaxis of HSV has been established. Barrier forms of contraception, especially condoms, may decrease transmission of disease, especially from episodes of asymptomatic infection. Condoms are probably less reliable when lesions are present. Clinical trials of HSV vaccines are expected in the near future.

ADDITIONAL READING

Ashley R et al.: Inability of enzyme immunoassays to discriminate between infections with herpes simplex virus types 1 and 2. *Ann Intern Med* 115:520, 1991

Bevilacqua F et al.: Acyclovir resistance/susceptibility in herpes simplex virus type 2 sequential isolates from an AIDS patient. *J Acquir Immune Defic Syndr* 4: 967, 1991

Brock BV et al: Frequency of asymptomatic shedding of herpes simplex virus in women with genital herpes. *JAMA* 263:418, 1990

Brown ZA et al.: Neonatal herpes simplex virus infection in relation to asymptomatic maternal infection at the time of labor. *N Engl J Med* 324: 1247, 1991

Hardy WD: Foscarnet treatment of acyclovir-resistant herpes simplex virus infection in patients with acquired immunodeficiency syndrome: Preliminary results of a controlled, randomized, regimen-comparative trial. *Am J Med* 92(2A):30S, 1992

Hook EW III et al: Herpes simplex virus infection as a risk factor for human immunodeficiency virus infection in heterosexuals. *J Infect Dis* 165:251, 1992

Kaplowitz LG et al: Prolonged continuous acyclovir treatment of normal adults with frequently recurring genital herpes simplex virus infection. The Acyclovir Study Group. *JAMA* 265:747, 1991

Koelle DM et al.: Asymptomatic reactivation of herpes simplex virus in women after the first episode of genital herpes. *Ann Intern Med* 116:433, 1992

Koutsky LA et al.: Underdiagnosis of genital herpes by current clinical and viral-isolation procedures. *N Engl J Med* 326:1533, 1992

Kulhanjian JA et al.: Identification of women at unsuspected risk of primary infection with herpes simplex virus type 2 during pregnancy. *N Engl J Med* 326:916, 1992

Mertz GJ et al.: Risk factors for the sexual transmission of genital herpes. *Ann Intern Med* 116:197, 1992

For a more detailed discussion, see Spear PG: Biology of the Herpesviruses, Chap. 34, p. 379; and Corey L: Genital Herpes, Chap. 35, p. 391, in STD-2.

Cytomegaloviruses (CMVs) are a group of viruses within the *Herpesviridae* family. They are widely distributed and have been isolated from humans, green monkeys, mice, and many other species. Infection with this group of viruses typically results in a characteristic enlargement of cells and the appearance of distinctive intranuclear and cytoplasmic inclusion bodies which has led to the common name of cytomegalovirus. These inclusions resemble those associated with herpes simplex virus (HSV) infection. In humans, CMV causes asymptomatic as well as severe infections which may be followed by either persistent or latent infections.

The isolation of CMV from cervical secretions and semen and the demonstration of an association between CMV infection and chronic cervicitis provided early evidence that CMV might be a sexually transmitted disease. The virus is also transmitted by nonsexual means. CMV infection is a particularly common and severe clinical problem in patients with the acquired immunodeficiency syndrome (AIDS).

VIROLOGY

Human CMV is a double-stranded DNA virus with a genome of 150 million daltons. It is the most complex of all the DNA viruses, and its genome is approximately 50 percent larger than the genome of HSV. Morphologically, CMV resembles other herpesviruses. The enveloped virion is approximately 200 nm in diameter. It consists of a naked virus containing a spherical DNA-protein-complex core, surrounded by a 110-nm icosahedral capsid with 162 capsomeres. The naked virion is surrounded by an envelope with a single or double membrane structure which is acquired during budding from the nuclear or cytoplasmic membrane of the infected cell.

EPIDEMIOLOGY

CMV infections are ubiquitous and usually asymptomatic. Viral transmission occurs by intimate person-to-person contact. Potential sources of virus include saliva, urine, semen, breast milk, blood, transplanted donor organs, and cervical and vaginal secretions. The prevalence of CMV infection in the adult population ranges from 40 percent in Europe to almost 100 percent in Africa and the far east. In general, the prevalence of CMV infection is related to the socioeconomic status of a population and, to a certain extent, to the geographic location.

Sexual Transmission

Sexual transmission is a significant mode of spread for CMV. Virus may be isolated from the uterine cervix, semen, and saliva, although the relative roles played by each of these potential sources of virus is not clear. Approximately 8 to 10 percent of women, either pregnant or nonpregnant, shed CMV from the cervix, and approximately 30 percent of asymptomatic homosexual men have CMV in their semen. The level of sexual activity is a stronger predictor of CMV infection than race, age, or socioeconomic status.

Viruses with identical DNA restriction patterns have been isolated from sexual partners. This sharing of identical DNA restriction patterns indicates the epidemiologic relatedness of virus strains among these partners and strongly implies sexual transmission of CMV.

Compared with heterosexual men, homosexual men are significantly more likely to be CMV culture positive. Infection in homosexual men is associated with increased age, number of sexual partners, and the practice of anal-receptive intercourse. Excretion of CMV in semen is significantly associated with HIV seropositivity in asymptomatic homosexual men. Independent of infection with HIV, CMV seropositivity and CMV excretion are associated with increased T-suppressor lymphocyte counts and reduced T-helper/T-suppressor ratios.

Maternofetal Transmission and Infection During Early Childhood

Maternal infections play an important role in transmission of CMV to neonates. Approximately 1 percent of all infants are congenitally infected. CMV can be reactivated during gestation, and the virus may be transmitted to the fetus in utero despite circulating maternal antibody. Congenital infections may follow primary, reactivated, or recurrent maternal infections. Following primary maternal infection, CMV is transmitted to 40 to 50 percent of the offspring, and 5 to 10 percent of these congenitally infected infants will become symptomatic. Although maternal immunity to CMV does not protect the fetus from intrauterine infection, first (primary) infection during pregnancy is most likely to result in severe disease of the infant.

Infants may also become infected during the first six months of life, probably as a result of acquiring infection during passage through the birth canal or through breastfeeding. The next wave of CMV infection occurs in day care centers or nursery schools. By puberty, approximately 40 to 80 percent of youths have been infected with CMV.

CMV Infection in Transfusion Recipients and Immunosuppressed Populations

In addition to sexual and maternofetal transmission, primary or recurrent CMV infection occasionally follows blood transfusions or organ transplantation. Transfusion of leukocyte-enriched blood products increases the risk of CMV infection, while use of leukocyte-depleted or cryopreserved red blood cells decreases the risk.

CMV infection is very common in immunosuppressed populations (such as organ transplant recipients) and in persons with AIDS. Male homosexuals or bisexuals with AIDS have extremely high rates of CMV infection, as almost 100 percent of them excrete CMV in body fluids. This phenomenon does not exist in other populations at high risk for AIDS, such as intravenous drug users or hemophiliac patients. The rate of CMV infection among these other groups is less than that in homosexual men with AIDS and is close to that of similar populations without AIDS.

CLINICAL MANIFESTATIONS

Neonatal Infection

Clinical manifestations of congenital CMV infection range from minimal involvement to severe disease with neurologic abnormalities, hepatosplenomegaly, jaundice, chorioretinitis, and petechiae. Most congenitally infected infants (≥90 percent) are asymptomatic at birth, however. Nonetheless, 5 to 20 percent of these infants may develop late manifestations of CMV infection such as hearing loss and poor intellectual performance. Congenital or perinatal CMV infections are usually persistent with chronic viral excretion over months or years.

Infection in Normal Hosts

Primary CMV infections in normal children and adults are usually asymptomatic but may be associated with a mononucleosis-like illness involving fever, lethargy, myalgias, headache, and mild hepatitis. CMV causes about 8 percent of all infectious mononucleosis syndromes. CMV mononucleosis often resembles mononucleosis due to Epstein-Barr virus (EBV), another member of the *Herpesviridae* family, but certain clinical features differ. CMV-infected patients are older, with a mean age of 28 years, compared with EBV-infected patients, who have a mean age of 19 years. With CMV mononucleosis, the duration of fever is longer (mean duration 18 days) than in patients with EBV (mean duration 10 days). Pharyngitis, tonsillitis, lymphadenopathy, and lymphocytosis with atypical lymphocytes are more commonly associated with EBV than with CMV. Other complications of CMV infections in normal hosts are rare and include rash, granulomatous hepatitis, Guillain-Barré syndrome, meningoencephalitis, myocarditis, pneumonitis, hemolytic anemia, and thrombocytopenia.

Infection in Immunocompromised Persons

In immunocompromised patients, CMV infection may be asymptomatic or may cause serious illness with high morbidity and mortality. Adverse effects of CMV infection following organ transplantation include syndromes directly related to the virus, such as severe mononucleosis-like syndromes, leukopenia, pneumonitis, retinitis, and gastrointestinal ulcerations. In addition, there may be indirect effects including superinfection and a possibly increased risk of graft rejection.

In AIDS, CMV causes variable clinical manifestations similar to those described following transplantation. CMV retinitis, characterized by retinal hemorrhages and exudates, is the most common cause of blindness in patients with advanced HIV infection. CMV also causes erosive esophagitis with symptoms similar to those caused by *Candida* and HSV. Colonic infection can result in severe diarrhea. The virus is often isolated from lung biopsies of AIDS patients with pneumonia, usually in association with other pathogens such as *Pneumocystis carinii.* Pulmonary symptoms usually improve following anti–*P. carinii* pneumonia therapy without specific treatment for CMV. Less commonly, however, CMV is the only isolate, and pathology specimens reveal inclusion bodies and evidence of invasive disease. These findings suggest true CMV pneumonia, which sometimes responds to ganciclovir. Adrenalitis and meningoencephalitis have also been documented in patients with AIDS.

LABORATORY DIAGNOSIS

A laboratory diagnosis of suspected CMV infection may be confirmed by several methods, including viral isolation, serologic examination, electron microscopy, histologic evaluation, immunohistochemical staining of tissues, and/or nucleic acid hybridization techniques. Of these methods, viral isolation and serologic examination are the most commonly used in the clinical setting. CMV infection may be demonstrated histopathologically by detection of characteristic large cells with intranuclear and occasional cytoplasmic inclusions in biopsy or autopsy materials. The presence of these cytomegalic cells suggests CMV infection, but virologic or serologic confirmation is still desirable.

Serologic Diagnosis

A serologic diagnosis may be made by comparing antibody titers present in acute-phase sera with those in convalescent-phase specimens obtained 2 to 3 weeks later. A seroconversion or fourfold or greater rise in titer is diagnostic of recent (but not necessarily primary) infection. Single serum samples are useful for seroepidemiologic studies but are of little value for diagnosis of CMV infections. Because IgM CMV antibodies may persist for months, detection of IgM in a single sample generally has limited usefulness in adults.

Common serologic methods include the complement fixation (CF) test, indirect immunofluorescent antibody (IFA) test, indirect hemagglutinin (IHA) test, anticomplement immunofluorescence (ACIF), latex agglutination, and the enzyme-linked immunosorbent assay (ELISA). Presently, the ELISA is the most extensively used because of its sensitivity and ease of performance.

Virus Isolation

CMV may be cultured from throat washings, urine, cervical swab, blood (buffy coat), or biopsy specimens. In the evaluation of immunocompromised patients, buffy coat cultures are a better indicator of symptomatic infection than positive CMV cultures from urine or throat washings. Positive isolates from urine should be interpreted cautiously because shedding may persist up to 2 years after initial infection. Human fibroblast cells best support the growth of CMV and are therefore routinely used for diagnostic purposes. The time required for isolation of virus depends somewhat on the quantity of virus present. If titers are high, cultures may become positive within 2 to 10 days. Other cultures may take up to 6 weeks to exhibit cytopathic effects consistent with CMV infection. Specific approaches permitting more rapid diagnosis are important, especially in the management of immunosuppressed patients with a potentially rapid progressive CMV disease such as retinitis. In such settings the centrifugation-culture technique is currently the diagnostic method of choice. This involves centrifugation of the specimen onto monolayer cell cultures and subsequent assay for early CMV antigens by either immunofluorescence, immunoperoxidase staining, or ELISA using monoclonal antibodies.

TREATMENT

CMV infection in a normal host rarely requires treatment. However, therapy is commonly required in AIDS patients and other immunosuppressed hosts who show signs of serious clinical disease. The most promising drugs currently available for the treatment of CMV disease are ganciclovir and foscarnet.

Ganciclovir is structurally related to acyclovir and has good in vitro activity against CMV. The drug reduces CMV replication by inhibition of DNA polymerase. Patients with CMV retinitis usually stabilize on therapy, but chronic maintenance is required as retinitis usually relapses after discontinuation of antiviral therapy. Data on the treatment of some other forms of CMV disease with ganciclovir are encouraging but largely uncontrolled. The drug is generally well tolerated, but reversible neutropenia is a frequent adverse reaction.

Foscarnet selectively inhibits CMV DNA polymerase and consequently reduces viral replication. It has been used successfully to treat CMV retinitis in AIDS patients and may offer a survival advantage over ganciclovir. The drug is relatively well tolerated, but has been associated with substantial nephrotoxicity and occasional electrolyte abnormalities. Ganciclovir remains the drug of choice for treatment of CMV retinitis in AIDS patients at this time.

Recommended therapy for CMV retinitis in patients with AIDS: ganciclovir 5 mg/kg IV every 12 h for 14 to 21 days followed by 6 mg/kg daily 5 days a week indefinitely. Complete blood count should be monitored closely.

Alternative therapy for CMV retinitis in patients with AIDS: foscarnet 60 mg/kg IV every 8 h for 2 to 3 weeks, followed by 90–120 mg/kg IV per day indefinitely. BUN, creatinine, and electrolyte levels should be closely followed.

The doses of ganciclovir and foscarnet must be adjusted if renal failure is present.

PREVENTION

There is a need for methods to prevent CMV disease following intrauterine transmission of virus, after transplantation procedures, or during the development of AIDS. Both passive and active immunization approaches are under investigation.

ADDITIONAL READING

Collier AC et al: Cytomegalovirus infection in women attending a sexually transmitted diseases clinic. *J Infect Dis* 162:46, 1990

Fowler KB, Pass RF: Sexually transmitted diseases in mothers of neonates with congenital cytomegalovirus infection. *J Infect Dis* 164:259, 1991

Fowler KB, et al: The outcome of congenital cytomegalovirus infection in relation to maternal antibody status. *N Engl J Med* 326:663, 1992

Heinemann ME: Characteristics of cytomegalovirus retinitis in patients with acquired immunodeficiency syndrome. *Am J Med* 92:12S, 1992

Hirsch MS: The treatment of cytomegalovirus in AIDS—More than meets the eye. *N Engl J Med* 326:264, 1992

Lamy ME et al: Prenatal diagnosis of fetal cytomegalovirus infection. *Am J Obstet Gynecol* 166:91, 1992

Sohn YM et al: Cytomegalovirus infection in sexually active adolescents. *J Infect Dis* 163:460, 1991

Studies of Ocular Complications of AIDS Research Group, in collaboration
  with the AIDS Clinical Trials Group: Mortality in patients with the
  acquired immunodeficiency syndrome treated with either foscarnet or
  ganciclovir for cytomegalovirus retinitis. *N Engl J Med* 326:213, 1992

For a more detailed discussion, see Smiley L and Huang E-S:
Cytomegalovirus as a Sexually Transmitted Infection, Chap. 36,
p. 415, in STD-2.

Papillomaviruses are small, nonenveloped viruses with an icosahedral capsid and a double-stranded circular DNA genome. More than 70 "genotypes" of human papillomaviruses (HPVs) have been identified, each differing from the others by DNA-DNA hybridization criteria. Over 20 different HPV types are characteristically found in genital epithelium. Of these, certain types (e.g., HPV 6 and 11) cause genital warts, while others (most commonly 16, 18, and 31) are strongly associated with severe forms of genital dysplasia and carcinomas.

Genital warts are epidermal tumors caused by HPV. Condylomata acuminata, "pointed condylomas," are warts with a particular clinical appearance (see below), and the term should not be used as a synonym for anal or genital warts.

EPIDEMIOLOGY

Prevalence and Incidence

Data on the prevalence of genital warts in the general population are limited. Five percent of married women in King County, Washington, reported a history of genital warts. Subclinical infection is common; studies of unselected cervical smears have revealed koilocytotic atypia, indicative of HPV infection, in 1 percent of women. Furthermore, HPV DNA has been identified in many people with no clinical signs of infection. Studies have found HPV DNA in about 6 percent of men and 10 percent of women without clinical signs of infection.

The incidence of genital warts has markedly increased during the last 2 decades. Genital warts are the most common viral STD, perhaps three times as common as symptomatic genital herpes; their incidence is exceeded only by gonorrhea and chlamydial infection. Most cases are diagnosed in young adults between the ages of 16 and 25 years.

Transmission

HPV infections are transmitted by direct sexual contact. Nearly two-thirds of sex partners of individuals with genital warts develop the disease after an average incubation period of 2 to 3 months. Genital lesions in sex partners are often inconspicuous, and careful examination may be needed to identify them. Transfer of HPV by fomites plays a role in the epidemiology of skin warts; how often this occurs with genital strains of HPV is not known.

Involvement of Nongenital Areas

Genital strains of HPV can also infect the anus, and occasionally the mouth. Warts occurring only in the anal canal are strongly associated with receptive anorectal intercourse, especially in men. Anal warts usually contain HPV 6 DNA. In homosexual men, anal warts are much more common than penile warts, suggesting that the anal epithelium is particularly susceptible to acquisition of HPV infection through anorectal intercourse, or to expression of visible warts on infected sites.

Condylomata acuminata have been recognized in the mouth with increasing frequency during the past few years; some patients give a history of oral sex with an infected partner. The genotypes involved have not yet been extensively characterized.

PATHOGENESIS

Warts are generally benign, self-limiting tumors which regress after a time. All the layers of the normal epithelium are represented in the wart, and the basement membrane is not breached. The initial event in wart formation is probably trauma to the epithelium and entry of virus into one or a few cells of the basal germinal layer. Infection with the virus stimulates cell growth, creating an irregularly thickened prickle cell layer and a granular layer that contains foci of cells with intranuclear HPV. These cells, termed koilocytes, show nuclear chromatin changes and perinuclear vacuolar halos and may be prominent on Papanicolaou (Pap) smears of exfoliated cervical cells from women with cervical HPV infection.

Exposure to HPV in adults usually occurs through sexual contact with a partner who has a clinical or subclinical infection. The risk of infection rises with increasing numbers of sex partners.

CLINICAL MANIFESTATIONS

Subclinical HPV Infection

The clinical spectrum of genital HPV infection is wide and ranges from complete absence of any epithelial abnormality identifiable by magnification or biopsy, through a variety of microlesions visible only by magnification (e.g., with a colposcope) after applying acetic acid, to macroscopic warts visible to the naked eye. This clinical spectrum appears related to several factors, including viral factors such as viral genotype; the site of infection (risks of severe dysplasia and of eventual invasive cancer are greatest at the area of transformation from squamous to columnar epithelium on the cervix); and ill-defined host factors or associated risk factors. HPV infection at one genital site (e.g., vulva) tends to be correlated with infection at other sites (e.g., vagina).

In the experience of the University of Washington, HPV DNA has been detected by sensitive polymerase chain reaction (PCR) assays in genital swab specimens from about 50 percent of male and female STD clinic patients, most of whom lack clear macroscopic or colposcopic evidence of HPV infection. The prevalence in college students is lower and is related to the number of previous sex partners, with no genital HPV detected even by PCR among sexually inexperienced female students.

Colposcopic examination after application of acetic acid shows certain site-specific lesions to be correlated with detection of HPV DNA. Greatest experience is with cervical colposcopy, which shows, for example, that lesions that appear opaquely white with sharp borders after applying acetic acid (opaque acetowhite epithelium with sharp borders) are associated with HPV. Similarly, leukoplakia and "satellite" lesions, discrete from the squamocolumnar junction, are associated with HPV. Colposcopic examination of the vulva and vagina also reveal lesions that are associated with HPV. These have been termed flat warts, acetowhite epithelium, "filaments," "droplets," or "asperities."

Genital Warts in Men

Genital warts in men are pleomorphic. Condylomata acuminata (exophytic condylomas) are the most commonly seen lesion (Fig. 13-1). These warts, are soft, fleshy, and vascular. They often appear

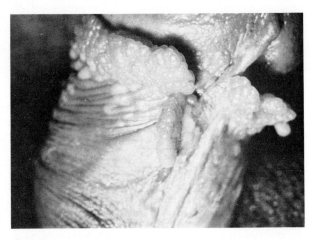

FIG. 13-1. Penile condylomata acuminata.

first on the frenum, coronal sulcus, glans penis, and the lining of the prepuce, areas susceptible to trauma during intercourse. They can also occur on the shaft of the penis and the scrotum. Papular warts appear on relatively dry areas, particularly the shaft of the penis; they are usually multiple and vary between 1 and 5 mm in diameter. Common warts occasionally appear on the shaft of the penis (Fig. 13-2), usually in association with similar lesions on nongenital skin. Exophytic condylomas may involve the urethra, either alone or in association with other lesions. They may cause urethral bleeding or discharge, or change in urinary stream, but usually cause no symptoms.

Flat condylomas affect the same areas as exophytic warts; they are usually multiple and may be confluent. They are generally subclinical, and the affected areas cannot be clearly identified unless acetic acid solution is applied and a colposcope or other source of magnification used.

Genital Warts in Women

Exophytic condylomas typically appear first on the fourchette and adjacent labia and may spread quite rapidly to other parts of the vulva; in about 20 percent of cases condylomas also appear on the perineum and perianal area. Any part of the vagina may be affected, and in a few women the vagina may be entirely occupied by condylomatous tissue (Fig. 13-3). Papular warts affect the outer parts of the genitals, such as the labia majora and perineum.

Exophytic condylomas of the cervix have been seen in about 6 percent of women with vulvar warts and occasionally occur alone.

Anal Warts

Perianal warts are usually condylomata acuminata. More than 50 percent of men with external anal warts have "internal" condylomas affecting squamous epithelium up to, but seldom beyond, the anal verge (the anorectal junction) as well.

Giant Condyloma

Genital and anal condylomata may reach a substantial size. Large vulvar condylomas occur in women with reduced cell-mediated immunity, such as occurs in pregnancy, Hodgkin's disease, or AIDS, or during receipt of immunosuppressive therapy. In this uncommon tumor an initial wartlike lesion enlarges relentlessly to form an extensive, destructive, but nonmetastasizing tumor. Despite its formidable clinical behavior, histologically it appears to be benign, consisting of condylomatous tissue.

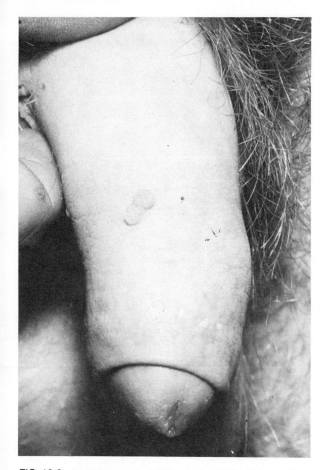

FIG. 13-2.   Penile common wart (verruca vulgaris). This lesion is unlikely to respond to podophyllin.

INTRAEPITHELIAL NEOPLASIA

It is now clear that much of the cytologic and histologic disease of the cervix, other genital squamous epithelium, and anus that has been termed *dysplasia* or *intraepithelial neoplasia* is in fact caused

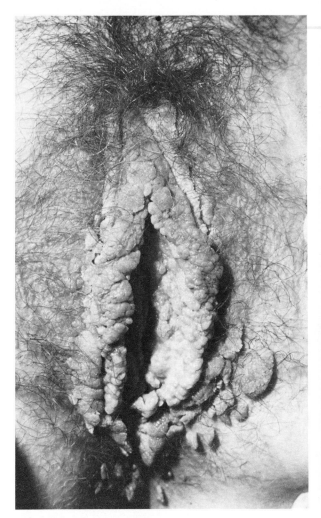

FIG. 13-3. Extensive condylomata acuminata of the labia and immediately adjacent sites. *(Courtesy of E. Stolz.)*

by recently acquired or reactivated HPV infection. The terms *mild, moderate,* or *severe* dysplasia (of the cervix) are synonymous with the terms *cervical intraepithelial neoplasia grades 1, 2,* or *3* (CIN1, CIN2, CIN3). Severe dysplasia (CIN3), is more or less synonymous with carcinoma in situ. The latest terminology, the Bethesda system, recognizes the difficulty of the cytopathologist in differentiating dysplasia—especially mild dysplasia—from active HPV infection. Thus, the three levels of severity recognized in the two previous terminologies are collapsed into two classifications, termed *mild squamous intraepithelial lesion/papilloma virus infection* (SIL/HPV), and *moderate to severe squamous intraepithelial lesion.* A recent University of Washington study showed that among women with cervical HPV type 16 or 18 infection but normal Pap smears who were enrolled in STD clinics, over one-third progressed to develop biopsy-confirmed moderate to severe squamous intraepithelial lesions within 2 years. There is a clinical consensus that among women with cervical Pap smears consistent with dysplasia (CIN), close follow-up and colposcopic exam are indicated, and that biopsy, plus some form of therapy, is necessary for those with moderate to severe squamous intraepithelial lesions. Some clinicians offer therapy for those with mild SIL/HPV as well. The role of specific testing for cervical HPV infection is still to be defined.

HPV AND GENITAL NEOPLASIA

Data implicating specific HPV types in the pathogenesis of genital epithelial neoplasia include the following:

1. As discussed above, of women experiencing cervical infection with HPV type 16 or 18, at least one-third develop moderate or severe dysplasia within 2 years.
2. Carcinoma of the cervix is associated with multiple sex partners and early age at first intercourse, suggesting a sexually transmitted etiological agent.
3. HPV DNA, usually from HPV type 16 or 18, can be found in about 90 percent of squamous cervical cancers, as well as in moderately severe or severe grades of CIN. This association is also present, although less consistently, with neoplasia of the vulva, vagina, penis, and anus.
4. HPV DNA is integrated into the genome of the host cell in invasive cancers but is usually episomal in lower grades of intraepithelial neoplasia.
5. HPV 16 or 18 DNA is found integrated into the genome of some (but not all) stable cell lines of cervical cancer (e.g., HeLa cells contain HPV 18).
6. Several papilloma viruses of animals are known to cause cancer. A human heritable disease, epidermodysplasia verruciformis

(EDV), involves depressed cellular immunity and development of squamous cell cancers at sites of HPV infection on areas of the body exposed to ultraviolet light.

7. At the molecular level, specific HPV oncogenes, termed $E6$ and $E7$, have been described and found to be very closely related to well-characterized oncogenes in SV 40 viruses and adenovirus. Expression of $E6$ and $E7$ is greater in "high-risk" HPV types (such as HPV 16 and 18) than in HPV types not strongly associated with genital cancers (e.g., HPV 6).

While HPV infection may indeed be a major factor in the pathogenesis of genital epithelial cancers, carcinogenesis is typically a complex multistep process involving several different factors at each stage of development. Much further work will be needed to clarify the precise role of HPV and of other cofactors in the pathogenesis of cervical cancers.

HIV Infection and HPV

Because immunosuppressed women (e.g., renal transplant recipients) have a greatly increased risk of cervical cancer, the effects of HIV infection on HPV infection and neoplasia are being studied. For both cervical and anal HPV infection, it appears that HIV infection increases reactivation and expression of latent HPV infection and increases the rate of severe dysplasia among those with HPV infection. These effects appear to increase as the level of HIV-related immunosuppression increases, suggesting that it is immunosuppression that affects HPV expression and the severity of dysplasia. However, a direct effect of HIV on HPV at the molecular level (i.e., transactivation of HPV by HIV) also has been demonstrated. Whether or not the effects of HIV infection on HPV infection will actually result in an increased risk of invasive cervical or anal cancer before the natural history of HIV infection results in death from other causes is uncertain. Nonetheless, it would be prudent to obtain cervical Pap smears at 6- to 12-month intervals from HIV-positive women and to perform colposcopy when the cytologic findings are abnormal. Anoscopy at regular intervals has been advocated for HIV-infected homosexual males to detect macroscopically visible neoplastic lesions.

DIAGNOSIS

Anal or genital warts must be differentiated from other papillomatous lesions, such as other infections, anatomical variants, and neoplasms. The most important infective lesions to be distinguished from anal or genital warts are the condylomata lata of secondary syphilis, which appear on moist areas such as the vulva and anus.

They are flatter or more smoothly rounded and transudative than warts and are associated with other signs of secondary syphilis. In the tropics, the chronic granulating lesions of donovanosis may be confused with anal or genital condylomata. The umbilicated tumors of molluscum contagiosum are usually easily distinguished from warts. Distinguishing warts from other neoplastic conditions is sometimes difficult. Any lesions which appear atypical should be biopsied.

Detection of subclinical HPV infections by Pap smear and colposcopy was discussed above. These methods are less sensitive than commercially available tests for detecting HPV DNA (e.g., VIRAPAP tests), and much less sensitive than PCR for detecting HPV. Certainly Pap smear is a well-established, though relatively insensitive, test for detecting cervical neoplasia; and colposcopy is an established method for localizing suspicious lesions for biopsy and for treatment (e.g., by excision, laser, or cryotherapy). There is also growing interest in the use of tests for detecting high-risk HPV types, but the utility of these tests in patient management remains to be defined.

TREATMENT OF GENITAL WARTS

The only therapies available are physically destructive or chemically cytotoxic, and none have been shown to eradicate HPV. The virus has been demonstrated in normal-appearing adjacent tissue after laser treatment of HPV-associated cervical intraepithelial neoplasia and after attempts to eliminate subclinical HPV by extensive laser vaporization of the surrounding anal or genital area. Presumably, the virus persists in deeper layers of basal epithelium, which must be preserved during laser therapy to prevent permanent scarring. The effect of genital wart treatment on HPV transmission and on the natural history of HPV is unknown. It is not known if visible lesions are more infectious than subclinical infection with a given HPV type, or whether treatment of visible lesions reduces infectivity. Therefore, the goal of treatment is removal of the warts for cosmetic reasons, and amelioration of signs and symptoms, not the eradication of HPV.

Expensive therapies, toxic therapies, and procedures that result in scarring should be avoided. Sexual partners should be examined for evidence of warts and other STDs. Patients with anal or genital warts should be made aware that they are contagious to uninfected sexual partners. Condom use is recommended to help reduce transmission, though condoms could be expected to be less effective in preventing transmission of HPV (which presumably requires only skin–skin contact which could occur even with partial covering of the penis by a condom) than in preventing gonorrhea, for example.

In most clinical situations, cryotherapy with liquid nitrogen or cryoprobe is the treatment of choice for external genital and perianal warts. Cryotherapy is nontoxic, does not require anesthesia, and if used properly, does not result in scarring. Podophyllin, trichloroacetic acid, and electrodesiccation/electrocautery are alternative therapies. The latter may be most effective in eliminating warts, but often results in scarring. Because of its relatively low efficacy, high incidence of toxicity, and high cost, treatment with interferon cannot be recommended for routine use.

The carbon dioxide laser and conventional surgery are useful only in the management of very extensive warts, particularly in those patients who have not responded to cryotherapy; these alternatives are not appropriate for treatment of limited lesions. Like more cost-effective treatments, these therapies do not eliminate HPV and are associated with appreciable rates of clinical recurrence.

External Genital/Perianal Warts

Recommended regimen: Cryotherapy with liquid nitrogen or cryoprobe.
Alternative regimens:
Podophyllin 10 to 25% in compound tincture of benzoin. To avoid systemic toxicity, the total volume of podophyllin solution applied should be limited to less than 0.5 ml per treatment session, and less than 10 cm^2 should be treated per session. The solution should be thoroughly washed off in 1 to 4 h. Applications may be repeated at weekly intervals and left on longer before washing, if initial applications are well tolerated. If the wart persists after three treatments, treatment should be switched to cryotherapy or electrodessication, and consideration given to biopsy. Mucosal warts are more likely to respond than highly keratinized warts on the penile shaft, buttocks, and pubic areas. *This podophyllin regimen is contraindicated in pregnancy.*

Trichloroacetic acid (85%). The solution should be applied only to warts. The area should be powdered with talc or sodium bicarbonate (baking soda) to remove unreacted acid. Application may be repeated at weekly intervals.

Electrodesiccation/Electrocautery. Electrodesiccation is contraindicated in patients with cardiac pacemakers, or for lesions proximal to the anal verge. Extensive or refractory disease should be referred to an expert.

Vaginal Warts

Recommended regimen: Cryotherapy with liquid nitrogen. (The use of a cryoprobe in the vagina is not recommended because of the risk of vaginal perforation and fistula formation.)
Alternative regimens:
Trichloroacetic acid (80 to 90%). See the instructions above in the section on external genital/perianal warts.

Podophyllin 10 to 25% in compound tincture of benzoin. The treatment area must be dry before removing speculum. Less than 2 cm² should be treated per session. Application may be repeated at weekly intervals. A square of gauze can be placed against the treatment area to protect the opposing vaginal wall from podophyllin. *This regimen is contraindicated in pregnancy.*

Urethral Meatus Warts

Recommended regimen: Cryotherapy with liquid nitrogen.
Alternative regimen: Podophyllin 10 to 25% in compound tincture of benzoin. The treatment area must be dry before contact with normal mucosa, and podophyllin must be washed off in 1 to 2 h. *This regimen is contraindicated in pregnancy.*

Anal Warts

Recommended regimen: Cryotherapy with liquid nitrogen.
   Alternative regimens:
      Trichloroacetic acid (80 to 90%).
      Surgical removal.

Oral Warts

Recommended regimen: Cryotherapy with liquid nitrogen.
   Alternative regimens:
      Electrodesiccation/electrocautery.
      Surgical removal.

Pregnant Patients and Perinatal Infections

Juvenile-onset recurrent respiratory papillomatosis is associated with maternal condyloma during parturition. Thirty to 50 percent of juvenile cases occur in the setting of overt maternal disease. In an individual mother with genital condyloma, however, the risk of delivering a child who develops papilloma appears relatively low, in the range of 1 to 400. Cesarean delivery for prevention of transmission of HPV infection to the newborn is not indicated, since the risk of transmission is low and cesarean delivery does not always prevent development of papillomatosis. However, in rare instances, cesarean delivery may be indicated for women with genital warts if the pelvic outlet is obstructed or if vaginal delivery would result in excessive bleeding.

PREVENTION

The most important strategy for the prevention of serious morbidity related to genital HPV infection is cervical cytologic screening. Among individuals with a history of known HPV infection, and those otherwise at high risk for STD, annual screening is recommended. Although empiric evidence is lacking, condoms may reduce the risk of HPV infection. The extraordinarily high prevalence of subclinical infection with HPV—including types related to genital cancers in sexually experienced young adults—represents a very strong case for health education that discourages multiple sex partners. From the perspective of the female, HPV ranks with chlamydial infection and HIV infection as a major health risk for women, often carried without symptoms by both sexes.

ADDITIONAL READING

Bauer HM et al: Genital human papillomavirus infection in female university students as determined by a PCR-based method. *JAMA* 265:472, 1991

de Villiers EM: Laboratory techniques in the investigation of human papillomavirus infection. *Genitourin Med* 68:50, 1992

de Villiers EM et al: Human papillomavirus DNA in women without and with cytological abnormalities: Results of a 5 year follow-up study. *Gynecol Oncol* 44:33, 1992

Franco EL: The sexually transmitted disease model for cervical cancer: Incoherent epidemiologic findings and the role of misclassification of human papillomavirus infection. *Epidemiology* 2:98, 1991

Horn JE et al: Genital human papillomavirus infections in patients attending an inner-city STD clinic. *Sex Transm Dis* 18:183, 1991

Kaufman RH: Human papillomavirus and cervical cancer: Risk to male partner. *JAMA* 265:1179, 1991

Kiviat N et al: Anal human papillomavirus infection among human immunodeficiency virus–seropositive and –seronegative men. *J Infect Dis* 162:358, 1990

Koutsky L et al: Cohort study of risk of cervical intraepithelial neoplasia grade 2 or 3 associated with cervical papillomavirus infection. *N Engl J Med* 327:1272, 1992

Laga M et al: Genital papillomavirus infection and cervical dysplasia—opportunistic complications of HIV infection. *Int J Cancer* 50:45, 1992

Palefsky J: Human papillomavirus infection among HIV-infected individuals. *Hematol Oncol Clin North Am* 5:357, 1991

Palefsky JM et al: Anal intraepithelial and anal papillomavirus infection among homosexual males with group IV human immunodeficiency virus disease. *JAMA* 263:2911, 1990

Vermund SH et al: High risk of human papillomavirus infection and cervical squamous intraepithelial lesions among women with symptomatic HIV infection. *Am J Obstet Gynecol* 165:392, 1991

For a more detailed discussion, see Shah KV: Biology of Human Genital Tract Papillomaviruses, Chap. 37, p. 425; and Oriel D: Genital Human Papillomavirus Infection, Chap. 38, p. 433, in STD-2.

DEFINITION

Molluscum contagiosum is a benign papular condition of the skin and mucous membranes which is often sexually transmitted in adults. It is caused by the molluscum contagiosum virus (MCV), a member of the poxvirus family.

EPIDEMIOLOGY

Because the lesions of MCV are usually sparse and self-limited, it is likely that many infected patients do not seek medical attention. There are few population-based data on those who do, since molluscum contagiosum is usually not a reportable disease.

Molluscum contagiosum appears to be spread by both sexual and nonsexual routes of transmission. In adults, lower abdominal, thigh, and genital lesions are more common than those in extragenital locations. Evidence for sexual transmission is further supported by a frequent history of contact with multiple sexual partners and prostitutes, the history and presence of other sexually transmitted diseases (STDs), the presence of genital lesions in sexual partners, and peak ages of occurrence (20 to 29 years) which are similar to those of other STDs. The nonvenereal form of disease occurs primarily in children on the face, trunk, and extremities and appears to be transmitted by direct contact with the skin of infected individuals and/or fomites.

ETIOLOGY

MCV has been purified from skin lesions and is considered to be a poxvirus. The virus is brick-shaped, approximately $300 \times 220 \times 100$ nm, with a biconcave viral core enclosed by an inner membrane and an outer envelope. The viral genome is a single molecule of linear double-stranded DNA. MCV yields a characteristic cytopathic effect in cell culture, but attempts at viral replication in cell culture have generally been unsuccessful.

CLINICAL MANIFESTATIONS

The incubation period of molluscum contagiosum averages 2 to 3 months, ranging from 1 week to 6 months. Most patients are asymptomatic, the diagnosis being made incidental to another problem; a minority complain of itching or tenderness. Lesions begin as tiny pinpoint papules which grow over several weeks to a diameter of 3 to 5 mm, occasionally enlarging to 10 to 15 mm,

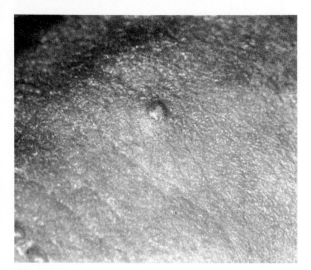

FIG. 14-1.   Solitary molluscum contagiosum lesion with typical dome shape and central umbilication. *(Courtesy of AC Cardozo.)*

producing the "giant molluscum." The smooth, firm, and dome-shaped papules have a highly characteristic central umbilication from which caseous material can be expressed (Fig. 14-1). They are usually flesh-colored but can appear gray-white, yellow, or pink.

In adults, lesions most often occur on the thighs, inguinal region, buttocks, and lower abdominal wall and less commonly on the external genitalia and perianal region, especially mucosal surfaces—a pattern contrasting with the distribution of genital warts. Lesions on the palms, soles, and mucous membranes are rare in children and adults. A linear distribution of lesions often occurs, suggesting autoinoculation by scratching. Lesions are usually more widespread in children than in adults, and while adults with genital molluscum contagiosum rarely develop extragenital lesions, 10 to 50 percent of children with molluscum contagiosum have lesions in the genital region.

In normal hosts, the number of lesions usually varies between 10 and 20, ranging from 1 to 100; patients with impaired host defenses, however, may develop hundreds of lesions. Extensive outbreaks of lesions can develop in patients with abnormal cell-mediated immunity—for example, in patients with sarcoidosis, Hodgkin's disease, and AIDS, and in those receiving immunosuppressive therapy. Of interest, the distribution of lesions in these patients, including homosexual men with AIDS, is usually over the face and trunk rather than the genital region.

The most frequent complication of molluscum contagiosum, bacterial superinfection, occurs in up to 40 percent of cases. Another common problem is "molluscum dermatitis," which appears 1 to 15 months after the onset of skin lesions in approximately 10 percent of patients. The dermatitis consists of a sharply bordered eczematoid reaction 3 to 10 cm in diameter around an individual lesion and usually disappears as the lesion resolves. Infection during pregnancy does not affect the outcome of pregnancy; no documented case of maternal–fetal transmission of infection has been reported.

The duration of untreated molluscum contagiosum averages approximately 2 years, ranging from 2 weeks to 4 years. Individual lesions usually resolve within 2 months. Recurrences of lesions after clearance have been noted in 15 to 35 percent of patients; whether these represent new infections or exacerbation of subclinical or latent infection is not clear.

DIAGNOSIS

The clinical diagnosis of molluscum contagiosum is usually made easily on the basis of the characteristic pearly, umbilicated papule with the caseous center, found on the face, trunk, extremities, or genital region. Lesions are most frequently misdiagnosed as common or genital warts or keratoacanthomas. Other considerations in the differential diagnosis include syringomas, plane warts, lichen planus, epithelial and intradermal nevi, seborrheic dermatitis, basal cell epithelioma, infection with herpes simplex or varicella zoster virus, and atopic dermatitis.

In atypical cases the diagnosis can be confirmed by demonstrating the pathognomonic enlarged epithelial cells with intracytoplasmic molluscum bodies on cytologic or histologic studies (Fig. 14-2). Thinly spread smears of material expressed from lesion cores stained by Wright, Giemsa, or Gram's stain demonstrate sheets of infected cells. Hematoxylin-and-eosin-stained sections of punch biopsies reveal characteristic epidermal histopathologic changes. Other diagnostic techniques include detection of MCV antigen with fluorescent antibody studies and visualization of the abundant viral particles by electron microscopy.

The possibility of an immunodeficiency, such as HIV infection, should be considered in the evaluation of those with widespread lesions.

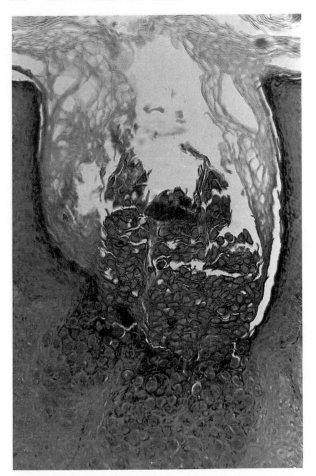

FIG. 14-2 Biopsy of a molluscum contagiosum lesion showing an area of epidermal hyperplasia surrounding a cystic lobule. Keratinocytes in the upper epidermis as well as those desquamated into the lobule demonstrate large round intracytoplasmic molluscum bodies. Hemotoxylin and eosin stain. *(Courtesy of BA Werness.)*

TREATMENT AND PREVENTION

Molluscum contagiosum is usually treated by eradicating lesions with mechanical destruction or techniques to induce local epidermal inflammation. While treatment hastens resolution of individual lesions and may therefore reduce autoinoculation and transmission to others, the high frequency of recurrences and the benign and self-limited nature of the infection must be weighed against the pain and potential for scarring induced by destructive therapies.

Controlled studies evaluating different therapeutic approaches have not been performed. The simplest and most widely used methods are excisional curettage or expression of the core of the lesion by direct pressure; these procedures are often followed by cauterization of the lesion base with electrodesiccation or a chemical agent such as silver nitrate, trichloroacetic acid, or iodine. Cryotherapy with liquid nitrogen is an alternative mode of direct destruction, often employed in patients with AIDS who have extensive lesions. For tiny lesions which may be difficult to curette or express, cryotherapy or topical application of irritating agents such as podophyllin, tretinoin, silver nitrate, phenol, or trichloroacetic acid have been recommended. No therapy is very effective in immunocompromised patients, presumably because of the increased occurrence of new lesions. Bacterial superinfection and molluscum dermatitis may require systemic antibiotics or topical corticosteroids, respectively.

ADDITIONAL READING

Billstein SA, Mattaliano VJJ: The "nuisance" sexually transmitted diseases: Molluscum contagiosum, scabies, and crab lice. *Med Clin North Am* 74:1487, 1990

Forghani B et al: Direct detection of molluscum contagiosum virus in clinical specimens by in situ hybridization using biotinylated probe. *Mol Cell Probes* 6:67, 1992

Radcliffe KW et al: Molluscum contagiosum: A neglected sentinel infection. *Int J STD AIDS* 2:416, 1991

Smith KJ et al: Molluscum contagiosum. Ultrastructural evidence for its presence in skin adjacent to clinical lesions in patients infected with human immunodeficiency virus type 1. *Arch Dermatol* 128:223, 1992

Smith MA, Singer C: Sexually transmitted viruses other than HIV and papillomavirus. *Urol Clin North Am* 19:47, 1992

For a more detailed discussion, see Douglas Jr JM: Molluscum contagiosum, Chap. 39, p. 443, in STD-2.

At least five distinctly different human viruses are now recognized as causative agents of acute viral hepatitis. Some of these organisms are sexually transmitted (Table 15-1).

Hepatitis A virus (HAV), hepatitis B virus (HBV), hepatitis delta virus (HDV), and at least two agents of what was formerly called non-A non-B hepatitis [hepatitis C virus (HCV) and hepatitis E virus (HEV)] share a remarkable predilection for involvement of the liver despite profound differences in physical structure, pathobiology, and epidemiology.

HAV is an RNA-containing picornavirus, similar in many respects to poliovirus, and known to cause only acute and not chronic hepatic disease. HBV, on the other hand, is a DNA-containing hepadnavirus, associated with both acute and chronic forms of hepatitis as well as hepatocellular carcinoma. HDV is a unique, defective RNA virus that is dependent on coinfection with HBV for replication and expression of disease. HCV and HEV, respectively, cause posttransfusion hepatitis and enterically transmitted disease. Many other infectious agents cause hepatitis, but since they either are seldom transmitted sexually or are discussed elsewhere in this text (e.g., cytomegalovirus), they are not mentioned here.

Sexual activity profoundly influences the transmission of both HAV and HBV, even though both viruses are also commonly transmitted by other means. Vaccines are available for prevention of hepatitis B (and may soon be available for hepatitis A), providing a unique means of prevention among sexually transmitted diseases. Their use must be considered in populations at risk for STD. The role played by sexual transmission in the spread of HDV, HCV, and HEV is much less certain and requires further investigation.

HEPATITIS A VIRUS

Pathobiology

The pathogenesis of hepatitis after natural infection with HAV is poorly understood. Infection of the hepatocyte, however, is central to the disease process, although the mechanisms responsible for hepatocellular damage are not known. It is found in the bile, and it is thought that this is the source of most virus shed in the feces. Viremia roughly parallels the shedding of virus in feces, but titer is of lower magnitude. At the onset of hepatic inflammation, the titer of infectious virus is greatest in liver, followed by feces, and then serum. Viral antigen may be detected in the feces as late as 2 weeks after the onset of symptoms, but chronic fecal shedding of virus has not been observed.

TABLE 15-1. Human Hepatitis Viruses

Designation	Virus type	Nucleic acid	Particle size, nm	Known antigens	Modes of transmission*	Acute disease	Chronic disease
Hepatitis A virus (HAV)	Picornavirus	ssRNA	27	HAV	ET ST PT (rare)	Yes	No
Hepatitis B virus (HBV)	Hepadnavirus	dsDNA	42	HBsAg HBcAg HBeAg	HT ST PT NT	Yes	Yes
Hepatitis delta virus (HDV)	Unclassified	ssRNA	36	HBsAg HDAg	PT ST(?)	Yes	Yes
Hepatitis E virus (HEV) (Enteric non-A non-B virus)	Unclassified	ssRNA(?)	30	HEV	ET	Yes	No
Hepatitis C virus (HCV)	Unclassified	ssRNA(?)	40(?)	HCV	PT, ST(?)	Yes	Yes

*Documented modes of transmission: ET, enterically transmitted; HT, horizontally transmitted; NT, perinatal transmission; PT, parenterally transmitted; ST, sexually transmitted.

181

Immunity

Antibody to the virus (anti-HAV) generally appears in the serum concurrent with the clinical onset of hepatitis (Fig. 15-1). Early antibody is comprised largely of IgM, although IgG may also be present shortly after the onset of symptoms. Both IgG and IgM antibody have viral neutralizing activity. IgG anti-HAV persists for life and confers protection against reinfection.

Epidemiology

Spread of HAV between individuals is almost uniformly due to fecal-oral transmission. Virus transmission is facilitated by conditions which favor fecal-oral spread, including sexual practices involving oral-anal contact. Saliva may contain very small amounts of infectious HAV, but it is likely that virus in saliva represents a trivial source of transmission in comparison with the much greater titers of virus present in the feces.

Potential for household transmission and even common-source outbreaks is enhanced by the extraordinary physical stability of the virus. Virus is concentrated from contaminated waters by filter-feeding shellfish; human hepatitis A infection may result if such shellfish are ingested uncooked. Parenteral transmission has occurred with

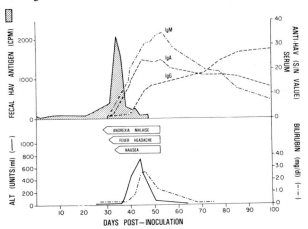

FIG. 15-1. Experimental HAV infection in a 21-year-old male volunteer. Fecal HAV and immunoglobulin-specific anti-HAV were measured by solid-phase radioimmunoassay. Feces from days 33 and 35 were shown to contain infectious HAV by passage to primates. *(Reprinted by permission from SM Lemon, N Engl J Med 313: 1059, 1985.)*

transfused blood, but such instances are rare because the viremia is relatively brief.

Although common-source outbreaks due to food or water contaminated with HAV may be highly dramatic and involve large numbers of patients, such outbreaks account for only a small proportion of all HAV infections. Infection of a food handler is commonly incriminated.

The vast majority of HAV infections occur sporadically, presumably as a result of person-to-person spread of virus, and in many cases may not be recognized as hepatitis. Preschool day care facilities, especially those enrolling children less than 2 years old, play a significant role in the spread of HAV. Most infected children under age 2 do not become icteric and are not recognized as having hepatitis. Subsequent transmission of infection to older siblings, parents, and babysitters (all of whom are more likely to develop classic signs of hepatitis) is common. HAV is also relatively common in intravenous drug users. This association probably reflects hygienic practices, but may also be due at least in part to occasional needle-borne transmission of virus.

HAV, like other predominantly enteric infections, may be transmitted during sexual activity. However, the importance of sexual transmission of HAV varies widely among different populations. Sexual transmission probably plays a greater role in the spread of HAV in industrialized nations which have good public health systems than in developing nations with inadequate sanitary and water systems. A number of studies suggest that HAV may be commonly transmitted among male homosexuals.

HAV differs from most other sexually transmitted pathogens, including other predominantly enteric organisms such as *Shigella,* in at least two important ways. First, infection with the virus produces solid immunity so that symptomatic reinfection occurs infrequently if ever. Second, the infected individual is infectious for a relatively brief period of time. There is no prolonged carrier state. Thus, to maintain sexual transmission of HAV within a population, several host conditions appear to be required. These include (1) a high degree of susceptibility among the population at risk, as defined by negative tests for anti-HAV, (2) multiple sexual contacts, so that numerous partners may be exposed during the relatively brief period when virus is shed, and (3) sexual practices facilitating fecal-oral spread of virus.

Clinical Manifestations of Hepatitis A

In the individual patient, acute illness due to HAV is indistinguishable from that due to HBV, HCV, or HEV. The incubation period of HAV is relatively short, averaging about 4 weeks (Fig. 15-1).

Under the age of 3 years, less than 10 percent of infected children develop symptoms of hepatitis, whereas most infected adults are symptomatic. Symptoms are often abrupt in appearance, although there may be a prodromal period of low-grade fever, malaise, headaches, and myalgias. Anorexia, nausea, and vomiting occur early in the illness, and diarrhea is not uncommon, especially among children. The specific diagnosis of viral hepatitis, however, is often not suggested until the occurrence of dark urine or jaundice.

Elevations of serum aminotransferase levels are similar in magnitude to those seen in acute hepatitis B, although they generally do not persist as long. Most infected individuals will have normal aminotransferase levels by 6 weeks after the onset of symptoms, although 10 to 20 percent of cases may have minor enzyme abnormalities persisting for up to 3 months.

Chronic hepatitis has yet to be documented following hepatitis A. Although jaundice may occasionally be prolonged for several weeks or more ("cholestatic hepatitis"), it is not indicative of severe hepatocellular disease and uniformly resolves with time. Hepatitis A accounts for less than 10 percent of all cases of fulminant hepatitis, and the mortality in acute symptomatic hepatitis A is probably less than 0.1 to 0.2 percent.

Diagnosis of HAV Infection

Diagnosis of hepatitis A rests entirely on serologic methods. Although anti-HAV may be detected by a variety of techniques, antibody is usually measured by solid-phase radioimmunoassay or enzyme-linked immunosorbent assay (ELISA). Absence of anti-HAV is strong evidence against current infection with HAV. However, the detection of anti-HAV in a patient with hepatitis does not prove that infection is recent or responsible for current symptoms. A specific serodiagnosis requires the demonstration of IgM anti-HAV, which is present in virtually all patients with acute hepatitis A and may be detected by sensitive antibody-capture immunoassays for as long as 6 months after the onset of symptoms.

Prevention of Hepatitis A

Immune globulin (IG), if administered 2 weeks before exposure, is 80 to 90 percent effective in protecting against illness associated with HAV infection. Infection is also probably prevented if IG is given soon enough after exposure. Postexposure prophylaxis (0.02 ml/kg intramuscularly) is recommended for all household and sexual contacts of patients with hepatitis A, as well as for individuals with exposure to day care centers or other institutional facilities within which significant transmission of HAV has been documented.

Postexposure prophylaxis is generally not recommended in the setting of a common-source outbreak because such outbreaks are usually recognized only well into their course when IG may no longer be effective in prevention of disease. However, it is difficult to exclude the possibility of a beneficial effect in individual cases. Preexposure IG prophylaxis (0.06 ml/kg body weight every 5 months) has been recommended for travelers to endemic areas in developing countries, especially when such travel is off the major tourist routes. Lesser doses of IG provide protection for shorter time periods.

Adverse reactions to IG are minimal and are generally limited to local and allergic manifestations which occur in about 1 percent of all recipients. There is good evidence that IG distributed commercially within the United States is not capable of transmitting HIV or other blood-borne agents such as HBV.

HEPATITIS B VIRUS

Virology

HBV is a hepadnavirus, one of a family of related DNA viruses infecting the livers of a variety of avian and mammalian species. The HBV virion (also known as the Dane particle) is a complex, double-shelled 42-nm spherical particle with an outer surface envelope surrounding a core structure containing a small DNA genome.

In addition to the genomic DNA, the HBV core contains a DNA polymerase which is thought to have reverse transcriptase activity, and possibly a protein kinase as well. The major core protein is a 21-kilodalton (kD) molecule with specific antigenic activity (hepatitis B core antigen, or HBcAg). Vigorous disruption of the virus core results in the release of another, antigenically distinct, soluble viral antigen (HBeAg).

The surface envelope surrounding the virus core is a complex structure containing as its major antigen a 24-kD glycoprotein (hepatitis B surface antigen, or HBsAg). HBsAg is usually produced in excess by infected hepatocytes and, in most carriers of HBV, incomplete 22-nm spherical or tubular HBsAg particles greatly outnumber intact HBV virion particles in the blood.

Pathobiology and Immunity

The HBsAg may appear in the blood as early as 6 days after parenteral exposure, although this interval is usually from 1 to 2 months after mucosal exposures. Shortly afterward, circulating virion particles, HBeAg, and DNA polymerase may be detected. This stage of detectable viremia is often brief. The synthesis of HBsAg is more abundant and typically more persistent, however,

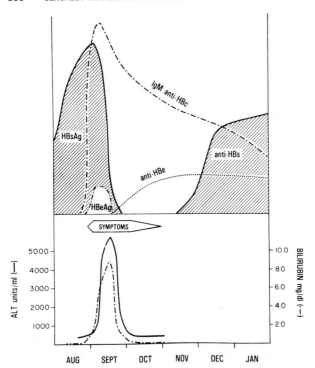

FIG. 15-2. Acute, self-limited HBV infection occurring in a 49-year-old laboratory technician. HBV-related antigens and antibodies were measured by solid-phase immunoassays.

and it may be detected for up to 5 months or in some cases even longer.

Most infections are self-limited (Fig. 15-2). The first humoral immune response to the virus, consisting of IgM antibody to HBcAg (IgM anti-HBc) develops shortly after the appearance of HBsAg. Following the disappearance of circulating DNA polymerase and HBeAg, antibody to HBeAg (anti-HBe) may also be detected. Over 95 percent of infected normal adults will eventually clear HBsAg from the circulation, and most, but not all, of these individuals develop antibody to HBsAg (anti-HBs). There may, however, be a delay of weeks to months prior to the first appearance of anti-HBs, even after the disappearance of HBsAg. During this so-called window period, anti-HBc and anti-HBe are the only serum markers of HBV infection. Symptoms of hepatitis usually develop after HBsAg has been circulating in the blood for 3 to 6 weeks, and usually occur while HBsAg is still present (approximately 90 percent of patients). Symptoms may develop during the "window period," however, or even after the appearance of anti-HBs. The appearance of anti-HBs signals the resolution of the infection. This antibody protects against reinfection. Anti-HBc and anti-HBs usually persist for years following infection.

A small proportion (probably <5 percent) of infected adults are not able to clear HBsAg from their blood and become chronic HBsAg carriers (Fig. 15-3). Such individuals frequently have little or no evidence of acute liver disease when initially infected. Development of the chronic carrier state is more frequently seen in individuals who are immunocompromised (e.g., previous HIV infection). Almost all infants who are infected neonatally become carriers. HBsAg may persist in the blood of these individuals for years in large and relatively constant amounts and may be associated with the presence of either HBeAg or anti-HBe. Carriers with HBeAg usually have circulating Dane particles and detectable DNA polymerase activity; such carriers should be considered to be especially infectious. Chronic HBsAg carriers typically have very high titers of anti-HBc and usually do not have anti-HBs.

While most persistent HBsAg carriers are asymptomatic and do not have evidence of significant liver disease, a minority have elevated levels of serum aminotransferases and the histologic picture of chronic active hepatitis. HDV plays an important role in promoting severe liver disease associated with HBV infection (see below). The presence of HBeAg correlates with significant liver disease, and seroconversion from HBeAg to anti-HBe in carriers with chronic hepatitis is frequently followed by resolution of liver function abnormalities. The carrier state itself may spontaneously resolve in some cases.

The mechanism of hepatocellular damage in either acute or chronic HBV infection is not known. Because immunosuppressed patients are less likely to develop overt signs of hepatitis and because replication of large quantities of virus occurs in many totally healthy carriers, it seems likely that the host immune response is intimately involved in the expression of liver disease.

There is a strong association between persistent HBV infection and primary carcinoma of the liver. Infection with HBV usually precedes the development of hepatocellular carcinoma by years, although the tumor occasionally develops during childhood. However, it remains uncertain whether HBV by itself is directly oncogenic, or only one of several important factors involved in tumorigenesis. The association of HBV with hepatocellular carcinoma

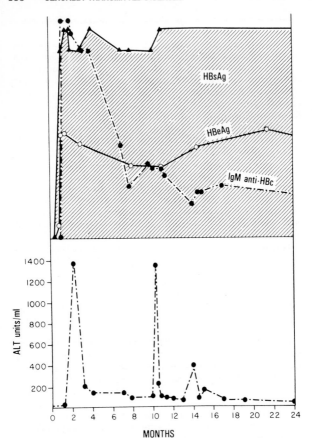

FIG. 15-3. Acute HBV infection progressing to the chronic HBsAg carrier state and chronic active hepatitis. HBsAg was measured by reverse passive hemagglutination, other HBV markers by solid-phase radioimmunoassay. *(Sera and HBsAg results courtesy of S Krugman.)*

is found worldwide, but hepatocellular carcinoma is a significant problem mainly in those countries where the HBsAg carrier rate is high and neonatal transmission of virus frequent.

Infection with HBV is marked by the development of antibody directed against each of the individual viral antigens: anti-HBs, anti-HBc, and anti-HBe. Of these, the antibody most clearly associated with a protective effect against reinfection is anti-HBs. Anti-HBc plays an uncertain role in protection. While the presence of anti-HBe in the blood of a HBsAg carrier suggests a relative lack of infectivity, there is no evidence that anti-HBe by itself has any protective effect. The role cell-mediated immunity plays in protection against reinfection is not known.

Epidemiology

Population Studies

Dramatic differences in HBV prevalence exist between various regions of the world. In parts of southeast Asia and Africa, >90 percent of the population may have serologic evidence of past or current HBV infection, and 10 to 20 percent of adults may be HBsAg-positive. In contrast, among New York City volunteer blood donors, less than 10 percent had past exposure to HBV, and less than 0.5 percent were HBsAg-positive. Striking differences in HBsAg carrier rates have also been noted between ethnically disparate groups living within the same geographic area. Within the United States, the seroprevalence generally increases with age and lower socioeconomic status and is higher among blacks and persons of Asian ancestry. In addition, health care workers are at increased risk of HBV infection, largely acquired through unapparent means but correlating with exposure to blood.

Transmission

Transmission of HBV may be categorized into four general modes: parenteral, sexual, perinatal, and horizontal (defined as occurring in the absence of recognized parenteral, sexual, or perinatal exposure). Transfusion has become an infrequent cause of hepatitis B since the introduction of sensitive methods for detecting HBsAg in donor units. While parenterally acquired HBV remains common among drug addicts, and needle-stick accidents are a source of infection for health care workers, HBV is much more commonly transmitted by nonparenteral means. HBsAg has been found in the saliva, vaginal secretions, and semen of infected individuals. The presence of virus in saliva and semen presumably reflects leakage from the circulation, and not the replication of virus at oro-pharyngeal or genital sites. Although studies directly examining the infectivity of various body fluids are limited, it is probably correct to state that any body fluid or secretion may be infectious.

Transmission of HBV to household members of HBsAg carriers is well documented, and multiple epidemiologic surveys suggest that horizontal transmission to young children is probably the most common means of transmission of this virus worldwide. The exact mechanism by which this occurs is not known, however. It is uncertain whether virus is commonly transmitted by oral exposure to infected secretions such as saliva. Most horizontal transmission within families and among young children is probably due to unrecognized parenteral exposures to saliva or blood. Such exposures may be relatively infrequent but are apt to occur over an extended period of household (or perhaps classroom) contact with a persistently infected virus carrier.

HBV is commonly transmitted from HBsAg carrier mothers to their infants and also following acute maternal HBV infection in the third trimester. Presence of maternal HBeAg is associated with an increased risk of virus transmission to the newborn. While intrauterine transmission has been noted, most infections probably occur at the time of birth or shortly thereafter.

Numerous studies indicate that both heterosexual and homosexual intercourse may transmit HBV. An increased prevalence of HBsAg and anti-HBsAg has been noted among prostitutes and individuals attending STD clinics, but such studies are difficult to control for possibly important socioeconomic variables. Primary risk factors for HBV among male homosexuals include rectal intercourse and exposure to large numbers of sexual partners. Another important factor is that HBsAg-positive male homosexuals are very likely to be HBeAg-positive, possibly reflecting their relatively recent acquisition of HBV as adults (Table 15-2). HBeAg is associated with an increased risk of transmission of virus following heterosexual and needle-stick exposures as well as with an increased risk of perinatal transmission, and its presence implies a high risk of infectivity for homosexual men.

The information above was derived from studies conducted in the years immediately preceding recognition of the AIDS epidemic. However, the subsequent adoption of safer sex practices by many homosexual men appears to have altered the epidemiology of HBV in this population. Although the overall incidence of hepatitis B increased within the United States from 1982 to 1987, the proportion of hepatitis B cases associated with homosexual activity fell from 20 to 9 percent in four sentinel counties studied by the Centers for Disease Control. In contrast, the proportion attributed to heterosexual contact increased from 15 to 22 percent during this same period.

There is considerable evidence to support the transmission of HBV by heterosexual contact as well. Sexual partners of individuals with acute hepatitis B are clearly at increased risk of acquiring infection when compared with other members of the household. The prevalence of HBV infection among heterosexuals attending STD clinics has been shown to be related to numbers of previous sex partners. At present, it is estimated that approximately one in

TABLE 15-2. Serum HBV Markers in Male Homosexuals

| Location | All individuals, % | | | HBsAg-positive only, % | | Reference |
	HBsAg	Anti-HBs	Anti-HBc*	HBeAg	Anti-HBe	
New York City	5.2	54	10	61	28	1,2
USA (multicenter)	6.1	52	3	65	16	3
London	5.2	38	Not done	Not done	Not done	4
Denmark	5.6	61	Not done	Not done	Not done	5

*Percentage shown is for those with only anti-HBc.
†All men had positive syphilis serologic tests.

191

five reported cases of acute hepatitis B in the United States may have been contracted through heterosexual exposure.

Clinical Manifestations

Many adults infected with HBV probably have silent infections which result in permanent and solid immunity. Compared with hepatitis A, however, acute hepatitis B is a more serious disease. The onset of illness is generally more insidious than that due to HAV, and evidence of hepatocellular disease resolves more slowly. The incubation period is usually from 40 to 110 days but may be shorter with large-inoculum parenteral exposures and may be prolonged by administration of globulin preparations. A small proportion (1 percent or less) of icteric adults develop acute hepatic failure, and about three out of four of these patients die as a result of their infection.

Approximately 15 to 20 percent of patients develop a transient serum sickness-like illness during the prodromal or early acute stage of hepatitis B. This syndrome is characterized by an erythematous macular or maculopapular, occasionally urticarial, skin rash, polyarthralgias, and frequently frank arthritis. The arthritis may be migratory, is frequently symmetrical, and may involve large joints of the extremities as well as the proximal interphalangeal joints of the hands. Serum aminotransferase levels are usually elevated and may be the best clue to the proper diagnosis.

A striking feature of hepatitis B is the development of persistent infection. Approximately 5 percent of persons with HBV infection become chronic carriers. Up to a third of chronic HBsAg carriers develop histologic evidence of chronic active hepatitis, while the remainder may have only a benign form of liver disease characterized by minimal inflammatory changes on liver biopsy. While chronic active hepatitis may progress to cirrhosis and death, it more frequently remits spontaneously even in moderately advanced cases.

Diagnosis

Approximately 90 percent of patients with acute hepatitis B have HBsAg detectable in their serum when they first present for medical care. About 10 percent of patients with acute HBV infection are HBsAg-negative, however, and these cases are more difficult to document. In such patients, anti-HBc is uniformly present while anti-HBs may be found in some. Both markers persist for many years after acute infection; their presence is not diagnostic of acute hepatitis B. IgM anti-HBc, however, is specific for acute HBV infection. It can be detected in almost all cases of acute hepatitis B and persists after acute infection for 6 to 24 months. While many

Table 15-3. Serologic Diagnosis of Hepatitis Virus Infections

Step 1 (patient has acute hepatitis):

		IgM anti-HAV	
		Positive	Negative
Anti-HBc	Positive	Acute hepatitis A hepatitis B, obtain HBsAg and IgM anti-HBc (step 2)	? hepatitis B, obtain HBsAg and IgM anti-HBc (step 2)
	Negative	Acute hepatitis A	Non-A non-B, rule out EBV and CMV

Step 2 (anti-HBc is positive):

		IgM anti-HBc	
		Positive	Negative
HBsAg	Positive	Acute hepatitis B, follow HBsAg to rule out development of carrier state	HBV carrier; get anti-HD to exclude delta superinfection
	Negative	Acute hepatitis B, obtain anti-HBs to confirm resolution of infection	Previous HBV; probable acute non-A non-B; rule out EBV and CMV

IgM anti-HAV:	IgM-specific antibody to HAV
Anti-HBc:	Antibody to HBV core antigen
IgM anti-HBc:	IgM-specific antibody to HBV core antigen
HBsAg	HBV surface (envelope) antigen
Anti-HBs:	Antibody to HBV surface antigen
Anti-HD:	Antibody to hepatitis delta antigen
Anti-HAV:	Antibody to HAV (useful to determine immunity)

chronic HBsAg carriers have persistent IgM anti-HBc, the titer is usually substantially lower than that found in acute infection, and it is seldom detected in commercial assays.

A useful approach for detecting the greatest possible number of HBV infections is to test first for anti-HBc (Table 15-3). If anti-HBc is absent, HBV infection is effectively ruled out. If anti-HBc is present, tests for HBsAg and IgM anti-HBc will establish whether or not the infection is active and recent. If HBsAg is not detectable, testing for anti-HBs will determine the immune status. Although in practice these tests are often carried out concurrently as part of a "hepatitis panel," such a staged approach to testing makes biological sense and ultimately may prove more economical. The presence of HBeAg in an HBsAg-positive individual should suggest a high degree of infectivity. Conversion of HBeAg to anti-HBe in a patient with chronic hepatitis B may signal a resolution of hepatocellular disease and in some cases even herald an end to the HBsAg carrier state. Overall, however, the clinical value of HBeAg or anti-HBe testing is questionable.

Prevention

Preexposure Vaccination

Preexposure vaccination should be the mainstay of any program to prevent hepatitis B. Vaccination is recommended for all infants and all persons with more than one sexual partner within the preceding 6 months. Users of illicit injectable drugs, homosexual or bisexual men, residents of correctional or long-term-care facilities, persons seeking treatment for STD, and prostitutes should also be vaccinated. Table 15-4 outlines other groups for whom immunization should be considered. Both plasma-derived and recombinant vaccines are safe and effective.

Among groups at high risk for hepatitis B (such as homosexual men), prevaccination screening for antibody to HBV is cost-effective. Testing in moderate risk groups (such as heterosexual persons with STD) is usually not indicated.

Recommendation for preexposure vaccination: HBV vaccine (several FDA-approved recombinant or plasma-derived preparations are available) in dosages as recommended by the manufacturer. The vaccination series requires an initial visit and two follow-up visits which are usually scheduled at 0, 1, and 6 months.

TABLE 15-4. Persons for Whom Hepatitis B Vaccination Is Recommended or Should Be Considered

---

Preexposure
  Persons for whom vaccine is recommended:
    Infants
    Health care workers having blood or needle-stick exposures
    Clients and staff of institutions for the developmentally disabled
    Hemodialysis patients
    Homosexually active men
    Heterosexuals with multiple sexual partners
    Users of illicit injectable drugs
    Recipients of certain blood products
    Household members and sexual contacts of HBV carriers
    Special high-risk populations
  Persons for whom vaccine should be considered:
    Inmates of long-term correctional facilities
    Heterosexually active persons with multiple sexual partners
    International travelers to HBV endemic areas
Postexposure
  Infants born to HBV-positive mothers
  Health care workers having needle-stick exposures to human blood

---

Vaccine should *not* be administered in the gluteal (buttocks) or quadriceps (thigh) muscle. Following vaccination, testing for antibody response is not routinely indicated unless the patient is infected with HIV.

Postexposure Prophylaxis

Prophylactic treatment with HBV IG should be considered in the following situations: sexual contact with a patient who has active hepatitis B or who develops hepatitis B; or sexual contact with an HBV carrier (blood test positive for HBsAg). Prophylactic treatment for sexual exposure should be given within 14 days of sexual contact. Assay for preexisting immunity to HBV may be cost-effective in individuals from populations at high risk for HBV infection.

Recommendation for postexposure prophylaxis: HBV IG (HBIG) 0.06 ml/kg IM in a single dose *followed by* initiation of HBV vaccine series as described above.

Passive immunization with globulin preparations, unlike vaccine, provides immediate but only temporary protection, and its use should be reserved for postexposure prophylaxis. HBIG is effective in preventing hepatitis B when given after percutaneous or mucosal exposure to HBV, while the efficacy of regular immune globulin (IG) is less certain. IG no longer has a role in postexposure prophylaxis of hepatitis B.

Postexposure prophylaxis should also be given after significant percutaneous or mucosal exposure to blood or other body fluids that might contain HBV. HBIG (0.06 ml/kg) must be given as soon as possible after exposure (preferably within 24 to 48 h). A second dose is recommended 1 month after the first unless concomitant immunization with HBV vaccine is begun. The decision to proceed with active immunization depends on the likelihood of continuing exposure to HBV-containing material.

Simultaneous administration of vaccine and HBIG to neonates born to HBsAg-positive mothers is highly effective in preventing perinatally transmitted HBV infection. HBIG (0.5 ml IM) should be given to such infants within 12 h of birth, with concomitant initiation of a three-dose vaccine series at an alternate site. All pregnant women should be screened in advance for HBsAg, as strategies restricting screening to high-risk groups miss a large proportion of carrier mothers.

HEPATITIS DELTA VIRUS

HDV is a defective virus whose replication is absolutely dependent on simultaneous HBV infection. Thus HDV infects only patients with active HBV infection. The HDV virion is a 35-nm particle found in the blood. It has an outer envelope consisting of HBsAg and an amorphous core containing delta antigen (HDAg) complexed with a small, circular, single-stranded RNA molecule. Because of its high G + C content and extensive intramolecular complementarity, this genomic RNA assumes a rodlike, predominantly double-stranded secondary structure.

HDV infection may occur as a coinfection with acute hepatitis B in an individual who was previously susceptible to HBV, or as a "superinfection" in an HBV carrier. Either type of infection may result in severe hepatitis with fulminant disease and death. Coinfections are often marked by a biphasic serum aminotransferase response, while superinfections may be associated with transient (at times permanent) suppression of HBV replication markers. Those who survive acute coinfections usually go on to complete recovery and do not seem to be at an increased risk of becoming chronic HBV carriers. On the other hand, HBV carriers surviving HDV superinfections frequently become carriers for HDV as well and often subsequently show evidence of significant chronic liver disease.

The diagnosis of HDV infection is generally dependent on demonstration of antibody to HDAg (anti-HD) as this is the only widely available test. However, the anti-HD response in coinfection is often transient and of low magnitude, and thus probably often missed. In superinfections, anti-HD typically rises to and persists at high levels, signifying persistent HDV infection. One of the most useful means of distinguishing acute HDV-HBV coinfection from HDV superinfection of a chronic HBsAg carrier is by measurement of IgM anti-HBc (Table 15-3). Indeed, persons presenting with what appears to be acute type B hepatitis who lack this serum marker should be suspected of having HDV superinfection.

HDV is found in the blood of anti-HD-positive HBsAg carriers, and the prevalence of anti-HD among American carriers is strongly associated with parenteral drug abuse, hemophilia, or a history of multiple transfusions. Geographic differences in the distribution of HDV are striking, however, and anti-HD is significantly more prevalent among HBsAg carriers from middle eastern and Mediterranean countries.

It is not clear whether HDV is sexually transmitted, but this is likely to be the case. Homosexually active males who are HBsAg-positive generally have a low prevalence of anti-HD compared with other carrier groups. However, HDV coinfection has been found in 14 percent of gay men presenting with HBsAg-positive hepatitis, and delta hepatitis occurs in such men in the absence of a history of transfusions or parenteral drug abuse. In some studies the presence of anti-HD was correlated with sexual activity as measured by numbers of previous sex partners, as well as intravenous drug use.

Although there is no specific means for prevention of HDV infection (particularly in the person who is already HBsAg-positive), immunization with HBV vaccine provides protection against HDV by preventing the necessary helper virus infection.

HEPATITIS C VIRUS

Diagnosis of non-A non-B (NANB) hepatitis requires exclusion of infection with HAV, HBV, cytomegalovirus, and Epstein-Barr virus. For many years the etiologic agent of this disease remained elusive. Recent studies, however, have revealed that HCV, an RNA virus, is the cause of most cases of posttransfusion NANB hepatitis.

The frequency with which HCV infection occurs in the absence of liver disease is not known. The incubation period of HCV hepatitis ranges from 2 to 15 weeks, with a mean of about 7 weeks. Recognized cases of posttransfusion hepatitis are usually milder than hepatitis associated with HAV or HBV, and most cases are anicteric. The most striking feature of HCV infection, however, is its strong association with chronic liver disease. Chronic active hepatitis develops in as many as 30 percent of posttransfusion NANB infections. Patients with this form of chronic active hepatitis appear to follow a relatively benign course, with most cases entering spontaneous biochemical remissions. However, cirrhosis may develop more frequently than previously thought.

The epidemiology of HCV hepatitis is that of a blood-borne virus and is in many respects very similar to that of HBV. Before the recent advent of HCV screening techniques, this virus was responsible for more than 80 percent of cases of posttransfusion hepatitis. However, HCV hepatitis occurs in the absence of transfusion or history of illicit self-injection, accounting for approximately 25 percent of sporadic cases of acute viral hepatitis in the United States. Moreover, 40 to 50 percent of patients with HCV hepatitis have no history of blood exposure.

Little is known about specific mechanisms of nonparenteral transmission of this agent, including the possibility of sexual transmission, and sexual contact appears to be a relatively inefficient means of spread. Nevertheless, a case control study by Alter el al. suggested that heterosexual transmission may play an important role in the spread of NANB hepatitis, as "significantly more patients with NANB hepatitis either had sexual or household contact with a person who had hepatitis in the past or had multiple heterosexual partners."[6] Further investigation of the role of sexual transmission of this virus is needed.

ENTERICALLY TRANSMITTED NON-A NON-B HEPATITIS (NANB-E)

Several large, apparently water-borne outbreaks of hepatitis have occurred in India and other developing countries. Clinical characteristics of the disease resemble hepatitis A, but it has been associated with a high mortality among infected pregnant women. The etiologic agent is a virus distinct from HAV, HBV, and HCV. The epidemiology is poorly understood. There is no information concerning the possibility that this virus might be sexually transmitted.

MANAGEMENT OF ACUTE VIRAL HEPATITIS

Most patients with acute hepatitis follow an uneventful course leading to complete recovery. Hospitalization is best avoided because of the risk of nosocomial spread but should be considered for patients over 40 years old, with underlying disease, or with severe illness (bilirubin level greater than 15 mg/dl or significant prolongation of the prothrombin time). No specific therapy is clearly beneficial, and the primary purpose of hospitalization is to ensure adequate supportive care and monitoring.

A careful attempt at virus-specific diagnosis should be made using available serologic techniques (Table 15-3). Sexual partners of patients with acute HBV infection should be tested for HBsAg, anti-HBs, and anti-HBC, and appropriate prophylaxis should be given susceptible contacts as previously outlined. Unless the partner has received appropriate prophylaxis, sexual intercourse is best avoided while the patient is HBsAg (and especially HBeAg) positive. Condom use may reduce the risk of sexual transmission of HBV and provide protection in addition to that afforded by HBIG and immunization, but the efficacy of condoms in this setting has not been studied.

REFERENCES

1. Szmuness W: Large-scale efficacy trials of hepatitis B vaccines in the USA: Baseline data and protocols. *J Med Virol* 4:327, 1979
2. Szmuness W et al: Prevalence of hepatitis B "e" antigen and its antibody in various HBsAg carrier populations. *Am J Epidemiol* 113:113, 1981
3. Schreeder MT et al: Hepatitis B in homosexual males: Prevalence of HBV infection and factors related to transmission. *J Infect Dis* 146:7, 1982
4. Coleman JC et al: Hepatitis B antigen and antibody in a male homosexual population. *Br J Vener Dis* 53:132, 1977
5. Kryger P et al: Increased risk of infection with hepatitis A and B viruses in men with a history of syphilis: Relation to sexual contacts. *J Infect Dis* 145:23, 1982
6. Alter MJ et al: Importance of heterosexual activity in the transmission of hepatitis B and Non-A, Non-B hepatitis. *JAMA* 262:1201, 1989

ADDITIONAL READING

Alter HJ: Descartes before the horse: I clone, therefore I am: The hepatitis C virus in current perspective. *Ann Intern Med* 115:644, 1991

Alter MJ et al: The changing epidemiology of hepatitis B in the US. Need for alternative vaccination strategies. *JAMA* 263:1218, 1990

Centers for Disease Control: Hepatitis A among homosexual men—United States, Canada, and Australia. *MMWR* 41:155, 1992

Centers for Disease Control: Protection against viral hepatitis: Recommendations of the Immunization Practices Advisory Committee (ACIP). *MMWR* 39:1, 1990

Eyster ME et al: Heterosexual co-transmission of hepatitis C virus (HCV) and human immunodeficiency virus (HIV). *Ann Intern Med* 115:764, 1991

Liaio YE et al: Heterosexual transmission of hepatitis delta virus in the general population of an area endemic for hepatitis B virus infection: A prospective study. *J Infect Dis* 162:1170, 1990

Smith MA, Singer C: Sexually transmitted viruses other than HIV and papillomavirus. *Urol Clin North Am* 19:47, 1992

For a more detailed discussion, see Lemon SM, Newbold JE: Viral Hepatitis, Chap. 40, p. 449, in STD-2.

The order Anaplura includes over 400 species of sucking lice, which are ectoparasites of mammals. Sucking lice are dorsoventrally compressed, wingless, and small, with retractable piercing-sucking mouth parts. One species is the cause of a common sexually transmitted disease: pubic lice, or "crabs."

Three species of lice infest human beings: *Phthirus pubis,* the crab louse; *Pediculus humanus humanus,* the body louse; and *Pediculus humanus capitis,* the head louse. This chapter focuses principally on pubic lice, but head and body lice will be briefly considered for purposes of comparison.

Lice have five stages in their life cycle: egg (or nit), three nymphal stages, and the adult stage. All stages occur on the host. Lice feed on human blood. When ready to feed, the louse anchors its mouth to the skin, stabs an opening through the skin, pours saliva into the wound to prevent clotting, and pumps blood from the wound into its digestive system.

A difference between the body and head louse and the pubic louse involves their grasping ability. The grasp of the pubic louse's claw matches the diameter of pubic and axillary hairs; hence it is not only found in the pubic area (Fig. 16-1) but also has been recovered from the axillae, bearded areas of the face, eyelashes (Fig. 16-2), and eyebrows. However, the diameter of the head louse's claw grasp seems to be uniquely adapted to the diameter of the scalp hair. Therefore, it is very difficult to transplant head lice to other areas of the body.

EPIDEMIOLOGY

It is estimated that more than 3 million cases of pediculosis are treated each year in the United States. Most cases are due to head and pubic lice infestations.

Human lice are transmitted from one person to another primarily by intimate contact. Both head and body lice are spread by sharing personal articles such as hairbrushes, combs, towels, or clothing. Pubic lice do not seem to spread as rapidly as other human lice when off the host. They have a shorter life span (24 h compared with several days for other lice), and their movements are more lethargic. Sexual transmission is considered to be the most important means of pubic lice transmission. However, there are documented cases of transmission from toilet seats, beds, and egg-infested loose hairs dropped by infested persons on shared objects.

The population with the highest incidence of pubic lice is similar to that of gonorrhea and syphilis: single persons, ages 15 to 25. Pubic lice infestation is rare in persons older than 35.

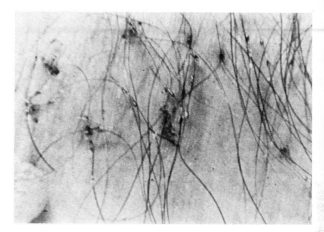

FIG. 16-1. Adult pubic lice and nits.

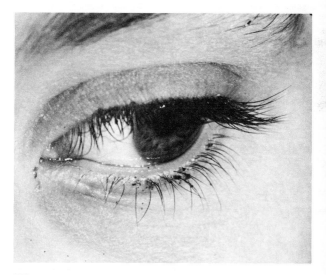

FIG. 16-2. Adult pubic lice and nits on eyelashes. *(Courtesy of E. Stolz.)*

CLINICAL MANIFESTATIONS

Sensitivity to the effect of louse bites varies with the individual. When previously unexposed persons are bitten, there may be no signs or symptoms or only slight sting with little or no itching or redness. At least 5 days must pass before allergic sensitization can occur. At that point, the main symptom is itching, which leads to scratching, erythema, irritation, and inflammation. An individual who has been bitten by a large number of lice over a short period of time may have mild fever, malaise, and increased irritability.

Apparently, many persons eventually develop some degree of immunity to the bite of the louse. Persons infested for a long time may even become oblivious to the lice on their bodies. The opposite may also occur. Excessive scratching may lead to superinfection. Characteristic small "blue spots" may appear in the skin, as the result of crab louse bites; these persist for several days.

DIAGNOSIS

Diagnosis of lice infestation is made by (1) taking a careful history from the patient, (2) considering lice infestation as a possible or probable cause of the patient's signs and symptoms, and (3) careful examination of the patient. Both adult lice and their eggs (nits) are easily seen by the naked eye (Figs. 16-1 and 16-2).

Head lice characteristically are found on the scalp surface with the nits attached to the hair. Most of the unhatched nits are within 5 mm of the scalp surface. Nits on scalp hair are usually cemented at an oblique angle. This helps to distinguish them from foreign material which slides up and down and frequently surrounds the hair.

Upon examination of the groin or pudendal area, pubic lice may be perceived as scabs over what first were thought to be "scratch papules," but if nits appear on the hairs, the proper diagnosis becomes obvious. If the "crust" is removed and placed on a glass slide for microscopic examination, the crust often walks away before the cover glass is in place. When no adult lice are available, demonstration of nits under the microscope will also confirm the diagnosis.

When white flakes on the hair are visible with the naked eye, other possible considerations are seborrheic dermatitis, hair casts, solidified globules of hair spray, and accretions on hair shafts.

MANAGEMENT

Ideally the regimen should employ a pediculocide which kills both the adults and the eggs. Also, partners and other household contacts of the patient should be examined so that both source and spread cases can be treated.

Recommended regimen

Permethrin (1%) creme rinse applied to affected area and washed off after 10 min *or*

Pyrethrins and piperonyl butoxide applied to the affected area and washed off after 10 min *or*

Lindane 1% shampoo applied for 4 min and then thoroughly washed off (not recommended for pregnant or lactating women).

Patients should be reevaluated after 1 week if symptoms persist. Re-treatment may be necessary if lice are found or eggs are observed at the hair-skin junction. Clothing or bed linen that may have been contaminated by the patient within the past 2 days should be washed and dried by machine (hot cycle in each), or dry-cleaned.

Pediculosis of the eyelashes should be treated by the application of occlusive ophthalmic ointment to the eyelid margins, 2 times a day for 10 days, to smother lice and nits. Lindane or other drugs should not be applied to the eyes.

Sex partners should be treated as above.

ADDITIONAL READING

Billstein SA, Mattaliano VJ: The "nuisance" sexually transmitted diseases: Molluscum contagiosum, scabies, and crab lice. *Med Clin North Am* 74:1487, 1990

Blondell RD: Parasites of the skin and hair. *Prim Care* 18:167, 1991

Burnett JW: Lice infestation. *Cutis* 48:32, 1991

Gillis D et al: Seasonality and long-term trends of pediculosis capitis and pubis in a young adult population. *Arch Dermatol* 126:638, 1990

For a more detailed discussion, see Billstein SA: Human Lice, Chap. 41, p 467, in STD-2.

Scabies, caused by the itch mite *Sarcoptes scabiei,* is characterized by pruritic skin lesions. The infestation is transmitted by sexual and other close personal contact.

BIOLOGY OF THE ORGANISM

The adult female itch mite is 400 μm long. It burrows into the horny layer of the skin to the boundary of the stratum granulosum. The burrow provides its home for life, approximately 30 days. Within hours of burrowing, it begins laying enormous eggs, which develop through larval and nymphal stages to form adult mites in 10 days. Infested patients harbor an average of 11 mites.

The mites concentrate mainly on the hands and wrists. However, since the eruption may be caused in part by immature stages of the mite and by sensitization, the distribution of adult female mites does not parallel that of the typical scabietic lesions. In primary infestation, itching or eruption does not occur for several weeks, the time required for sensitization.

IMMUNOLOGY AND PATHOGENESIS

Epidemics of scabies occur in 30-year cycles with a 15-year gap between the end of one epidemic and the beginning of the next; the epidemics usually last about 15 years. The cause of the current pandemic is probably multifactorial. A number of factors (poverty, poor hygiene, increased numbers of sexual partners, misdiagnosis, increased travel, and demographic and ecological considerations) promote development of scabies.

Immunologic factors probably play an important role in the pathogenesis of scabies. Among some patients there appears to be a relationship between scabies and atopic dermatitis. It can be difficult to differentiate scabies from variations of atopic dermatitis (especially papular urticaria). Moreover, in a significant number of patients the two conditions occur together and dermatitis persists after the scabies has cleared. A high incidence of scabietic hypersensitivity sequelae (nodular scabies, dyshidrosiform syndrome) have been noted in patients with an atopic background.

EPIDEMIOLOGY

The socioeconomic characteristics of patients with this infestation are representative of those of the general population. The frequency of scabies in African-Americans appears to be significantly lower than that in white Americans and in some other racial groups.

Transmission of scabies usually is associated with close personal contact. The long incubation period associated with an individual's first infestation may make it difficult to trace the source. If one member of the household becomes infested, multiple members or the entire family may eventually be affected unless specific treatment is instituted. When several members of a family or group complain of a pruritic eruption, scabies is a likely diagnosis.

Sexual transmission of scabies, particularly in sexually active young adults, is common. This infestation is frequently seen at venereal disease clinics and may coexist with gonorrhea, syphilis, pediculosis pubis, and other sexually transmissible conditions. A diagnosis of scabies, particularly when penile lesions are present, should prompt a search for coexisting sexually transmitted disease, beginning with culture for gonorrhea and serologic test for syphilis. The prevalence of asymptomatic gonorrhea is high in female patients with scabies, particularly in the 15- to 29-year age group. The chancre of syphilis is sometimes seen in a cutaneous lesion of scabies. Although syphilis and gonorrhea are frequently transmitted by brief sexual contact, scabies is more likely to be transmitted during more prolonged exposure, such as when the partners spend the night together.

Scabies is one of the few sexually transmitted diseases which is also commonly transmitted in households by nonsexual contact to individuals of all ages. Scabies is frequent in school-age children but is unlikely to be transmitted in schools. Outbreaks occur in nursing homes, hospitals, and other institutions. People with high parasite loads are more likely to transmit infestation to others.

CLINICAL MANIFESTATIONS

Classic Scabies

(See Table 17-1.) In classic scabies, itching is characteristically nocturnal. Lesions are symmetrical. The hands are often the first areas involved, and lesions occur mainly on the finger webs and the sides of the digits (Figures 17-1, 17-2). Flexor surfaces of the wrist, anterior axillary folds, and extensor surfaces of the elbows are commonly involved. Lesions may be nodular, but more often are dry and eczematous. Papular lesions are usually present on the abdomen, particularly around the umbilicus, in a spoke-like arrangement. The disease may affect the lower portion of the buttocks in the crease where they join the upper part of the thighs. Penile involvement is characteristic: nodules may dominate, or chancriform changes or pyoderma may be present. In adults, the upper back, neck, face, scalp, palms, and soles are seldom involved.

The pathognomonic burrow is a short, wavy, dirty-appearing line

TABLE 17-1. Diagnosis of Scabies

1. Suggestive
    a. Distribution: Hands, wrists, elbows, anterior axillary folds, areolae of female breasts, abdomen, genitals, buttocks.
    b. Morphology: Typically polymorphic. Burrows are pathognomonic.
    c. Nocturnal pruritus.
    d. Contact cases (highly suggestive).
    e. Response to "specific" therapy.
    f. Skin biopsy in inflammatory or nodular lesions.
2. Diagnostic: Identification of the mite (success rate varies with experience and persistence).
    a. Microscopic study: Skin scrapings or other techniques.
    b. Skin biopsy (performed in difficult cases): Sections may reveal mites or fecal pellets.

which often crosses skin lines; it is most common on the fingerwebs (Fig. 17-2), volar wrists, elbows, and penis. Examination reveals small, erythematous, often excoriated papules. Secondary eczematization and infection may overshadow other features, making diagnosis more difficult.

Special Forms of Scabies

In the current epidemic cycle, presentations of scabies which vary from the classic form are common.

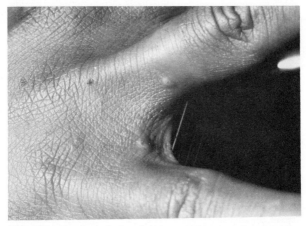

FIG. 17-1. Papules in the interdigital area, highly suggestive of scabies. *(Courtesy of E. Stolz.)*

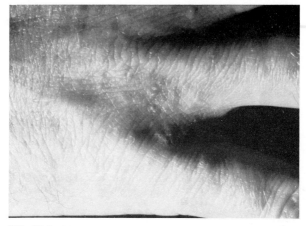

FIG. 17-2. Multiple scabietic burrows and papules are present on the fingerwebs. *(Courtesy of A. Hoke.)*

The incidence of scabies has increased among persons who bathe often. The disease is easily misdiagnosed in these cases because lesions and burrows may be difficult to find. The person presumably removes many mites with frequent bathing (soap destroys many mite life forms). Meticulous physical examination suggests the diagnosis, which is confirmed by identification of the mite.

Administration of topical or systemic corticosteroids may ameliorate signs and symptoms of scabies while the infestations and transmissibility persist. This frequently results in unusual clinical presentations, atypical distribution, and unusually extensive involvement, which sometimes mimics other diagnoses.

Nodular scabies is an uncommon form of the disease. Nodules are reddish brown and pruritic and occur on covered areas, most frequently male genitalia, groin, and axillary regions. Mites are seldom identified in nodules present for more than a month. The nodules probably develop as a hypersensitivity reaction. The disease frequently remains misdiagnosed for long periods; its histologic features are similar to those of lymphoma and arthropod bites.

Scabies is also frequently misdiagnosed when it occurs in infants and young children. Widespread secondary eczematous changes may occur, as well as atypical distribution with involvement of head, neck, palms, and soles. Secondary bacterial infection is common.

Crusted (Norwegian) scabies is highly contagious, even on casual contact, because of the myriad of mites in the exfoliating scales. In hospitals or other institutions, local or regional epidemics of more typical forms of scabies can result from patients with this form of scabies. Crusted scabies is a psoriasiform dermatosis of the hands and feet, with dystrophy of the nails and a variable erythematous, scaling eruption that may become generalized. Pruritus is minimal. The disease has a predilection for persons with mental retardation, physical debilitation, or immunosuppression.

DIFFERENTIAL DIAGNOSIS

Scabies is a great imitator. Differential diagnosis includes nearly all pruritic dermatoses, including atopic dermatitis, contact dermatitis, prurigo, papular urticaria, pyoderma, pruritus due to systemic disease, pruritic dermatoses of pregnancy, infectious eczematoid dermatitis, insect bites, excoriations, lichen planus, dermatitis herpetiformis, mastocytosis, urticaria, and pediculosis, as well as syphilis, keratosis follicularis, and vasculitis.

DIAGNOSIS

A variety of techniques are available for diagnosis of scabies (Table 17-2).

Skin Scrapings

Locate recently developed, unexcoriated papules or burrows. Place mineral oil on a sterile scalpel blade and allow it to flow into the lesions. Remove the top of burrows or papules by vigorous scraping with the scalpel blade. Transfer the oil and scraped material to a glass slide, and apply a cover slip. Diagnosis is confirmed by visualization of any stage of the mite or typical fecal pellets (Fig. 17-3).

Needle Extraction of Mite

Use a needle to perforate the burrow at the site of the mite (the "dark point" in white patients and the "white point" in black patients). Move the needle tangential to the skin from side to side. The mite will grip the end of the needle and should then be transferred to a slide.

TABLE 17-2.   Laboratory Techniques for Microscopic Study

1. Skin scrapings
2. Needle extraction of mite
3. Epidermal shave biopsy
4. Burrow ink test (BIT)
5. Curettage of burrows
6. Swab technique with clear cellophane adhesive
7. Topical tetracycline, then Wood's light
8. Punch biopsy

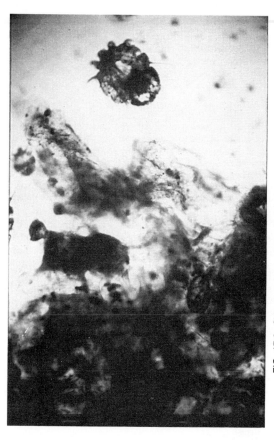

FIG. 17-3. Skin scrapings of unexcoriated papules fortuitously disclose adults, larva, eggs, and fecal pellets, any of which would be diagnostic.

Epidermal Shave Biopsy

Locate a suspicious papule or burrow, elevate the papule between the thumb and forefinger, and gently "saw" off the top of the lesion with a 15 scalpel blade held parallel to the skin surface. The biopsy is so superficial that bleeding should not occur nor should local anesthesia be necessary. Place the biopsy material on a slide and examine with a light microscope.

Burrow Ink Test (BIT)

Gently rub the scabietic papule with the underside of a fountain pen, covering the papule with ink. Immediately wipe off the surface ink from the lesion with an alcohol pad. In the BIT-positive lesion the ink will track down the mite burrow by forming a characteristic dark zigzag line running across and away from the papule. Although BIT is relatively insensitive, the technique is painless and more useful than the superficial shave biopsy in a child or uncooperative patient.

Curettage of Burrows

Superficially curette the long axis of a burrow or the summit of a papule and deposit the curetting on a clean slide with the aid of a scalpel, then place one to two drops of mineral oil on the curetting and cover with a cover slip. This technique is particularly valuable in infants, small children, and uncooperative patients.

Skin-Swab Technique with Clear Cellophane Adhesive Tape

Clean the skin with ether, then apply cellophane tape to the lesion and remove with brisk movement. Stick strips of adhesive tape to the slide, and examine the slide microscopically.

Topical Tetracycline

Apply topical tetracycline, wipe off, and examine area with Wood's light.

Punch Biopsy

Use punch biopsies to demonstrate mites or products if necessary.

TREATMENT

Adults and older children

Recommended regimen: lindane (1%) 1 oz of lotion or 30 g of cream applied thinly to all areas of the body from the neck down and washed off thoroughly after 8 h. (This regimen is not recommended for pregnant or lactating women.)

   Alternative regimen: crotamiton (10%) applied to the entire body

from the neck down for 2 nights and washed off thoroughly 24 h after the second application.

Infants, Children 2 Years or Less, Pregnant and Lactating Women

In these groups lindane is contraindicated. The **crotamiton** regimen (above) should be used.

Contacts

Sex partners and close household contacts should be treated for scabies as outlined above.

Special Considerations

Pruritus may persist for several weeks after adequate therapy. A single re-treatment after 1 week may be appropriate if there is no clinical improvement. Additional weekly treatments are warranted only if live mites can be demonstrated.

Clothing or bed linen that may have been contaminated by the patient within the past 2 days should be washed and dried by machine (hot cycle in each), or dry cleaned.

ADDITIONAL READING

Amer M, El-Gharib I: Permethrin versus crotamiton and lindane in the treatment of scabies. *Int J Dermatol* 31:357, 1992

Billstein SA, Mattaliano VJJ: The "nuisance" sexually transmitted diseases: Molluscum contagiosum, scabies, and crab lice. *Med Clin North Am* 74:1487, 1990

Donabedian H, Khazan U: Norwegian scabies in a patient with AIDS. *Clin Infect Dis* 14:162, 1992

Elgart ML: Scabies. *Dermatol Clin* 8:253, 1990

Head ES et al: *Sarcoptes scabiei* in histopathologic sections of skin in human scabies. *Arch Dermatol* 126:1475, 1990

Inserra DW, Bickley LK: Crusted scabies in acquired immunodeficiency syndrome. *Int J Dermatol* 29:287, 1990

Kolar KA, Rapini RP: Crusted (Norwegian) scabies. *Am Fam Physician* 44:1317, 1991

O'Donnell BF, et al: Management of crusted scabies. *Int J Dermatol* 29:258, 1990

Purvis RS, Tyring SK: An outbreak of lindane-resistant scabies treated successfully with permethrin 5% cream. *J Am Acad Dermatol* 25:1015, 1991

Roth WI: Scabies resistant to lindane 1% lotion and crotamiton 10% cream. *J Am Acad Dermatol* 24:502, 1991

Schultz MW et al: Comparative study of 5% permethrin cream and 1% lindane lotion for the treatment of scabies. *Arch Dermatol* 126:167, 1990

For a more detailed discussion, see Orkin M, Maibach H: Scabies, Chap. 42, p. 473, in STD-2.

Trichomoniasis, an infection with a flagellated protozoon, *Trichomonas vaginalis,* is a common sexually transmitted disease. When symptomatic, the infection results in vaginitis in women and urethritis in men. Many infected persons, however, remain asymptomatic.

MICROBIOLOGY

Trichomonas vaginalis grows best in vitro under moderately anaerobic conditions and reproduces by binary fission. The organism is generally ovoid, but in specimens obtained directly from patients, its shape may be less regular, with ameboid properties. In fresh preparations, *Trichomonas* can be recognized by its jerky, swaying motion. At higher magnification ($\geq \times 400$) one can see its undulating membrane and beating flagella (Fig. 18-1).

Differences among strains and isolates of *T. vaginalis* have been clearly defined. Strains of different sizes and rates of growth have been identified, and these characteristics might be related to virulence. Isolates differ in their ability to produce inflammation in a variety of experimental systems.

EPIDEMIOLOGY

Because in most countries trichomoniasis is not reportable, incidence figures are sketchy, and those existing are often outdated. Before the advent of metronidazole in the 1950s, trichomoniasis was so common that it was erroneously regarded by some as a normal part of the vaginal flora, and the associated discharge was often taken for granted. Currently, in industrialized countries, trichomoniasis has become quite uncommon in women with good access to health care—the prevalence being under 1 percent in all European countries and in college students in the United States. However, in female STD clinic patients in the United States, prevalence rates still reach 15 percent or more, and in male STD clinic patients, prevalence rates of 5 to 10 percent are seen. However, information on the prevalence of trichomoniasis in men is limited because of the large fraction of cases which are asymptomatic, the frequently self-limited nature of the infection, and the difficulty of diagnosis. In some developing countries, trichomoniasis remains extraordinarily prevalent, with rates as high as 15 to 30 percent among pregnant women, and even higher in some groups of prostitutes.

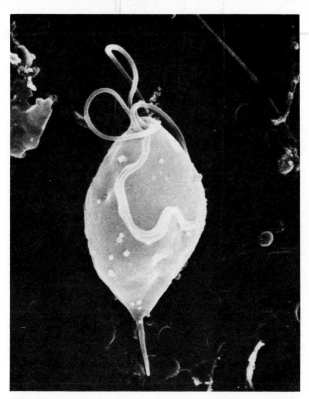

FIG. 18-1. Scanning electron micrograph of *Trichomonas vaginalis*. Three of the four anterior flagella (and the origin of the fourth), the undulating membrane with its trailing flagellum, and the axostyle protruding at the end of the body are clearly seen. × 6000 magnification. *(From A Warton, BM Honigberg, J Protozool 26:56, 1979.)*

The method of contraception used has been associated with the prevalence of trichomoniasis. Trichomoniasis has been less common in women who use barrier methods and those who use oral contraceptives. Estrogens have no direct effect on trichomonad growth but may act by changing the vaginal environment. Although contraceptive foam is highly active against trichomonads in vitro, a clinical protective effect has not been documented.

Sexual Transmission

Several lines of evidence document the importance of the sexual acquisition of trichomoniasis. Trichomoniasis is most prevalent among sexual partners of patients with documented infection. The organism is usually demonstrated in 30 to 40 percent of the male sexual partners of infected women and at least 85 percent of the female partners of infected men. Asymptomatically infected men and women are important reservoirs of infection; eventual control of trichomoniasis depends on effective treatment of men as well as women. Several studies have shown an increased cure rate in women following treatment of their regular sexual partners.

Women with trichomoniasis frequently have gonorrhea. The prevalence of gonorrhea is 1.4 to 3 times higher among women with trichomoniasis than among women without this infection. Trichomonads have been isolated from 16 to 20 percent of men with gonococcal urethritis. Because of these associations, patients with trichomoniasis should be evaluated for the presence of other sexually transmitted diseases.

Nonvenereal Transmission

Perinatal acquisition has been reported in about 5 percent of female babies born of infected mothers.

Nonvenereal acquisition of *T. vaginalis* by adults is infrequent. The site specificity of the organism means that infection can follow only intravaginal or intraurethral inoculation. The organism is very sensitive to desiccation, but if not desiccated it can survive for several hours in various body fluids (urine, semen, vaginal exudates). In spite of the possibility of transmission via objects contaminated with body fluids, no well-documented cases have been reported. Nonetheless, the age distribution of reported cases of trichomoniasis in women in some series has been somewhat older than for most STDs, suggesting either prolonged chronicity, unusual susceptibility of older women, fomite transmission, or perhaps biased oversampling of older women.

PATHOGENESIS

The mechanisms by which *T. vaginalis* causes disease are mostly undefined.

Urogenital Infection

Trichomoniasis is an infection almost exclusively of the urogenital tract.

In adult women with trichomoniasis, the organisms are isolated from the vagina in over 95 percent and from the urinary tract alone in less than 5 percent. Only areas covered by squamous but not by columnar epithelium are involved. Although the exterior of the cervix shares in the vaginal inflammatory response, trichomonads are isolated from the endocervix in the minority of infected women.

The urethra and Skene's glands have been infected in up to 90 percent of cases studied. Dysuria and discharge from the urethra or Skene's ducts may result, and a wet mount examination of material recovered from the urethra shows organisms in more than half of infected women. Organisms have occasionally been isolated from bladder urine. The significance of these extravaginal genitourinary sites of infection may be that organisms can persist there even after they have been eliminated from the vagina by local therapy.

In men the urethra appears to be the most common site of infection. Involvement of other parts of the urogenital tract, such as the epididymis, is much less frequently documented.

Host–parasite Relationships

Trichomonal infection of women ranges from an asymptomatic carrier state to profound, acute, inflammatory disease. About one-third of asymptomatically infected women became symptomatic within 6 months in one study, suggesting that changes in the host may contribute to pathogenic expression. Symptoms may appear or exacerbate during or immediately following the menstrual period. This observation suggests that the vaginal microenvironment affects the pathogenicity of trichomonads and may vary from time to time in the same patient. Other factors in the vaginal microenvironment, including menstrual blood, pH, oxidation–reduction potential, hormonal levels, or other microbes, may contribute to the expression of pathogenicity.

Infected male sexual partners of women with florid disease are often but not always asymptomatic. The absence of an inflammatory response in the male urethra to infection with the same strain of trichomonads producing severe disease in the vagina further supports the argument that the pathogenicity of trichomonads is dependent on features of the site of infection. Nonetheless, male urethral trichomoniasis has been demonstrated to be significantly associated with symptoms and signs of mild urethritis in a recent STD clinic study.

Pathology

Trichomonal infection in women usually elicits an acute inflammatory response resulting in a vaginal discharge containing large numbers of polymorphonuclear neutrophils (PMNs). The number of PMNs in the discharge correlates roughly with the degree of the patient's symptoms. Trichomonads are found in the vaginal cavity or adhering to the epithelial surfaces; there is no invasion of the mucosa. Colposcopy reveals proliferation and characteristic double cresting of mucosal capillaries and microhemorrhages. Only squamous epithelium is involved.

Immunity and Immune Response

Repeated trichomonal infections are common, and clinically significant protective immunity does not appear to occur in trichomoniasis. There are no data suggesting that trichomoniasis is more severe or becomes disseminated in neutropenic or immunocompromised patients.

CLINICAL MANIFESTATIONS

Disease in Women

The percentage of women harboring trichomonads who have symptoms varies with the manner in which cases are selected and ranges from 50 to 90 percent. Infected women often have insufficiently severe symptoms to prompt them to seek medical attention but on questioning indicate some mild urogenital complaints. Trichomonad infection, as mentioned above, is often accompanied by infections with other organisms; thus it is often difficult to attribute the symptoms and signs observed to *T. vaginalis* alone. Table 18-1 summarizes clinical aspects of disease in women.

History

Vaginal discharge has been noted by 50 to 74 percent of women diagnosed in STD clinics as having trichomoniasis. Only about 10 percent of patients describe the discharge as malodorous. Malodorous discharge, particularly when associated with relatively little vulvovaginal irritation, is more suggestive of bacterial vaginosis. Vaginal pruritus is described by one-quarter to one-half of patients and is often severe, resembling that of vulvovaginal candidiasis. Up to one-half of infected patients note some degree of dyspareunia. Dysuria and, more rarely, urinary frequency are mild, but the former suggests urethritis.

Lower abdominal pain is not a common complaint but has been described by 5 to 12 percent of women. It is possible that this discomfort results from pelvic lymphadenitis. The clinician must, however, always be suspicious that lower abdominal pain actually represents coincident salpingitis due to other sexually transmitted organisms.

Most investigators have found incubation periods varying from 3 to about 28 days in experimental and natural infections.

TABLE 18-1. Prevalence of Clinical Features among Women with Trichomoniasis

Symptoms, signs, and laboratory findings	Prevalence, %
Symptoms:	
None	9–56
Discharge	50–75
Malodorous	10–67
Irritating, pruritic	23–82
Dyspareunia	10–50
Dysuria	30–50
Lower abdominal discomfort	5–12
Signs:	
None	~15
Diffuse vulvar erythema	10–37
Excessive discharge	50–75
Yellow, green	5–42
Frothy	8–50
Vaginal wall inflammation	20–75
Strawberry cervix	
Naked eye	1–2
Colposcopy	~45
Laboratory findings:	
pH > 4.5	66–91
Positive whiff test	~75
Wet mount	
Excess PMNs	~75
Motile trichomonads	40–80
Fluorescent antibody	80–90
Gram stain	<1
Acridine orange	~60
Giemsa stain	~50
Papanicolaou smear	56–70

SOURCE: MF Rein, in *Trichomonads Parasitic in Humans*, BM Honigberg (ed), New York, Springer, 1989, with data added from P Wolner-Hanssen et al, *JAMA* 264:571, 1989.

Physical Examination

The vulva is diffusely erythematous or excoriated in less than one-tenth to one-third of patients. Vaginal discharge may be copious enough to run out onto the vulva even before a speculum is introduced. The labia range from pallid in mild disease to markedly erythematous and even edematous with more severe infection, although edema is more likely to be seen in candidiasis. On insertion of the speculum, excessive discharge is observed in one-half to three-quarters of infected women. The typical discharge of trichomoniasis is often described as yellow and frothy, but such typical discharge is seen in a minority of patients. The discharge is often grayish and is visibly frothy in only a small proportion of infected women. A frothy discharge is also seen in bacterial vaginosis.

The vaginal walls are erythematous in 20 to 75 percent of symptomatic patients, and in more severe cases, they may have a granular appearance. Punctate hemorrhages of the cervix (colpitis macularis) may result in a strawberry appearance which is observed by the naked eye in only about 1 to 2 percent of cases, but in nearly half by colposcopy. Its presence strongly suggests trichomoniasis.

Some patients with trichomoniasis show no evidence of vaginal inflammation on physical examination.

Disease in Men

Many men with trichomonal infection remain asymptomatic and come to treatment only because they are the sexual partners of women with symptomatic disease.

Urethritis

It is reasonably well established that *T. vaginalis* is one cause of nongonococcal urethritis (NGU). Trichomonal infection is more closely associated with NGU that fails to respond to treatments active against more common causes of NGU, such as *Chlamydia trachomatis* and *Ureaplasma urealyticum.* Subsequent response to metronidazole supports the diagnosis.

Most symptomatic men describe a discharge which is usually scant and clear and may be intermittent. Less than one-quarter of men report dysuria, and another quarter note mild meatal pruritus.

For most men, trichomonal urethritis appears to be self-limited. The organism can be recovered from 70 percent of men who have had sex with infected women within 48 h, but the prevalence drops with increasing time after the last sexual exposure. It is possible that antitrichomonal properties of prostatic fluid contribute to the rate of spontaneous resolution, or that usual methods of testing men (e.g., first-voided urine sediment cultures) underestimate higher rates of persistent infection.

Urethral stricture of any cause may make it difficult to cure trichomonal urethritis. About 10 percent of men with relapsing or persistent infection have some degree of stricture; urologic evaluation is recommended for patients with relapsing trichomonal urethritis.

Other Conditions

A few cases of acute, nongonococcal epididymitis or prostatitis have been allegedly attributable to trichomonal infection. The prostate is said to be involved in up to 40 percent of infected patients, but such involvement is usually asymptomatic, and it is hard to prove the prostate is the site of infection.

COMPLICATIONS

Few late complications of trichomoniasis are known. However, the 1980s NIH Multicenter Vaginal Infection in Pregnancy study showed that vaginal trichomoniasis in midpregnancy was significantly associated with preterm delivery. In addition researchers in Zaire found that women with trichomoniasis had increased susceptibility to subsequent heterosexual acquisition of HIV infection. Further medical significance derives primarily from the high incidence and the physical and emotional discomfort caused by trichomoniasis.

DIAGNOSIS

Although certain signs and symptoms are predictive of trichomoniasis, these are insufficient to establish the diagnosis, which requires detection of the parasite either by direct microscopic examination or by culture.

Microscopic Examination

Women

With the speculum in place, material can be recovered for examination by sweeping the anterior and posterior fornices with a cotton or Dacron swab. The cotton swab can be agitated in 1 ml of saline in a test tube and a drop of the resulting suspension transferred to a microscope slide. Alternatively, a drop of saline can be put on the microscope slide and vaginal material mixed in the drop directly on the slide. In either case, the preparation is covered with a coverslip and then examined while warmed to body temperature at low (×100) and then medium (×400) magnification. Phase contrast or dark field microscopy is rarely used but makes evaluation of the wet mount easier. Potassium hydroxide preparation destroys the organisms.

Wet mounts from women with symptomatic trichomoniasis typically reveal increased numbers of PMNs (more than one PMN per epithelial cell), which cause the yellow color of the discharge noted in severely affected women. Absence of PMNs, however, does not rule out infection.

Bacteria often are easily recognized in the wet mount and are either rods or coccobacilli. Concurrent infection with *Candida albicans* or *Gardnerella vaginalis* is common, and these organisms should be sought on the wet mount.

The diagnosis of trichomoniasis by microscopy is made by observing the typical, motile parasites. Ovoid and slightly larger

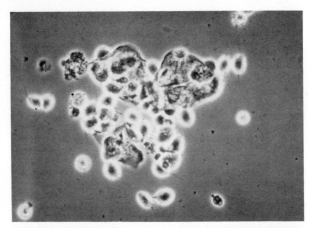

FIG. 18-2. Phase photomicrograph of vaginal wet mount showing epithelial cells, polymorphonuclear neutrophils, and trichomonads. *(Courtesy of Centers for Disease Control, Atlanta.)*

than PMNs, they are best recognized by their motility (Fig. 18–2). By phase or dark field microscopy, the individual flagella and undulating membrane are easily identified. Visualization of a single trichomonad establishes the diagnosis, since motile trichomonads are easily recognized when present in sufficient numbers. Unfortunately, the wet mount reveals trichomonads in only 40 to 80 percent of cases. Thus at least one-quarter of women with trichomoniasis will not be diagnosed correctly if the wet mount is used alone.

Trichomonads are often reported on Papanicolaou (Pap) smears from the cervix. Pap smears have a sensitivity of about 60 to 70 percent, equivalent to the wet mount, although false positives are common by Pap smear, so diagnosis should be confirmed by direct visualization or culture.

Men

Demonstration of *T. vaginalis* in male urine or genital secretions can be difficult. Men should be examined before their first-voided urine. Urethral discharge should be examined in a manner similar to that of vaginal discharge. In addition, examination of the sediment of the first-voided portion of a urine specimen should be examined microscopically and by culture. Finally, culture of ejaculated semen sometimes reveals *T. vaginalis* when urine sediment cultures are negative.

Culture

A variety of media for the diagnosis of trichomoniasis have been studied and are roughly comparable. Culture is more sensitive than microscopy, especially for asymptomatic men and women. Cultures should be incubated anaerobically. Most isolates grow within 48 h, but negative cultures are held for 7 days and reexamined periodically for motile trichomonads.

TREATMENT

Recommended regimen
Metronidazole 2 g orally in a single dose.
Reported cure rates among women range between 82 and 88 percent with this regimen. When sexual partners are treated simultaneously the cure rate is often greater than 95 percent.

Alternative regimen
Metronidazole 500 mg twice daily for 7 days.
If failure occurs with either regimen, the patient should be retreated with metronidazole 500 mg twice daily for 7 days. If repeated failure occurs, the patient should be treated with a single 2-g dose of metronidazole daily for 3 to 5 days.

Isolates of *T. vaginalis* with relatively high levels of resistance to metronidazole have been obtained from patients who were not cured by repeated courses of the drug. Evaluation of such cases should include determination of the susceptibility of *T. vaginalis* to metronidazole.

Treatment of Sexual Partners

Sexual partners should be treated with either the single-dose or the 7-day metronidazole regimen.

Trichomoniasis during Pregnancy

Metronidazole is contraindicated in the first trimester of pregnancy, and its safety in the rest of pregnancy is not established. However, no other adequate therapy exists. Local therapy has poor efficacy but may reduce symptoms to a tolerable level. Vinegar douches (2 tablespoons of vinegar in a quart of water daily and then twice weekly) may palliate symptoms for some women. For patients with severe symptoms after the first trimester, treatment with 2 g of metronidazole in a single dose may be considered.

Toxicity of Metronidazole

In certain individuals, metronidazole has a disulfiram-like effect; thus it can produce a variety of systemic symptoms including nausea and flushing. Patients should be cautioned concerning consumption of alcohol while on treatment. High doses of metronidazole given for prolonged periods (e.g., for resistant trichomoniasis) must be closely monitored, because they can cause peripheral neuropathy, which is sometimes not reversible. This is not a problem with doses recommended above.

ADDITIONAL READING

Borchardt KA, Smith RF: An evaluation of an InPouch TV culture method for diagnosing *Trichomonas vaginalis* infection. *Genitourin Med* 67:149, 1991

Cotch MF et al: Demographic and behavioral predictors of *Trichomonas vaginalis* infection among pregnant women. The Vaginal Infections and Prematurity Study Group. *Obstet Gynecol* 78: 1087, 1991

Grossman JH 3, Galask RP: Persistent vaginitis caused by metronidazole-resistant *Trichomonas*. *Obstet Gynecol* 76:521, 1990

Kiviat NB et al: Histopathology of endocervical infection caused by *Chlamydia trachomatis,* herpes simplex virus, *Trichomonas vaginalis,* and *Neisseria gonorrhoeae*. *Hum Pathol* 21:831, 1990

Krieger JN et al: Characteristics of *Trichomonas vaginalis* isolates from women with and without colpitis macularis. *J Infect Dis* 161:307, 1990

Livengood CH 3, Lossick JG: Resolution of resistant vaginal trichomoniasis associated with the use of intravaginal nonoxynol-9. *Obstet Gynecol* 1991

Lossick JG, Kent HL: Trichomoniasis: Trends in diagnosis and management. *Am J Obstet Gynecol* 165:1217, 1991

Roy S: Nonbarrier contraceptives and vaginitis and vaginosis. *Am J Obstet Gynecol* 1991

Saxena SB, Jenkins RR: Prevalence of *Trichomonas vaginalis* in men at high risk for sexually transmitted diseases. *Sex Transm Dis* 18:138, 1991

For a more detailed discussion, see Rein MF and Muller M: *Trichomonas vaginalis* and Trichomoniasis, Chap. 43, p. 481, in STD-2.

EPIDEMIOLOGY

Vulvovaginal candidiasis (VVC), also called candidal vaginitis, is found throughout the world. In the United States VVC is second only to bacterial vaginosis in frequency and is three times more frequent than trichomonas vaginitis. Although VVC is not a reportable disease, most authors feel that it is increasing in frequency, the most likely explanation being the widespread use of systemic and topical vaginal antimicrobial agents.

Candida species may be isolated from the genital tract of approximately 20 percent of asymptomatic, healthy women of childbearing age. The natural history of asymptomatic colonization is unknown, although both animal and limited human studies suggest that vaginal carriage may continue for several months and perhaps years. Several factors are associated with increased prevalence of asymptomatic vaginal colonization with *Candida.* These include pregnancy, use of high-estrogen-content oral contraceptives, uncontrolled diabetes mellitus, and attendance at STD clinics. The rarity of *Candida* isolation in premenarchal females and the lower prevalence of *Candida* vaginitis after menopause emphasize the hormonal dependence of the infection.

Three subpopulations of women may be identified. Some women never develop symptomatic VVC throughout their lives; a second group has infrequent isolated episodes; and a third population suffers from repeated, recurrent, and often chronic infection. It has been estimated that approximately 75 percent of all women will experience at least one episode of VVC during their lifetime.

MICROBIOLOGY

Between 85 and 90 percent of yeasts isolated from the vagina are *Candida albicans* strains. The remainder are other *Candida* spp., and *Torulopsis glabrata,* the latter being the commonest next to *C. albicans.* Nonalbicans *Candida* spp. are capable of inducing vaginitis and are often more resistant to conventional therapy. Uniquely virulent strains have not been identified.

Candida organisms are dimorphic, in that they may be found in different phenotypic phases in humans. In general, blastospores (blastoconidia) are the phenotypic form responsible for transmission or spread, including the bloodstream phase, as well as the form associated with asymptomatic colonization of the vagina. In contrast, germinated yeast which produce mycelia are the most common tissue-invasive form and are usually identified in the presence of symptomatic disease.

PATHOGENESIS

Candida organisms gain access to the vaginal lumen and secretions predominantly from the adjacent perianal area. Candidal vaginitis is seen predominantly in women of childbearing age, and in the majority of cases a precipitating factor can be identified to explain the transformation from asymptomatic carriage to symptomatic vaginitis.

Two fundamental questions are critical in understanding the pathogenesis of VVC. The first relates to the mechanism whereby asymptomatic colonization of the vagina changes to symptomatic VVC. The second concerns the mechanism whereby some women suffer from repeated and chronic vulvovaginal candidal infections. It appears that *C. albicans* may be either a commensal or a pathogen in the vagina, and that changes in the host vaginal environment are usually necessary before the organism induces pathologic effects.

Predisposing Factors

Pregnancy

The vagina during pregnancy shows an increased susceptibility to vaginal infection by *Candida* spp., resulting in both a higher prevalence of vaginal colonization and a higher rate of symptomatic vaginitis. The rate of symptomatic vaginitis is maximally increased in the third trimester, and symptomatic recurrences are also common during pregnancy.

The mechanism by which reproductive hormones increase vaginal susceptibility to *Candida* infection is unclear. It is generally thought that the high levels of hormones—by providing a higher glycogen content in the vaginal environment—provide an excellent carbon source for *Candida.* A more complex mechanism is probably likely, in that estrogens enhance adherence of *Candida* to vaginal epithelial cells, possibly by increasing expression of epithelial cell receptors for the organism. Not surprisingly, rates of cure of candidal vaginitis are significantly lower during pregnancy.

Oral Contraceptives

Several studies have shown increased vaginal colonization with *Candida* following high-estrogen-content oral contraceptive use. Almost certainly, the same mechanism operative in pregnancy applies to these subjects. Investigations of low-estrogen-content oral contraceptives have not found an increase in candidal vaginitis.

Diabetes Mellitus

Vaginal colonization with *Candida* is more frequent in diabetic women. Although uncontrolled diabetes predisposes to symptomatic vaginitis, most diabetic patients do not have repeated infection. It has become traditional to perform glucose tolerance tests in all women with recurrent VVC. The yield of these expensive studies is extremely low; testing, therefore, is not justified in premenopausal women.

Antibiotics

Onset of symptomatic VVC is frequently observed during courses of oral systemic antibiotics. Not only is symptomatic vaginitis frequently precipitated, but vaginal colonization rates increase from approximately 10 to 30 percent. Antibiotics, both systemic and topical agents, are thought to act by eliminating the protective vaginal bacterial flora. The most important protective normal bacterial flora may be hydrogen peroxide–producing lactobacilli. Thus the natural flora is thought to provide colonization resistance as well as preventing germination and superficial mucosal invasion by *Candida*.

Miscellaneous

Among the factors that may have contributed to the increased incidence of VVC in western societies has been the use of tight, restricting, poorly ventilated clothing and nylon underclothing with increased local, perineal moisture and temperature. The use of well-ventilated clothing and cotton underwear may be of value in preventing infection. Anecdotal evidence suggests that the use of commercial douches, perfumed toilet paper, chlorinated swimming pools, or feminine hygiene sprays contributes to symptomatic vaginitis. Chemical contact, local allergy, or hypersensitivity reactions may alter the vaginal milieu and permit the transformation from asymptomatic colonization to symptomatic vaginitis.

Source of Infection

The gastrointestinal tract may well be the initial source of *Candida* colonization of the vagina. The source of vaginal reinfection, however, remains unclear. There is considerable controversy regarding the role of the intestinal tract as a focus of reinfection in women with recurrent VVC, but some vaginal relapses or apparent reinfections may be due to recolonization of the vagina by *Candida* residing in an intestinal site.

Circumstantial evidence implicates sexual transmission as a possible means of acquiring *Candida* infection, but direct confirmation that sexual transmission occurs is lacking.

Vaginal relapse is probably responsible for many recurrent infections. After systemic and topical antibiotic therapy, negative vaginal cultures once more become positive for *Candida* within 30 days in 20 to 25 percent of women. Small numbers of *Candida* might persist temporarily within superficial cervical or vaginal epithelial cells following treatment, only to reemerge some weeks or months later. However, there is no evidence that *Candida* undergoes latency analogous to cytomegalovirus, herpes simplex virus, or other intracellular pathogens.

Mechanisms Involved in Invasion and Inflammatory Response

During the symptomatic episode germinated or filamentous forms of *Candida* appear. Germinated organisms not only enhance colonization but represent the dominant invasive phase capable of penetrating intact epithelial cells and invading the vaginal epithelium, although only the very superficial layers are involved.

The mechanism whereby *Candida* induces inflammation is not yet established. Yeast cells are capable of producing several extracellular proteases as well as phospholipases. Both blastoconidia and pseudohyphae are capable of destroying superficial cells by direct invasion.

Based on the clinical spectrum, which varies from an acute florid exudative form with thick white vaginal discharge and large numbers of germinated yeast cells to the other extreme of absent or minimal discharge, fewer organisms, and yet severe pruritus, it appears that more than one pathogenic mechanism may exist.

CLINICAL MANIFESTATIONS

Acute pruritus and vaginal discharge are the usual presenting complaints, but neither symptom is specific to VVC, and neither is invariably associated with disease. The most common symptom is vulvar pruritus, which is present in virtually all symptomatic patients. Vaginal discharge is not invariably present and is frequently minimal. Although described as typically cottage cheese–like, the discharge may vary from watery to homogeneously thick. Vaginal soreness, irritation, vulvar burning, dyspareunia, and external dysuria are commonly present. Odor, if present, is minimal and inoffensive. Examination frequently reveals erythema and swelling of the labia and vulva, often with discrete pustulopapular peripheral lesions. The cervix is normal, and vaginal mucosal erythema is present together with adherent whitish discharge. Characteristically, symptoms are exacerbated in the week preceding the onset of menses, and some relief accompanies the onset of menstrual flow.

A clinical spectrum of candidal vaginitis exists. In some patients a more exudative picture is apparent with copious discharge and white vaginal plaques satisfying the traditional description of vaginal thrush. At the other end of the spectrum are those with minimal discharge and severe erythema with extensive vulvar involvement often extending into the inguinal and perianal regions.

Although *Candida* spp. occasionally cause extensive balanoposthitis in male partners of women with vaginal candidiasis, a more frequent event is a transient rash, erythema, and pruritus or a burning sensation of the penis which develops minutes or hours after unprotected intercourse. The symptoms are self-limiting and frequently disappear after showering.

DIAGNOSIS

The relative lack of specificity of symptoms and signs precludes diagnosis of a first episode based only on history and physical examination. Neither clinical signs and symptoms alone nor culture confirmation of the presence of *Candida* should be regarded as a satisfactory basis for diagnosis. The most *Candida*-specific symptom is pruritus without discharge, and even this criterion correctly predicts VVC in only 38 percent of patients.

Most patients with symptomatic vaginitis may be readily diagnosed by simple microscopic examination of vaginal secretions (Fig. 19-1). Figure 19-2 outlines an algorithm for diagnosis and treatment of VVC. A wet-mount or saline preparation should routinely be done, not only to identify yeast cells and mycelia but also to exclude the presence of "clue cells" and motile trichomonads. Large numbers of white cells are also invariably absent and when present should suggest a mixed infection. The 10% potassium hydroxide preparation is even more sensitive in diagnosing the presence of germinated yeast. Vaginal pH indicators reveal a normal pH (4.0 to 4.5) in candidal vaginitis, and the finding of a vaginal pH greater than 5.0 should strongly alert clinicians to the possibility of bacterial vaginosis, trichomoniasis, or a mixed infection.

Despite the value of direct microscopy, several studies have revealed that up to 50 percent of patients with culture-positive symptomatic candidal vaginitis (responding to antimycotic therapy) have negative microscopic findings. Thus, although cultures are unnecessary if the wet-mount or potassium hydroxide preparations show yeast and mycelia, vaginal culture should be performed in the presence of negative microscopic findings if VVC is suspected because of symptoms or signs. Although vaginal culture is the most sensitive method currently available for detecting *Candida*, a positive culture does not necessarily indicate that *Candida* is responsible for the vaginal symptoms.

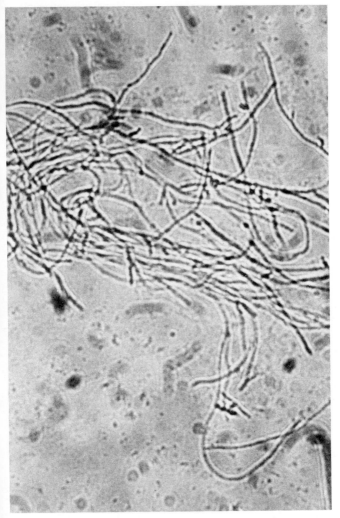

FIG. 19-1. Wet-mount examination of vaginal discharge from a woman with VVC, showing mycelia. 1000 × magnification.

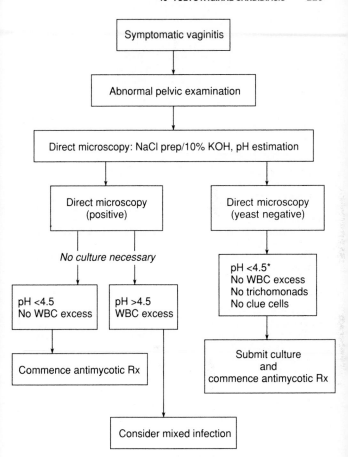

*Useful indication for Candida latex agglutination slide test.

FIG. 19-2. Algorithm for diagnosis and treatment of vulvovaginal candidiasis.

TREATMENT

Acute Vaginitis

At the outset, clinicians should attempt to differentiate those women with infrequent episodes from those with chronic, recurrent, or recalcitrant VVC. This differentiation influences the duration of therapy. In general, most physicians advise against treatment of asymptomatic vaginal carriage or colonization with *Candida*. Many effective treatment regimens exist, but 3- and 7-day regimens are superior to single-dose topical therapy.

Recommended Treatment

Examples of effective regimens include the following:

Miconazole nitrate (vaginal suppository 200 mg), intravaginally at bedtime for 3 days or

Clotrimazole (vaginal tablets 200 mg), intravaginally at bedtime for 3 days or

Butoconazole (2% cream 5 g), intravaginally at bedtime for 3 days (6 days if pregnant) or

Terconazole (80-mg suppository or 0.8% cream 5 g), intravaginally at bedtime for 3 days.

Alternative Treatment

Miconazole nitrate (vaginal suppository 100 mg or 2% cream 5 g), intravaginally at bedtime for 7 days or

Clotrimazole (vaginal tablets 100 mg or clotrimazole 1% cream 5 g), intravaginally at bedtime for 7 days.

Nystatin and single-dose therapy are less effective than the recommended therapies and are not recommended. Studies have also demonstrated efficacy of fluconazole 150 mg orally, given as a single dose.

Treatment of sexual partners is not necessary unless candidal balanitis (which responds to local anticandidal preparations) is present.

Treatment of Recurrent and Chronic VVC

The management of women with recurrent and chronic VVC remains problematic. There has been considerable confusion primarily because of the lack of a clear, concise definition of what constitutes recurrent disease. A definition which appears reasonable is that of at least four mycologically proven symptomatic episodes in the previous 12 months, with exclusion of other common vaginal pathogens.

The first step the clinician should take is to identify and eliminate possible underlying or predisposing causes. Uncontrolled diabetes must be controlled. Corticosteroids, other immunosuppressive agents, and hormones such as estrogens should be stopped where possible. Discontinuation of oral contraceptives should also be considered. The possibility of HIV infection should be considered. The yield of performing a glucose tolerance test in otherwise asymptomatic healthy premenopausal women to diagnose latent or chemical diabetes mellitus is extremely low and is not worthwhile. Tight-fitting clothing and synthetic underwear should be avoided. Douching with commercial preparations and vinegar is of no value and should be discouraged. Unfortunately, in the majority of women with recurrent or chronic VVC, no underlying or predisposing factor can be identified.

Therapeutic choices include patient self-diagnosis and early initiation of self-treatment with topical therapy, or long-term maintenance suppressive prophylaxis with either topical or low-dose systemic therapy (e.g., 100 mg of ketoconazole daily). However, the benefits of successful suppressive therapy must be weighed against the potential toxicity of long-term oral therapy. Hilton et al. reported a decrease in the incidence of VVC following daily ingestion of yogurt containing *Lactobacillus acidophilus*.[1]

Prophylactic antifungal medication is not routinely recommended to accompany antibiotic therapy in most women. However, in women with recurrent VVC in whom antimicrobial agents have been identified as a frequent and inevitable precipitating factor, it may be prudent to simultaneously administer topical antimycotic therapy together with antibiotics.

Finally it is necessary to emphasize the importance of reassurance, support, and counseling in dealing with patients with chronic or recurrent VVC. Chronic vaginitis results in chronic dyspareunia, and inevitably sexual and marital relations suffer, often irreversibly. Patients should be reassured that today virtually all women with chronic VVC can be adequately controlled if not cured.

REFERENCE

1. Hilton E, et al: Ingestion of yogurt containing *Lactobacillus acidophilus* as prophylaxis for candidal vaginitis. *Ann Intern Med* 116:353, 1992

ADDITIONAL READING

Boag FC et al: Comparison of vaginal flora after treatment with a clotrimazole 400 mg vaginal pessary or a fluconazole 150 mg capsule for vaginal candidosis. *Genitourin Med* 67:232, 1991

Drutz DJ: Lactobacillus prophylaxis for *Candida* vaginitis. *Ann Intern Med* 116:419, 1992

Hillier SL et al: The relationship of hydrogen peroxide-producing lactobacilli to bacterial vaginosis and genital microflora in pregnant women. *Obstet Gynecol* 79:369, 1992

Horowitz BJ: Mycotic vulvovaginitis: A broad overview. *Am J Obstet Gynecol* 165:1188, 1991

Imam N et al: Hierarchical pattern of mucosal candida infections in HIV-seropositive women. *Am J Med* 89:142, 1990

Kent HL: Epidemiology of vaginitis. *Am J Obstet Gynecol* 165:1168, 1991

For a more detailed discussion, see: Sobel JD: Vulvovaginal Candidiasis, Chap. 45, p 515, in STD-2.

Infections of the lower genital tract cause substantial morbidity
among women. Many of the disease patterns caused by STD
pathogens in women are complex. Organisms such as *Neisseria
gonorrhoeae, Chlamydia trachomatis,* and herpes simplex virus
(HSV) have a predilection for simultaneous infection of the urethra,
cervix, and rectum. Symptom patterns are variable, and each has a
wide range of differential diagnostic possibilities. Infection at any
one site can produce symptoms that are poorly localized and easy
to erroneously attribute to involvement of a contiguous site.
Infections of the bladder, vulva, or urethra, for example, can all
produce dysuria or dyspareunia, and infections of the cervix and
vagina both produce vaginal discharge.

CYSTITIS AND URETHRITIS

EPIDEMIOLOGY AND ETIOLOGY

Acute bacterial cystitis is most common in women 20 to 25 years
of age, especially among those who are sexually active. The
traditional criterion of greater than or equal to 100,000 organisms
per milliliter of urine is insensitive for diagnosis of acute cystitis in
women with dysuria, because from one-third to one-half have
"low-count" bacteriuria, with cultures yielding 100 to less than
100,000 organisms per milliliter. Common pathogens include *Escherichia coli, Staphylococcus saprophyticus, Proteus mirabilis,
Klebsiella pneumoniae,* and *Enterobacter* species.

Dysuria and frequency in women whose urine has fewer than 100
organisms per milliliter constitute the "urethral syndrome" or, in
the presence of pyuria, the "dysuria–sterile pyuria syndrome."
Chlamydia trachomatis appears to be an important pathogen among
university students who present with the urethral syndrome and
sterile bladder urine. Chlamydia is also common among female
contacts of men with nongonococcal urethritis. However, both *N.
gonorrhoeae* and *C. trachomatis* may be important causes of the
urethral syndrome among indigent women who are at high risk of
gonorrhea as well as chlamydial infection.

Other pathogens can also cause dysuria. HSV infections can
produce urethritis, dysuria, and pyuria and can be mistaken for
bacterial cystitis if vulvar lesions are not noted. Dysuria in women
who have neither bacteriuria nor urethral infections with STD
pathogens is often attributable to vulvar inflammation caused by
genital herpes or vulvovaginitis. Dysuria may be caused by vaginitis

more frequently than by cystitis because vaginitis is so much more common than cystitis.

DIAGNOSIS

Characteristic features of syndromes causing dysuria in women are outlined in Table 20-1. Figure 20-1 illustrates an algorithm for workup. "Internal" dysuria is felt inside the body and correlates better with UTIs than "external" dysuria, which is felt on the vaginal labia and correlates with periurethral or vulvar inflammation caused by *Candida albicans* or HSV. In all patients with dysuria a speculum exam should be performed to rule out vaginitis or mucopurulent cervicitis.

TABLE 20-1. Characteristic Features Which Differ in the Three Major Causes of Dysuria in Women

	Acute bacterial cystitis	Urethritis	Vulvitis
Predisposing factors	Previous cystitis Diaphragm use Onset of symptoms within 24 h after intercourse	New sex partner	History of genital herpes Partner with genital herpes Antibiotic use History of recurrent vulvovaginal candidiasis
Symptoms	Internal dysuria Duration of symptoms ≤4 days Frequency and urgency Gross hematuria	Internal dysuria Duration of symptoms often ≥7 days with chlamydial urethritis	External dysuria Vaginal discharge Vulvar irritation, burning, pruritis, or lesions
Signs	Suprapubic tenderness	Mucopurulent cervicitis Vulvar lesions	Vulvar lesions Vulvitis Curdlike vaginal exudate
Laboratory	Pyuria Microscopic hematuria Rapid nitrite test Urine Gram stain Urine culture	Pyuria Urethral discharge or bartholinitis Endocervical exudate Cervical and urethral tests for *C. trachomatis* and *N. gonorrhoeae* Test lesion for HSV	No pyuria Test lesion for HSV Test vaginal discharge for *C. albicans*

Urinalysis should be performed on a midstream specimen collected by the clean-catch method. The most sensitive and specific test for pyuria involves use of a hemocytometer or calibrated chamber, but leukocyte count can also be determined with relative accuracy by resuspending centrifuged sediment in 1 ml of urine and counting 1 to 2 drops of this solution on a microscope slide under a cover slip. Dipsticks for detection of leukocyte esterase are also useful screening tests for detection of pyuria.

Once the presence of pyuria has been determined, bacteriuria can be assessed by (1) Gram stain of a fresh, midstream, clean-catch, uncentrifuged urine specimen and examination with an oil-immersion lens (the presence of 1 organism per field is correlated with quantitative isolation of greater than or equal to 100,000 bacteria per milliliter of urine), or (2) examination of unstained, centrifuged urinary sediment under the high-dry objective (detection of 100 organisms per field also correlates well with isolation of greater than or equal to 100,000 bacteria per milliliter). Because bacterial concentrations of fewer than 100,000 organisms per milliliter are not readily visualized by Gram stain, this technique is insensitive for detection of bacteriuria in symptomatic women. Urine culture is essential for confirmation of bacteriuria in women with pyuria and no microscopic evidence of bacteriuria, and for identification and susceptibility testing of uropathogens in patients with recurrent bacterial cystitis. The patient with pyuria and no bacteriuria who is at risk for STDs or has evidence of mucopurulent endocervicitis should be cultured for *N. gonorrhoeae* and tested for *C. trachomatis* infection at both the endocervix and urethra.

TREATMENT

Women with microscopic evidence of bacteriuria and clinical findings consistent with bacterial cystitis should be treated with short courses (preferably 3 days) of an appropriate oral antimicrobial agent unless the temperature exceeds 101°F, symptoms have been present for longer than 1 week, or there is costovertebral angle pain or tenderness, as these findings suggest pyelonephritis. Acceptable drugs include trimethoprim-sulfamethoxazole, amoxicillin-clavulanic acid, or one of the newer quinolones.

Recommendations for duration of therapy of uncomplicated cystitis vary among authors from a single dose to a 10-day regimen. Longer courses have more side effects, and single-dose treatments have lower rates of cure. Thus, an intermediate length of therapy, such as 3 days, appears optimal at this time.

Women with pyuria and no bacteriuria who are suspected of having chlamydial urethritis should be treated with a tetracycline such as doxycycline 100 mg twice daily for 7 days while urine

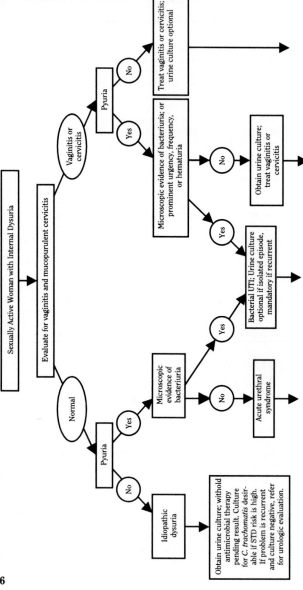

FIG. 20-1 Algorithm for management of sexually active woman with dysuria.

236

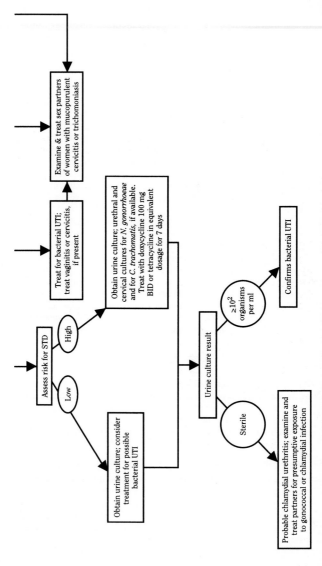

Assess risk for STD

High →
Obtain urine culture; urethral and cervical cultures for *N. gonorrhoeae* and for *C. trachomatis*, if available. Treat with doxycycline 100 mg BID or tetracycline in equivalent dosage for 7 days

Low →
Obtain urine culture; consider treatment for possible bacterial UTI

Urine culture result

≥10² organisms per ml → Confirms bacterial UTI

Sterile → Probable chlamydial urethritis; examine and treat partners for presumptive exposure to gonococcal or chlamydial infection

Treat for bacterial UTI; treat vaginitis or cervicitis, if present

Examine & treat sex partners of women with mucopurulent cervicitis or trichomoniasis cultures are pending. Male sex partners of women with suspected or confirmed gonococcal or chlamydial urethritis should be examined and tested to exclude urethral infections, or should be treated for exposure to these agents.

VAGINAL INFECTIONS IN WOMEN

Vaginal infections in adult women are extremely common. The three most common types of vaginal infections are vulvovaginal candidiasis, trichomoniasis, and bacterial vaginosis. See Chaps. 18, 19, and 21 for a discussion of each. Human papillomavirus is another cause of vulvovaginal infection (see Chap. 13). Other causes of vaginitis in adults include a destructive type of ulcerative vaginitis attributed to toxin produced by *Staphylococcus aureus* in women with toxic shock syndrome, vaginal ulceration associated with the use of vaginal tampons or cervical caps, infections associated with other intravaginal foreign bodies, and miscellaneous uncommon vaginal infections.

In postmenopausal women, vaginal symptoms are common, and a distinction must be made between vaginal infection and vaginal atrophy, which is negatively correlated with frequency of intercourse and with circulating concentrations of gonadotrophins and androgens. In older women a number of poorly understood syndromes are seen. These include desquamative inflammatory vaginitis (also known as "erosive vaginal lichen planus"), vulvar vestibulitis, purulent vaginitis (not attributable to trichomoniasis or candidiasis), recurrent bacterial vaginitis, and essential vulvodynia. The etiology of these syndromes is unknown. Treatment is empirical and should be as conservative as possible.

ENDOCERVICITIS

Endocervicitis or mucopurulent cervicitis is usually caused by *C. trachomatis, N. gonorrhoeae,* or HSV and should be distinguished from ectocervicitis. Cervical infection is a reservoir for sexual and perinatal transmission of pathogenic microorganisms, and ascending infection may lead to two complications: (1) ascending intraluminal spread of pathogenic organisms from the cervix, resulting in endometritis and salpingitis, or (2) ascending infection during pregnancy, resulting in chorioamnionitis, premature rupture of membranes, premature delivery, amniotic fluid infection, and puerperal infection. Because endocervicitis produces symptoms less often than urethritis does in males, careful clinical assessment and appropriate use of laboratory tests for detection of subclinical infection in women are of paramount importance in the control of gonococcal and chlamydial infections.

The lack of widely recognized objective signs of cervical inflammation has led to much clinical confusion and a proliferation of terms. In this book the term *mucopurulent cervicitis* refers to the appearance of the inflamed endocervix on physical examination—optimally by colposcopy—with visualization of edema, erythema at the zone of ectopy, easily induced endocervical bleeding, and yellow endocervical discharge on a white cotton-tipped swab of endocervical secretions. These findings are associated with infection due to *C. trachomatis* and *N. gonorrhoeae*. The presence of greater than or equal to 30 neutrophils per 1000× microscopic field (oil immersion) is also associated with chlamydial or gonococcal infection, but the predictive value of this finding varies in different settings.

ECTOCERVICITIS

Colposcopic examination can be valuable in determining the cause of an ectocervical infection. Cervical HSV infection correlates with cervical ulcers or necrotic lesions, while trichomoniasis correlates with colpitis macularis ("strawberry cervix"), and both *C. trachomatis* and cytomegalovirus infection of the cervix are associated with the presence of immature metaplasia. *Candida albicans* and *T. vaginalis* can produce ectocervicitis; they are also associated with inflammation of the contiguous stratified squamous vaginal epithelium.

DIAGNOSTIC PROCEDURES FOR CERVICITIS

Cervicitis can be confirmed by a variety of supplementary diagnostic procedures such as Gram's stain of endocervical mucus, cervical cytologic examination, colposcopy, and cervical biopsy.

The presence of greater than or equal to 30 neutrophils per 1000× Gram-stained field supports the diagnosis of endocervicitis unless the slide is heavily contaminated by vaginal squamous cells (e.g., greater than 100 squamous cells per slide) and vaginal flora (e.g., greater than 100 bacteria per 1000× field overlying cervical mucus). The ectocervix should therefore be wiped clean with a large swab before endocervical mucus is obtained. Contamination by vaginal cells or flora suggests that any neutrophils present may have originated in the vagina rather than the endocervix and can also obscure microscopic detection of gonococci in endocervical mucus. Detection of gram-negative diplococci within neutrophils in properly collected endocervical mucus is highly specific, but relatively insensitive for diagnosis of gonorrhea; gonococci can be identified by Gram's stain in only about 50 to 60 percent of women with cervical gonococcal infection.

Cytopathologic examination is widely used to detect cervical neoplasia and may also be useful in identifying women with cervicitis. Certain infections correlate with specific cytologic patterns. Human papillomavirus infection correlates with cervical intraepithelial neoplasia (also known as dysplasia or squamous intraepithelial lesion). *Chlamydia trachomatis* infections are associated with certain other epithelial changes and inflammatory cell patterns. Use of cytopathologic examination to identify cervical inflammation may be an important tool for control of chlamydial infection in the future.

Colposcopy and cervicography (photographing the cervix with a greater depth of field than seen with colposcopy) also have potential utility for detection of cervical infection. Further evaluation is needed to determine clinical utility.

Confirmatory microbiological studies can be invaluable in making a specific diagnosis. *Neisseria gonorrhoeae, C. trachomatis,* and HSV can be isolated, or detected by the presence of microbial antigens. Even if gram-negative intracellular diplococci are present on Gram stain, a culture for *N. gonorrhoeae* should be obtained to test for antimicrobial susceptibility. Because patients with gonococcal cervicitis are also frequently infected by chlamydia, a confirmatory test for *C. trachomatis* should also be performed. The development of methods for immunologic detection of *C. trachomatis* in endocervical specimens has made diagnostic testing more widely available. If cervical ulcers or other lesions suggestive of HSV are present, culture can be used to obtain isolates for typing as HSV-1 or HSV-2; the distinction is clinically important because HSV-1 is less likely to recur than HSV-2. If colpitis macularis is seen, wet mount examination for motile trichomonads is usually positive.

TREATMENT FOR MUCOPURULENT CERVICITIS

Patients with proven or suspected gonococcal cervicitis should be treated with **one 250-mg IM dose of ceftriaxone and doxycycline 100 mg twice a day orally for 7 days,** as coinfection with chlamydia is extremely common. It is reasonable to treat mucopurulent cervicitis with both drugs while tests for gonorrhea and chlamydial infection are pending. Women with negative *N. gonorrhoeae* cultures may receive doxycycline alone (100 mg daily for 7 days).

DIFFERENTIAL DIAGNOSIS AND MANAGEMENT OF VAGINAL DISCHARGE

Signs and symptoms of abnormal vaginal discharge may be caused by either vaginal infection or cervicitis. Therefore, evaluation of vaginal infections must first exclude cervicitis, the more serious condition. Mucopurulent endocervicitis caused by *C. trachomatis* or *N. gonorrhoeae* must be differentiated from ectocervicitis, cervical HSV infection, HSV, or simple cervical ectopy. Ectopy occurs when columnar epithelium lies in an exposed position on the ectocervix;

it is a normal finding and requires no therapy in the absence of cervicitis.

The presence of mucopurulent cervicitis raises the possibility that endometritis, with or without salpingitis, may also be present. Distinguishing features of endometritis include midline abdominal tenderness or menorrhagia, often with elevation of the erythrocyte sedimentation rate or peripheral white count, and characteristic histopathologic features. With salpingitis, additional findings include adnexal tenderness and cervical motion tenderness. Further extension of infection from the salpinges to the pelvic peritoneum can result in signs of pelvic peritonitis, with low abdomen rebound tenderness, and nausea and vomiting. However, the absence of findings of endometritis and salpingitis does not rule out these conditions, which may be subclinical.

Once the presence or absence of cervicitis is determined, the likelihood of vaginal infection should be assessed. Cervicitis often coexists with vaginal infections, especially bacterial vaginosis and trichomonal vaginitis (see Table 20-2 for diagnostic features and management). The amount, consistency, and location of discharge within the vagina should be noted. A sample of discharge should be removed from the vaginal wall, its pH should be determined, and its color should be noted in comparison with the white color of the swab. Separate specimens should be mixed with KOH and saline and examined for detection of the presence and quantity of normal epithelial cells, clue cells, neutrophils, motile trichomonads, or fungal forms. Chapters 18, 19, and 21 contain a discussion of evaluation and therapy of vaginal infection.

GYNECOLOGIC COMPLICATIONS OF LOWER GENITAL TRACT INFECTIONS

Although the pathogenesis of pelvic inflammatory disease (PID) is not completely understood, gonococcal and chlamydial cervicitis predispose patients to endometritis and salpingitis and other upper tract complications. It is also suspected that bacterial vaginosis plays a role in the development of some PID cases. Moreover, a great deal of attention has focused on defining the importance of cervical infection and bacterial vaginosis in causing complications of pregnancy, such as chorioamnionitis and premature delivery. These potential complications should be kept in mind when evaluating and treating women with lower genital tract infections.

PREVENTION

Correct use of the condom is an effective way to decrease infection due to sexually transmitted agents of vaginitis and mucopurulent cervicitis. Other intravaginal barrier contraceptives, such as the

TABLE 20-2. Diagnostic Features and Management of Vaginal Infection in Premenopausal Adults

	Normal vaginal exam	Yeast vaginitis	Trichomonal vaginitis	Bacterial vaginosis (NSV)
Etiology	Uninfected; *Lactobacillus* predominant	*Candida albicans* and other yeasts	*Trichomonas vaginalis*	Associated with *Gardnerella vaginalis*, various anaerobic bacteria, and mycoplasma
Typical symptoms	None	Vulvar itching and/or irritation, increased discharge	Profuse purulent discharge, vulvar itching	Malodorous, slightly increased discharge
Discharge:				
Amount	Variable; usually scant	Scant to moderate	Profuse	Moderate
Color*	Clear or white	White	Yellow	Usually white or gray
Consistency	Nonhomogeneous, floccular	Clumped; adherent plaques	Homogeneous	Homogeneous, low viscosity; uniformly coating vaginal walls
Inflammation of vulvar or vaginal epithelium	None	Erythema of vaginal epithelium, introitus; vulvar dermatitis common	Erythema of vaginal and vulvar epithelium; colpitis macularis	None
pH of vaginal fluid†	Usually ≤4.5	Usually ≤4.5	Usually ≥5.0	Usually ≥4.7
Amine ("fishy") odor with 10% KOH	None	None	May be present	Present

(continued)

242

Microscopy‡	Normal epithelial cells; lactobacilli predominate	Leukocytes, epithelial cells; yeast, mycelia, or pseudomycelia in up to 80%	Leukocytes; motile trichomonads seen in 80–90% of symptomatic patients, less often in the absence of symptoms	Clue cells; few leukocytes; lactobacilli outnumbered by profuse mixed flora, nearly always including G. vaginalis plus anaerobic species, on Gram stain
Usual treatment	None	Miconazole or clotrimazole intravaginally each 100 mg daily for 7 days	Metronidazole or tinidazole 2.0 g orally (single dose) Metronidazole 500 mg orally twice daily for 7 days	Metronidazole 500 mg orally twice daily for 7 days
Usual management of sex partners	None	None; topical treatment if candidal dermatitis of penis is present	Examine for STD; treat with metronidazole, 2 gm p.o.	Examine for STD; no treatment if normal

*Color of discharge is determined by examining vaginal discharge against the white background of a swab.
†pH determination is not useful if blood is present.
‡To detect fungal elements, vaginal fluid is digested with 10% KOH prior to microscopic examination; to examine for other features, fluid is mixed (1:1) with physiologic saline. Gram's stain also is excellent for detecting yeasts and pseudomycelia and for distinguishing normal flora from the mixed flora seen in bacterial vaginosis but is less sensitive than the saline preparation for detection of T. vaginalis.

diaphragm, especially when used with antiseptic spermicides, may also be expected to reduce the risk of cervical infection with *N. gonorrhoeae* and *C. trachomatis.*

ADDITIONAL READING

Foxman B: Recurring urinary tract infection: Incidence and risk factors. *Am J Public Health* 80:331, 1990

Foxman B, Chi JW: Health behavior and urinary tract infection in college-aged women. *J Clin Epidemiol* 43:329, 1990

Hilton E et al: Ingestion of yogurt containing *Lactobacillus acidophilus* as prophylaxis for candidal vaginitis. *Ann Intern Med* 116:353, 1992

Hooton TM, Stamm WE: Management of acute uncomplicated urinary tract infection in adults. *Med Clin North Am* 75:339, 1991

Kent H L: Epidemiology of vaginitis. *Am J Obstet Gynecol* 165:1168, 1991

Knud HCR et al: Surrogate methods to diagnose gonococcal and chlamydial cervicitis: Comparison of leukocyte esterase dipstick, endocervical gram stain, and culture. *Sex Transm Dis* 18:211, 1991

Malotte CK et al: Screening for chlamydial cervicitis in a sexually active university population. *Am J Public Health* 80:469, 1990

McKay M: Vulvitis and vulvovaginitis: Cutaneous considerations. *Am J Obstet Gynecol* 165:1176, 1991

Measley REJ, Levison ME: Host defense mechanisms in the pathogenesis of urinary tract infection. *Med Clin North Am* 75:275, 1991

Raz R, Boger S: Long-term prophylaxis with norfloxacin versus nitrofurantoin in women with recurrent urinary tract infection. *Antimicrob Agents Chemother* 35:1241, 1991

Roy S: Nonbarrier contraceptives and vaginitis and vaginosis. *Am J Obstet Gynecol* 165:1240, 1991

Stapleton A et al: Postcoital antimicrobial prophylaxis for recurrent urinary tract infection. A randomized, double-blind, placebo-controlled trial. *JAMA* 264:703, 1990

For a more detailed discussion, see Holmes KK: Lower Genital Tract Infections in Women: Cystitis, Urethritis, Vulvovaginitis, and Cervicitis, Chap. 46, p 527, in STD-2.

Bacterial vaginosis (BV) is the most prevalent cause of vaginal symptoms among women of childbearing age. BV, previously called nonspecific vaginitis, is characterized by slightly increased quantities of malodorous vaginal discharge. By convention, the diagnosis of bacterial vaginosis is made after excluding other causes of vaginal discharge. However, many of these other conditions, such as trichomoniasis, vulvovaginal candidiasis, and cervicitis, can coexist with BV. No single organism is responsible for this syndrome; it appears to have a polymicrobial etiology. Examination of vaginal fluid reveals decreased amounts of lactobacillus (a component of normal vaginal flora) and a preponderance of anaerobes, genital mycoplasmas, and *Gardnerella vaginalis.* Because vaginal inflammation is not associated with bacterial vaginosis, the condition appears to represent a disturbance in the vaginal microbial ecosystem rather than a true infection. Recent work has demonstrated an increased risk for prematurity and chorioamnionitis among pregnant women with BV and suggests that BV may be a risk factor for pelvic inflammatory disease.

EPIDEMIOLOGY

The prevalence of BV varies with the population studied. It is lowest among women undergoing routine annual examinations (5 percent) and highest among those attending STD clinics (up to 37 percent). Among pregnant women, the prevalence is lowest among private patients and highest among patients visiting a teaching clinic or requesting termination of pregnancy.

The two lines of evidence support the sexual transmission of BV, but the data are by no means conclusive. First, some studies have found a higher prevalence of BV among very sexually active women than among those who are sexually inexperienced. Second, BV-associated organisms, particularly *G. vaginalis,* can be isolated from the male partners of women with BV. However, not all studies are in agreement, and more research is required to determine whether BV is sexually transmitted.

ETIOLOGY

Gardnerella vaginalis is highly associated with BV. However, this organism can also be isolated, occasionally in high concentrations, from women with no signs of vaginal discharge. Though once thought to be the sole agent of this condition, *G. vaginalis* is now believed to interact with anaerobic bacteria and genital mycoplasmas, especially *Mycoplasma hominis,* to cause vaginosis. The anaerobes most commonly isolated are the new genus *Mobiluncus* and the black-pigmented *Bacteroides* spp. (*B. asaccharolyticus, B. intermedius, B. melaninogenicus, B. corporis*), *B. bivius,* and *B. ureolyticus.* Members of the *B. fragilis* group, which are common in the gastrointestinal tract, are less commonly isolated from the vagina and are not associated with BV. Other anaerobic bacteria implicated include fusobacteria, anaerobic *Lactobacillus* spp., *Bifidobacterium* spp., *Eubacterium* spp., anaerobic gram-positive cocci (primarily peptostreptococci), *Veillonella* spp., and *Mobiluncus.*

In summary, no single organism is responsible for BV. However, four organisms, *Mobiluncus* spp., *Bacteroides* spp., *G. vaginalis,* and *M. hominis,* have been independently associated with BV. The prevalence of these organisms is significantly higher among women with BV than among normal women. In addition, when these organisms are found in the vaginas of normal women, they are present at 100- to 1000-fold lower concentrations than are found in BV.

PATHOGENESIS

BV results from replacement of the normal vaginal flora *(Lactobacillus)* with a mixed flora consisting of *G. vaginalis,* anaerobes, and *M. hominis.* So far, no host factor has been definitely identified that increases susceptibility to BV. There is evidence that use of an intrauterine device increases susceptibility to BV, but the mechanism by which this may occur is unknown.

Amines produced by the microbial flora may account for the characteristic abnormal fishy odor produced when vaginal fluid is mixed with 10% KOH. However, it is still unknown which, if any, organisms produce these amines.

CLINICAL MANIFESTATIONS

Symptoms most indicative of BV include vaginal malodor and vaginal discharge. Abdominal pain, pruritus, and dysuria are not associated with this condition. Examination typically reveals a nonviscous, white, homogeneous vaginal discharge which is uniformly adherent to the vaginal walls and often visible on the labia and fourchette before insertion of a vaginal speculum.

POSSIBLE COMPLICATIONS OF BACTERIAL VAGINOSIS

Several studies suggest that BV during pregnancy increases the risk of obstetric complications, such as chorioamnionitis, amniotic fluid infection, postpartum and post-cesarean endometritis and bacteremia, premature rupture of the membranes, and premature delivery. There is also some evidence that BV may predispose nonpregnant women to develop pelvic inflammatory disease.

DIAGNOSIS

Symptoms alone are not reliable for the diagnosis of BV. Diagnosis is based on the presence of three of the following four signs: (1) characteristic homogeneous white adherent discharge, (2) vaginal fluid with pH greater than 4.5, (3) release of a fishy amine odor from vaginal fluid mixed with 10% KOH, and (4) presence of clue cells (usually representing at least 20 percent of vaginal epithelial cells). The most useful single office procedure for the diagnosis of BV is the microscopic finding of clue cells.

The discharge of BV is white, nonfloccular, adherent to the walls of the vagina, and only moderately increased over that normally seen. Care must be taken in evaluating the discharge because it can be obscured by recent douching or intercourse.

The vaginal fluid pH should be measured using pH paper having appropriate range (pH 4.0 to 6.0). Vaginal pH is best determined by swabbing the lateral and posterior fornices of the vagina and then placing the sample directly on the pH paper. Alternatively, the pH paper can be placed on the surface of the speculum after it has been removed from the vagina. The cervical mucus must be avoided since it has a higher pH (pH 7.0) than the vaginal fluid. The vaginal fluid pH is less than or equal to 4.5 in most normal women, and greater than or equal to 4.7 in most women with BV (and also in most women with trichomoniasis). Elevated vaginal fluid pH has the greatest sensitivity of the four clinical signs, but the least specificity for detection of BV.

Vaginal malodor is the most common symptom of women with BV. Release of "fishy" amines from the vaginal fluid after addition of 10% KOH (the "whiff test") greatly increases detection of this sign in BV. A drop of vaginal fluid should be placed on a glass slide and a drop of KOH added. The amines are released immediately, and the odor dissipates quickly. A cover slip may be placed over this preparation for microscopic exam of hyphal forms associated with candidiasis.

Clue cells are squamous vaginal epithelial cells which are covered with vaginal bacteria, giving them a stippled or granular appearance (Fig. 21-1). The borders are obscured or fuzzy due to adherence of the many small bacterial forms (*Gardnerella, Mobiluncus,* and others). Although lactobacilli in the normal vagina can bind to epithelial cells, they seldom do so in high enough concentration to create the fuzzy border. Clue cells are found by mixing a sample of vaginal fluid with a drop of normal saline on a glass slide. Ten fields of this suspension should be examined under high power (400×). We recommend that at least 20 percent of the vaginal epithelial cells present be noted as clue cells to establish the diagnosis of BV. The

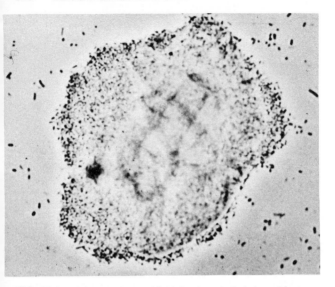

FIG. 21-1. Wet mount of vaginal fluid showing a typical clue cell from a woman with bacterial vaginosis. Note that the cell margins are obscured, × 1000 magnification.

presence of clue cells is the finding most closely associated with the diagnosis of BV by Gram stain.

LABORATORY TESTS FOR DIAGNOSIS OF BACTERIAL VAGINOSIS

The most useful confirmatory test for diagnosis of BV is the Gram-stained smear of vaginal fluid. A pathologic smear is defined as the presence of *Gardnerella* (small pleiomorphic, gram-negative rods) plus anaerobic bacterial morphotypes and no more than 5 lactobacillus morphotypes per oil-immersion field (Figs. 21-2 and 21-3). This method has been reported to have a sensitivity of 93 percent and a specificity of 79 percent. The vaginal smear for Gram-stain evaluation can be prepared at the same time that the wet mount is prepared by rolling (not streaking) the swab across the surface of a glass slide. The slide should be air-dried, heat-fixed, and stained as usual in the clinical lab. The advantages of Gram stain for diagnosis are that the smear can be interpreted using standardized criteria by a microbiolo-

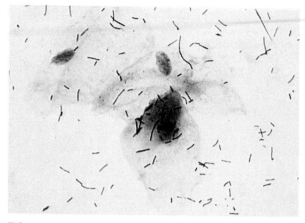

FIG. 21-2. Gram stain of normal vaginal fluid, showing gram-positive rods with blunt ends consistent with lactobacilli, × 1000 magnification.

gist, it is suitable for quick screening, and it can be stored for batch reading or later confirmation.

Culture of *G. vaginalis* has limited usefulness because although this organism can be recovered from almost all women with BV, it can also be recovered from more than half of women without other criteria for BV. Therefore, a positive vaginal culture for *G. vaginalis* in the absence of clinical signs of BV should not be used as a basis for therapy.

TREATMENT

Recommended Treatment

Metronidazole 500 mg orally, 2 times daily for 7 days, is recommended for treatment of nonpregnant women with BV. Though metronidazole is not active against *M. hominis* or *Mobiluncus*

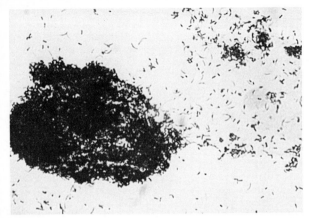

FIG. 21-3. Gram stain of vaginal fluid from a woman with bacterial vaginosis showing absence of lactobacilli and large numbers of gram-negative or gram-variable coccobacilli. Curved gram-variable rods are consistent with *Mobiluncus*. Note that epithelial cell on the left is a clue cell, while the epithelial cell to the right has clear margins, × 1000 magnification.

curtisii, metronidazole or its hydroxy metabolite is active against anaerobes and *G. vaginalis*.

Alternative Treatment

Clindamycin cream, 2%, 5g, intravaginally at bedtime for 7 days.
[*or*]
Metronidozole gel, 0.75%, 5g, intravaginally, 2 times a day for 5 days
[*or*]
Metronidazole, 2 g orally, once
Clindamycin 300 mg orally, 2 times daily for 7 days.
The penicillin agents are less effective than metronidazole against BV. This may be attributable not only to the poorer activity of penicillins against *Bacteroides* spp., but also to peni-

cillin's activity against the normal lactobacilli. Erythromycin and tetracycline are not effective. Other alternative therapies which are ineffective include acetic acid gel, sulfonamide-containing vaginal preparations, dienoestrol cream, and povidone-iodine vaginal tablets.

UNRESOLVED ISSUES IN PATIENT MANAGEMENT

Relapse rates for BV are as high as 80 percent within 9 months after therapy. It is not known why the relapse rate is so high but it may be related to reinfection by colonized male partners, failure to eradicate causative microorganisms which are inhibited but not killed, failure to establish normal vaginal flora, or persistence of an unidentified host susceptibility factor.

More research is needed concerning whether treatment of male partners would reduce rates of recurrence. Because placebo-controlled trials of treatment of male partners has usually not reduced the rate of recurrent BV, we do not recommend routine treatment of male partners.

Current over-the-counter preparations for recolonizing vaginal flora with *Lactobacillus* appear to be of little benefit. These include acidophilus milk, yogurt, or various *Lactobacillus*-containing capsules and powders. The commercial strains present in these products adhere poorly to vaginal epithelial cells and probably do not successfully colonize the vagina. Many of the products are also contaminated with other bacteria.

Other therapeutic questions concern treating asymptomatic and pregnant women with BV. Both issues require more information before a general recommendation can be made. Asymptomatic women with BV should be informed of their diagnosis, and treatment should be offered if requested. However, without information about whether bacterial vaginosis increases the risk of upper tract infection, it is impossible to recommend routine treatment for all asymptomatic women with BV. As mentioned earlier, pregnant women with BV may be at increased risk for certain adverse outcomes. However, before a recommendation to screen and treat all pregnant women with BV is made, carefully controlled trials must be conducted and must show benefit exceeding cost and risk of treatment. Currently, the decision whether to treat all pregnant women is left to the discretion of the patient and her clinician.

PREVENTION

Since the microbiological and host risk factors for acquisition of BV are poorly understood, it is difficult to design effective prevention strategies. Because BV is associated with sexual activity, abstinence or condom use may provide the best means of prevention.

ADDITIONAL READING

Barbone F et al: A follow-up study of methods of contraception, sexual activity, and rates of trichomoniasis, candidiasis, and bacterial vaginosis. *Am J Obstet Gynecol* 163:510, 1990

Cook RL et al: Clinical, microbiological, and biochemical factors in recurrent bacterial vaginosis. *J Clin Microbiol* 30:870, 1992

Fredricsson B et al: Could bacterial vaginosis be due to the competitive suppression of lactobacilli by aerobic microorganisms? *Gynecol Obstet Invest* 33:119, 1992

Hillier S et al: Microbiologic efficacy of intravaginal clindamycin cream for the treatment of bacterial vaginosis. *Obstet Gynecol* 76:407, 1990

Hillier SL et al: Microbiological, epidemiological and clinical correlates of vaginal colonization by *Mobiluncus* species. *Genitourin Med* 67:26, 1991

Hillier SL et al: The relationship of hydrogen peroxide–producing lactobacilli to bacterial vaginosis and genital microflora in pregnant women. *Obstet Gynecol* 79:369, 1992

Hillier SL et al: Characteristics of three vaginal flora patterns assessed by Gram stain among pregnant women. Vaginal Infections and Prematurity Study Group. *Am J Obstet Gynecol* 166:938, 1992

Joesoef MR et al: Reproducibility of a scoring system for Gram stain diagnosis of bacterial vaginosis. *J Clin Microbiol* 29:1730, 1991

Jones BM, Willcox LM: The susceptibility of organisms associated with bacterial vaginosis to spermicidal compounds, in vitro. *Genitourin Med* 67:475, 1991

Klebanoff SJ et al: Control of the microbial flora of the vagina by H_2O_2-generating lactobacilli. *J Infect Dis* 164:94, 1991

Larsson PG, Platz CJJ: Enumeration of clue cells in rehydrated air-dried vaginal wet smears for the diagnosis of bacterial vaginosis. *Obstet Gynecol* 76:727, 1990

Larsson PG et al: Is bacterial vaginosis a sexually transmitted disease? *Int J STD AIDS* 2:362, 1991

Moi H: Prevalence of bacterial vaginosis and its association with genital infections, inflammation, and contraceptive methods in women attending sexually transmitted disease and primary health clinics. *Int J STD AIDS* 1:86, 1990

Nugent RP et al: Reliability of diagnosing bacterial vaginosis is improved by a standardized method of Gram stain interpretation. *J Clin Microbiol* 29:297, 1991

Rotimi VO et al: Direct Gram's stain of vaginal discharge as a means of diagnosing bacterial vaginosis. *J Med Microbiol* 35:103, 1991

Schmitt C et al: Bacterial vaginosis: Treatment with clindamycin cream versus oral metronidazole. *Obstet Gynecol* 79:1020, 1992

Sheiness D et al: High levels of *Gardnerella vaginalis* detected with an oligonucleotide probe combined with elevated pH as a diagnostic indicator of bacterial vaginosis. *J Clin Microbiol* 30:642, 1992

Thomason JL et al: Bacterial vaginosis: Current review with indications for asymptomatic therapy. *Am J Obstet Gynecol* 165:1210, 1991

Watts DH et al: Bacterial vaginosis as a risk factor for post-cesarean endometritis. *Obstet Gynecol* 75:52, 1990

Watts DH et al: Upper genital tract isolates at delivery as predictors of post-cesarean infections among women receiving antibiotic prophylaxis. *Obstet Gynecol* 77:287, 1991

For a more detailed discussion, see Hillier S, Holmes KK: Bacterial Vaginosis, Chap. 47, p 547, in STD-2.

DEFINITIONS

Pelvic inflammatory disease (PID) is caused by ascending spread of microorganisms from the vagina or cervix to the endometrium, fallopian tubes, and/or contiguous structures. Thus, PID includes endometritis, parametritis, salpingitis, oophoritis, pelvic peritonitis, and tubal or tuboovarian abscess. (Figure 22-1 illustrates normal anatomy of the female pelvis.) The classic view of PID is that of an acute syndrome of low abdominal pain and adnexal tenderness. An emerging view is that ascending uterine infection may produce no symptoms, or only subtle symptoms and signs such as abnormal menses or uterine tenderness, in the absence of adnexal tenderness.

MICROBIAL ETIOLOGY

General Aspects

Most cases of PID are caused by *Neisseria gonorrhoeae* and/or *Chlamydia trachomatis.* In addition, certain bacteria which colonize the vagina—particularly those associated with bacterial vaginosis— cause some cases. Finally, no pathogen can be identified in up to 20 percent of all cases of clinical acute PID with laparoscopically documented tubal inflammation.

Neisseria Gonorrhoeae

Neisseria gonorrhoeae causes many cases of PID in populations with high incidence rates of gonorrhea (e.g., many developing countries, indigent urban U.S. populations), but causes few cases where gonorrhea is coming under control (most industrialized countries other than the United States). In the United States, gonorrhea has remained particularly common among young inner city women and continues to cause many cases of PID. Among women with cervical gonorrhea, 10 to 20 percent or more develop symptoms of acute PID.

Chlamydia Trachomatis

Chlamydia trachomatis is now established as an important cause of PID. Chlamydial PID has become far more common than gono-coccal PID in Europe and predominates among patients of middle to upper socioeconomic status with PID in the United States. Combined results from many European studies reveal that *C. trachomatis* is the causative agent in at least 60 percent of cases. However, in regions where chlamydia control programs have been initiated (e.g., Sweden and the Pacific northwest United States), the incidence of PID attributed to chlamydia has been declining.

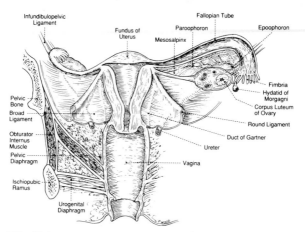

FIG. 22-1. Coronal section of pelvis illustrating broad ligament, endopelvic space, pelvic diaphragm, and urogenital diaphragm.

Mixed Infections with STD Agents

It is common to isolate more than one sexually transmitted pathogen from the lower genital tract of patients with PID. When both *N. gonorrhoeae* and *C. trachomatis* are isolated simultaneously from the cervix of a women with PID, it is difficult to know whether one or both organisms are present in the upper genital tract. Women with long-standing symptoms of PID, those with repeated episodes of PID, and women who develop PID while using an intrauterine device (IUD) are often found to have multiple organisms in the upper genital tract, pelvic cavity, and cul-de-sac. These organisms are often the same as those present in the vagina in bacterial vaginosis. They include facultative and anaerobic streptococci, *Mycoplasma hominis, Gardnerella vaginalis,* and vaginal *Bacteroides* species. In addition, facultative pathogens such as *Escherichia coli,* group B streptococci, or *Haemophilus influenzae* are found.

In rare instances, *Clostridia* and *Actinomyces* species or viruses such as coxsackievirus B5, echovirus 6, and herpes simplex virus type 2 (HSV-2) have been isolated from the genital tract of patients with PID. Group A streptococci are occasionally isolated. Parasitic causes include *Enterobius vermicularis, Trichomonas vaginalis, Schistosoma,* and the agents of filariasis. *Mycobacterium tuberculosis* is still an important cause of chronic pelvic infection in developing countries, but this form of PID is not considered in this chapter.

RISK FACTORS

Risk factors for PID can be divided into those which determine risk of acquiring sexually transmitted cervical or vaginal infections and those which determine the risk of infection ascending from the cervix or vagina into the endometrium and endosalpinx and causing PID.

Sexual Activity

The risk of acquiring an STD and, hence, an STD-associated PID, is correlated with the number of sexual partners. In women with only one sexual partner, the risk of PID is correlated with coital frequency. PID is rare in the celibate.

Age

Among sexually active women, the highest risk for developing PID is in those aged 15 to 19. If this age group is assigned a relative risk of 1, women aged 20 to 24 have a relative risk of 0.7, those aged 25 to 29 have a relative risk of 0.4, and those aged 30 to 34 have a relative risk of 0.2.

Contraception

Most available data indicate that (1) use of combined oral contraceptive pills decreases the risk that a lower genital tract infection, especially one caused by chlamydia, will ascend and cause PID, (2) use of oral contraceptives is associated with a milder course of PID, (3) use of an IUD increases the risk of PID, especially during the first few weeks after insertion, (4) tubal ligation greatly decreases the risk of salpingitis, and (5) use of condoms, diaphragms with spermicide, or sponges containing nonoxynol-9 reduces risk of acquiring an STD and subsequent PID.

Vaginal Douching

Vaginal douching is associated with about a twofold increase in the risk of PID.

Iatrogenic PID

Operative procedures such as cervical dilatations, curettage, tubal insufflation, hysterosalpingography, IUD insertion, and legal abortion have been associated with about 10 percent of PID cases. A reduced rate of postoperative PID has been observed after prophylaxis with doxycycline.

Repeated Infections

Up to one-third of women who have had one episode of PID suffer from repeated bouts. Among young women, the second and subsequent episodes of PID are often not STD-associated. A second episode usually appears within one year of the first.

Postpartum Infection

Intrapartum gonorrhea and chlamydial infection, and possibly bacterial vaginosis as well, are risk factors for postpartum endometritis and secondary infertility (infertility which follows childbearing). The risk of postpartum endometritis is greatly increased following Cesarean section.

CLINICAL MANIFESTATIONS AND DIAGNOSIS

General

The diagnosis of acute PID is usually made on the basis of clinical criteria and results of laboratory procedures. Conventional criteria for clinical diagnosis include lower abdominal pain with bilateral adnexal and cervical motion tenderness. Additional criteria useful for diagnosis of PID include purulent cervical or vaginal discharge, oral temperature greater than 38°C, increased erythrocyte sedimentation rate (ESR) or levels of C-reactive protein, and evidence of cervical infection with *N. gonorrhoeae* or *C. trachomatis*. The presence of one or more of these findings increases the probability of the diagnosis of PID, but some women with salpingitis lack all these findings. Furthermore, there is some evidence that a substantial subset of women with PID, especially those with endometritis, but no salpingitis, may lack some of the classic symptoms and adnexal signs. Endometritis can be suspected when abdominal pain or menometrorrhagia are present with signs of mucopurulent cervicitis and uterine tenderness. More definitive diagnosis depends on laparoscopy, histopathologic evidence on endometrial biopsy, and tuboovarian abscess on sonography. Cervical culture for *N. gonorrhoeae* and a culture or nonculture test for *C. trachomatis* should be performed on all women with suspected PID; demonstration of either infection supports the clinical diagnosis. Clinically, acute PID can vary from asymptomatic to a life-threatening condition, but the majority of patients with PID are not considered seriously ill at presentation.

Symptoms

See Table 22-1. The pain associated with PID is usually dull and subacute in onset. Pain is located in the low abdomen or pelvis and

TABLE 22-1. Correlation of Clinical and Laboratory Abnormalities with Laparoscopic Findings in 2220 Cases Given a Clinical Diagnosis of Acute Salpingitis

Clinical and laboratory abnormalities	Laparoscopic diagnosis		Percentage of women with salpingitis presenting the symptoms or signs
	Salpingitis, %	Normal or other %	
Low abdominal pain *plus* signs of an LGTI* *plus* motion tenderness	61	39	16
As above plus one or more of the following: ESR ≥ 15 mm/h; temperature > 38.0°C; palpable adnexal mass:			
+ Plus one of the above abnormalities	78	22	28
+ Plus two of the above abnormalities	90	10	39
+ Plus all three abnormalities	96	4	17

*LGTI = lower genital tract infection, as defined by the presence of inflammatory cells outnumbering other cellular elements on wet mount examination of vaginal fluid.

SOURCE: WHO Scientific Group, *WHO Tech Rep Ser* 660:95, 1981.

typically but not invariably bilateral. It tends to begin within 1 week of the first menstrual day when PID is caused by chlamydia or gonorrhea but is often premenstrual in other cases. Brief duration of abdominal pain (fewer than 3 days) has been associated with gonococcal PID, while symptoms of abdominal pain may be milder and tolerated for a longer period before seeking care when PID is caused by chlamydia.

Menorrhagia or metrorrhagia are commonly reported in PID and are probably attributable to endometritis. Dysuria occurs in about one-fifth of patients with PID and is presumably related to urethral infection by chlamydia or gonococci. Only about half of the patients with PID actually notice an increased or changed vaginal discharge.

Nausea and vomiting are infrequent unless peritonitis is present or PID is of long duration. In one study, 7 percent of patients described symptoms of proctitis such as frequent stools and/or passage of mucus. Dyspareunia is common. Pleuritic pain or tenderness in the right upper quadrant, attributable to perihepatitis in some cases, occurs in about 5 percent and could mislead the clinician to pursue a diagnosis of cholecystitis or pleuritis.

These various symptoms can occur among patients with normal laparoscopic examinations. However, when considering differential diagnoses such as appendicitis, tubal pregnancy, urinary tract infection, or proctocolitis, it is useful to be aware that such symptoms are consistent with PID.

Physical Examination and Readily Available Laboratory Tests

Mucopurulent Cervicitis

PID often results from ascending cervical infection by *N. gonorrhoeae* or *C. trachomatis;* uterine infection by these organisms often produces cervicitis, as well as endometritis and salpingitis. Careful inspection of the cervix usually (about 80 percent of confirmed PID cases) reveals yellow endocervical exudate (if the patient is not still menstruating). Microscopic examination of Gram-stained endocervical exudate usually shows greater than 30 neutrophils per $1000\times$ oil-immersion field within strands of cervical mucus. Gram-negative diplococci can be identified intracellularly within neutrophils or extracellularly within the mucus in about 50 percent of cervical mucus specimens from women with gonococcal PID. Since cervical exudate eventually mixes with vaginal fluid, it is also possible to enumerate neutrophils in vaginal fluid (even when the patient is menstruating); if neutrophils outnumber the polygonal vaginal epithelial cells, the diagnosis of cervicitis is supported (although trichomoniasis also causes purulent vaginal exudate). Because bacterial vaginosis is regarded as a risk factor for PID, it is possible that detecting bacterial vaginosis would support the clinical diagnosis of PID. However, this has not yet been ascertained.

Adnexal Swelling

Adnexal swelling is palpable in about 50 percent of women with laparoscopically confirmed salpingitis. Palpable swelling correlates with severity of salpingitis, but is not highly specific; in one large study, one-fourth of women with visually normal tubes at laparoscopy were considered by gynecologic experts to have adnexal swelling.

Fever, Leukocytosis, and Acute-Phase Reactants

The presence of fever, leukocytosis, and elevation of acute-phase reactants is more common with PID than with uncomplicated gonococcal or chlamydial infection. However, they are relatively insensitive predictors of upper tract infection. Furthermore, in women with abdominal pain they do not differentiate PID from other diagnoses, such as appendicitis or pyelonephritis.

Laparoscopy reveals salpingitis in 6 of 10 women meeting the criteria of lower abdominal, bilateral adnexal, and cervical motion tenderness. Though the probability of salpingitis increases with additional signs and symptoms of the disease, the classic picture of PID (low abdominal pain, pelvic tenderness, adnexal mass, fever, and elevated ESR) was present in only about 17 percent of patients with salpingitis in a classic Swedish study (Tables 22-1 and 22-2). Rectal temperature of more than 38°C is recorded in one-third of laparoscopically verified cases of salpingitis. Acute-phase reactants such as C-reactive protein are more common in patients with PID than in those with lower genital infection alone. The presence of an increased concentration of inflammatory cells in peritoneal fluid obtained by culdocentesis or laparoscopy supports the diagnosis of suspected PID, but these cells could result from blood contamination of the peritoneal fluid or from other causes of peritonitis.

Etiologic Diagnosis

It is often difficult to determine the microbial cause in the individual patient with PID because upper genital tract cultures require laparoscopy or endometrial aspiration, and because polymicrobial upper tract infection is common. Demonstration of *N. gonorrhoeae* or *C. trachomatis* in the cervix suggests but does not prove the presence of endometrial or tubal infections with the same pathogen in the patient with PID and does not exclude the presence of upper tract infections with vaginal microorganisms as well.

CONFIRMATORY DIAGNOSTIC PROCEDURES

Human Chorionic Gonadotropin

Before a diagnosis of PID is made, ectopic pregnancy must be ruled out by using a sensitive pregnancy test which detects human chorionic gonadotropin (HCG) in urine or blood. In women with unilateral adnexal findings and those who have missed a menstrual period, serum or urine β-HCG assay should be performed to exclude tubal pregnancy and avoid endometrial biopsy if there is an intrauterine pregnancy.

Laparoscopy

Laparoscopy is the gold standard for diagnosis of acute salpingitis and should be done when the case is ambiguous and differential diagnosis includes appendicitis, salpingitis, or ectopic pregnancy. For routine clinical diagnostic work, however, the expense and risks of laparoscopy must be considered. In very experienced hands the risks of laparoscopy are small. One large series describes 3000 procedures, no mortality, and three laparotomies, with all patients recovering uneventfully. In less experienced hands, risks are greater and the interpretation of laparoscopic findings may be less reliable.

TABLE 22-2. Percentage Prevalence of Symptoms, Signs, and Laboratory Abnormalities among 807 Women Subjected to Laparoscopy Because of Clinically Suspected Salpingitis; All Women Had (as Inclusion Criteria) Abdominal Pain, Adnexal Tenderness, and Objective Evidence of Purulent Vaginal Discharge

Symptoms	Laparoscopic diagnosis		Signs and laboratory abnormalities	Laparoscopic diagnosis	
	Salpingitis, %	No salpingitis, * %		Salpingitis, %	No salpingitis,† %
Abnormal discharge	55	51	Temperature > 38.0°C	41	20
Irregular bleeding	36	43	Palpable mass	49	25
Dysuria	19	20	ESR ≥ 15 mm/h	76	53
Vomiting	10	9	WBC > 10,000/ml blood†	59	33
Anorectal symptoms	7	3	Acute-phase reactants‡	79	24
			Decreased isoamylases§	90	20

*Normal intraperitoneal findings; assumed to have lower genital tract infection or endometritis.
†WBC was determined in 240 cases.
‡ Antichymotrypsin, orosomucoid, or acute-phase reactants including CRP, determined in 95 cases.
§Determined in peritoneal fluid in 95 cases.

SOURCE: Jacobson L, Westrom L, *Am J Obstet Gynecol* 105: 1088, 1969; Westrom L, *Diagnosis, Aetiology, and Prognosis of Acute Salpingitis* (Thesis). Lund, Sweden, Studentlitteratur, 1976; Svensson L et al, *Am J Obstet Gynecol* 138:1017, 1980.

The findings of redness and edema in the tubes may be mild and resemble normal changes seen at menstruation, but exudate is always pathologic and must be diligently sought. Cultures should be obtained during laparoscopy from the tubal mucosa, cul-de-sac exudate, or abscesses in order to determine the cause.

Endometrial Biopsy

Endometrial biopsies are abnormal in approximately 90 percent of those with laparoscopic evidence of salpingitis. In addition, up to one-third of women with suspected PID who have normal laparoscopic exams actually have histopathologic evidence of endometritis. Histopathologic criteria include the presence of plasma cells in the endometrial stromal tissue, together with neutrophils within the endometrial epithelium. In cases of chlamydial endometritis, immunocytochemical stains show chlamydial inclusions within endometrial epithelial cells.

Endovaginal Ultrasonography (EVUS)

Abdominal sonography is useful for detecting and following adnexal abscesses. Although this procedure has not proved useful for the diagnosis of less severe salpingitis, recent preliminary data suggest EVUS may be more useful. Criteria for the diagnosis of salpingitis by EVUS include (1) tubal dilation, (2) intratubal fluid, and (3) tubal wall thickening.

Clinical Syndromes in Relation to Etiologic Diagnosis

The clinical picture is of limited use in determining the cause of PID. However, gonorrhea-associated PID occurs most often in a young patient of lower socioeconomic status with short duration of abdominal pain. Findings often include fever and adnexal swelling.

Chlamydia-associated PID is most commonly seen in a young patient who seeks consultation after a longer (7 to 9 day) period of abdominal pain; she often appears well and is afebrile. The ESR is often elevated to 30 to 50 mm/h, but clinical findings may be unimpressive. Laparoscopy often reveals inflammation disproportionate to the clinical findings. Onset of abdominal pain during or immediately after menstrual bleeding is most consistent with gonococcal or chlamydial infection.

The patient with mixed infection is usually older, and it is often not her first infection. She is more likely to be an IUD user. Clinical course is variable, but she may be very ill and actually prostrate. Palpable adnexal swelling, febrile illness, and peripheral blood leukocytosis are common.

DIFFERENTIAL DIAGNOSIS

Confirmatory diagnostic procedures, discussed above, are necessary to definitively differentiate salpingitis from other pelvic problems (see Table 22-3). It is critical to promptly distinguish appendicitis and ectopic pregnancy from PID because both require urgent surgical intervention.

Acute appendicitis is usually associated with a shorter period of abdominal pain, more prominent gastrointestinal symptoms, and a greater likelihood of prostration. Pain is usually diffuse at the onset of illness and then shifts to the right lower quadrant. The ESR is more often normal. Nonetheless, at surgery, visualization of an inflamed appendix requires close scrutiny of nearby adnexal structures to ensure that the appendicitis is not secondary to a tubal infection.

THERAPY

Though PID is often a self-limited disease even without treatment, chronic infection, persistent or recurrent symptoms, and decreased fertility are common if the patient and her sexual partner are not treated appropriately. Women with severe infections should be treated in the hospital until the diagnosis is established and the patient is afebrile and improving. Outpatient treatment is probably best limited to compliant, parous women with mild to moderately severe disease. If treated at home, the patient should rest, avoid

TABLE 22-3. Differential Diagnosis of Acute Salpingitis: Erroneous Clinical and Laparoscopic Diagnoses

Clinical diagnosis salpingitis before laparoscopy		Laparoscopic diagnosis salpingitis	
Laparoscopic diagnosis, %		Clinical diagnosis before laparoscopy, %	
Acute salpingitis	65.4	Ovarian tumor	22.0
Normal findings	22.6	Acute appendicitis	19.8
Acute appendicitis	2.9	Ectopic pregnancy*	17.6
Pelvic endometriosis	2.0	"Chronic PID"	11.0
Corpus luteum bleeding	1.5	Acute peritonitis	6.6
Ectopic pregnancy*	1.4	Pelvic endometriosis	5.5
"Chronic PID"	0.7	Fibroids	5.5
Ovarian tumor	0.9	Unclear pelvic pain	5.5
Mesenteric lymphadenitis	0.7	Miscellaneous	6.5
Miscellaneous	1.9		

N = 814   *N* = 91

*Study performed 1960–1967.
SOURCE: Jacobson L, Westrom L, *Am J Obstet Gynecol 105:* 1088, 1969.

coitus, and record body temperature twice a day. Follow-up pelvic examinations and ESR determinations can usually be limited to once a week. Monitoring wet mounts of the vagina can be helpful. Correct antibiotic treatment should lead to resolution within 14 days. It is imperative to examine and treat the patient's sexual partners. If the patient is using an IUD, it should be removed and contraceptive counseling should be given.

In most cases, antibiotic therapy is instituted before culture results are available. Patients who are severely ill, undergoing operative diagnosis, or unable to take oral medication reliably (e.g. because of nausea or poor anticipated compliance) should be started on parenteral therapy. There are two main options when initiating therapy:

(1) **Outpatient management:** Young women with mild or moderately severe infection most often have STD-associated PID, and therapy should be selected to eradicate *N. gonorrhoeae* and *C. trachomatis.* When the patients are treated as outpatients, the following antibiotics are recommended:
Cefoxitin 2.0 g IM with probenecid 1.0 g by mouth *or* **ceftriaxone 250 mg IM**
plus
Doxycycline 100 mg by mouth twice daily for 14 days.
Alternative outpatient regimen:
Ofloxacia, 400 mg orally 2 times a day for 14 days
plus
either clindamycin, 450 mg orally 4 times a day *or* **metronidazole 500 mg orally 2 times a day for 14 days**

(2) **Inpatient management:** Patients with severe infections (prostration, fever, and evidence of tuboovarian mass) often have PID caused by mixed anaerobic-facultative bacteria (with or without gonorrhea or chlamydial infection) and may require surgery. Treatment should be initiated immediately with one of the following regimens:
Cefoxitin 2.0 g IV four times a day *or* **cefotetan 2 g IV every 12 h**
plus
Doxycycline 100 mg IV twice a day.

Intravenous treatment should continue for at least 48 h after the patient improves, and it is followed by oral doxycycline 100 mg twice daily to complete 14 days of therapy. An alternative regimen is:
Clindamycin 900 mg IV every 8 h
plus
Gentamicin or tobramycin 2.0 mg/kg followed by 1.5 mg/kg 3 times a day parenterally in patients with normal renal function.

Intravenous therapy should be continued for at least 48 h after the patient improves. After the patient is discharged from the hospital, doxycycline 100 mg orally two times daily should be given to complete 14 days of therapy. Continuation of clindamycin 450 mg orally four times daily may be considered as an alternative to doxycycline, although doxycycline remains the treatment of choice for chlamydial disease.

Operative procedures are indicated for life-threatening disease, abscesses, and failure of conservative antimicrobial treatment. Diagnostic laparoscopy is contraindicated in patients for whom a laparotomy is clearly indicated.

PROGNOSIS

Mortality

Death is a rare outcome; fatality rates for PID are very low, about 6 per 100,000 in Sweden between 1970 and 1980 for women under 40. Rupture of a tuboovarian abscess with generalized peritonitis has had a mortality of 6 to 8 percent and is the most common cause of death.

Infertility

Current estimates attribute one-half to one-third of all infertility to STD-related PID. Infertility rates increase dramatically both with number of episodes of PID and with increasing age. One study revealed that after one episode of salpingitis, 11 percent of women became infertile from postsalpingitis damage. After two episodes, 23 percent were infertile, and after three or more episodes, 54 percent of women were unable to conceive. There is conflicting evidence as to whether certain pathogens are more implicated in the development of infertility, but *N. gonorrhoeae* and *C. trachomatis* appear to play a substantial role.

Chronic Abdominal Pain

Abdominal pain of greater than 6 months' duration led 18 percent of women to seek medical advice after an episode of PID in a large Swedish study. Chronic pain is more common among infertile women who have had multiple episodes of PID. Pelvic adhesions are the most common finding; pain sometimes responds to continuous progesterone or danazol therapy.

Ectopic (Tubal) Pregnancy

Risk factors for ectopic pregnancy are believed to be increased age, postinfection or postoperative tubal damage or other tubal abnormality, and the use of an IUD. It is estimated that women who have had PID have a seven- to tenfold increased risk for ectopic pregnancy compared with women who have never had the disease.

PREVENTION

As is evident from the above, acute PID is most often a complication of a sexually transmitted infection. The strategy for preventing the late sequelae of PID therefore must follow two main lines: (1) controlling PID-producing sexually transmitted infections, and (2) preventing lower genital infection from ascending to the upper genital tract. Prevention efforts must focus mainly on chlamydial infection and gonorrhea, especially the former. Examinations for chlamydial infection should be performed frequently on all high-risk persons of both sexes who undergo checkups, regardless of symptoms or findings. The use of condoms should be encouraged. Sexual partners of women with PID should be examined and treated; partners of young women with PID should be considered for treatment with a tetracycline, even if the woman is not found to have gonococcal or chlamydial infection.

Women at risk for gonococcal or chlamydial infection should be screened for cervical infection before operative or diagnostic procedures involving penetration of the cervical mucus barrier in order to prevent introduction of these organisms into the endometrium.

"ATYPICAL" PID

The term *atypical PID* has been used to refer to PID which does not cause acute abdominal pain. However, we believe that "atypical" PID may really be the most typical form of PID. As described above, most cases of uterine and tubal infection and inflammation may not cause abdominal pain sufficient to lead to a diagnosis of acute PID. Thus, most infertile women who have tubal adhesions do not report a prior history of PID. Histopathologic and morphologic examination of tubal biopsies from women with tubal infertility sometimes show no difference between those with and without history of PID. Retrospective serologic examination suggests that *N. gonorrhoeae* and chlamydia may play a role in the development of atypical PID and subsequent infertility and ectopic pregnancy.

Many IUD users have chronic endometritis and endosalpingitis; subclinical IUD-related salpingitis also appears to be a risk factor for tubal infertility.

The absence of abdominal pain in women with upper genital tract infection may be partly related to absence of peritonitis, but this hypothesis requires confirmation. Development of peritonitis may be related to the causal pathogen, size of the infecting inoculum, virulence of the pathogen, effectiveness of the host immune response, and patency of the fallopian tubes. Some hypothesize that oral contraceptive pills promote atypical presentations of PID, but further studies are needed to substantiate this theory.

FITZ-HUGH–CURTIS SYNDROME

Definition and Etiology

Fitz-Hugh–Curtis syndrome (FHC) consists of perihepatitis in the presence of salpingitis. The cause of FHC was originally believed to be *N. gonorrhoeae* alone. However, since the 1970s, both *C. trachomatis* and *N. gonorrhoeae* have been recognized as the major causes of this syndrome. Antibody titres to *C. trachomatis* are exceptionally high in FHC even when compared with those in patients with PID alone.

Pathogenesis

Factors predisposing to the development of FHC are not clear, and only 3 to 5 percent of women who develop salpingitis develop FHC syndrome. Some serologic evidence suggests that reinfection with a new serovariant of *C. trachomatis* may be a risk factor. Oral contraceptive use may reduce the risk of FHC.

The mechanism by which infection spreads from the pelvis to the surface of the liver is obscure. Three mechanisms are possible: (1) direct intraperitoneal spread, (2) lymphatic spread, and (3) hematogenous spread. Though some support can be found for any of these routes, no completely convincing evidence supports any one above the others.

Incidence

The frequency of perihepatitis among women with salpingitis depends upon the stringency of the criteria used to diagnose it. When the findings of right upper quadrant tenderness and/or hepatic enlargement and elevated levels of serum glutamine phosphotransferase are used to diagnose perihepatitis, FHC occurs in up to 20 percent of women with acute salpingitis. Using strict laparoscopic criteria, occurrence is about five percent.

Clinical Manifestations

A clinical diagnosis of perihepatitis should be suspected whenever a sexually active female presents with right upper quadrant pain. Gonococcal and chlamydial perihepatitis occur almost exclusively in women, although on rare occasions men have developed hepatitis with gonococcemia. Onset of upper quadrant pain, most commonly right-sided, can be sudden and dramatic, although it is typically less acute than with acute cholecystitis. Pain often radiates to the top of the shoulder, and less commonly the back. The pain is exacerbated by breathing, coughing, or movement of the torso. Symptoms of lower abdominal pain are often present, but upper abdominal pain is often so severe that the lower abdominal pain is frequently not mentioned by the patient, and the diagnosis of salpingitis may be overlooked unless a careful pelvic examination is performed. Other symptoms include findings such as fever, nausea, vomiting, increased vaginal discharge, menorrhagia, dysmenorrhea, or dyspareunia. In about 60 percent of cases, onset of upper and lower abdominal pain is simultaneous. In about 30 percent, lower abdominal pain precedes upper abdominal pain by up to 14 days. Upper abdominal pain precedes lower abdominal pain by up to 6 days in the remainder.

Diagnosis

Findings of salpingitis are present, including fever over 38°C in approximately 40 percent of patients. Signs of generalized peritonitis may also be present and may be so severe that it is impossible to localize pain to the hepatic area. When generalized peritoneal signs are not present, liver tenderness is usually appreciated.

Although slight elevations in the levels of bilirubin and serum enzymes occur in 25 to 50 percent of patients with perihepatitis, scleral icterus suggests other causes of hepatic disease. White blood cell count and sedimentation rate are elevated in about one-third. The chest x-ray may reveal a small pleural effusion. Occasionally perihepatitis causes nonfilling of the gall bladder on oral cholecystogram, making this test unreliable to distinguish between biliary disease and FHC syndrome. However, ultrasound examination of the biliary tree is normal in patients with FHC syndrome. Other laboratory findings are identical to those of salpingitis.

Successful endocervical culture of *N. gonorrhoeae* or *C. trachomatis* is useful and supports the diagnosis, but negative culture does not rule it out.

Laparoscopic examination of the liver and pelvis confirms the diagnosis.

Differential Diagnosis

Differential diagnosis is of great importance because of the gravity of many syndromes that present as upper quadrant pain. Perihepatitis most commonly simulates cholecystitis, but patients with FHC have an average age of 15 to 25 years; this is younger than the usual patient with gallstones. Viral hepatitis also can resemble FHC syndrome, and women with liver tenderness and liver enzyme elevations should be tested serologically for hepatitis A, B, and C as well as for mononucleosis. Other causes of right upper quadrant tenderness such as drug- and alcohol-related hepatitis, toxic shock syndrome, or hepatitis secondary to bacteremias should also be ruled out.

When pain is referred to the right shoulder and is pleuritic, pleuritis, pneumonia, or pleurodynia must also be considered. If posterior back pain is present, acute pyelonephritis or abscess should be excluded. Other diagnoses that may warrant consideration include perforated gastric or duodenal ulcer, and acute pancreatitis; liver or subdiaphragmatic abscess and other primary intraabdominal infections, such as appendicitis, also need to be excluded.

Treatment

Treatment is identical to that for PID. Acute pain should resolve rapidly with initiation of therapy. Occasionally, the course is complicated by development of right upper quadrant adhesions resulting in chronic pain which requires laparoscopic lysis for relief.

ADDITIONAL READING

Aral SO et al: Self-reported pelvic inflammatory disease in the United States, 1988. *JAMA* 266:2570, 1991

Bulas DI et al: Pelvic inflammatory disease in the adolescent: Comparison of transabdominal and transvaginal sonographic evaluation. *Radiology* 183:435, 1992

Centers for Disease Control: Pelvic inflammatory disease: Guidelines for prevention and management. *MMWR* 40:No.RR-5, 1991

Farley TM et al: Intrauterine devices and pelvic inflammatory disease: An international perspective. *Lancet* 339:785, 1992

Kiviat NB, et al: Endometrial histopathology in patients with culture-proved upper genital tract infection and laparoscopically diagnosed acute salpingitis. *Am J Surg Pathol* 14:167, 1990

Landers DV et al: Combination antimicrobial therapy in the treatment of acute pelvic inflammatory disease. *Am J Obstet Gynecol* 164:849, 1991

Larsson PG et al: Incidence of pelvic inflammatory disease after first-trimester legal abortion in women with bacterial vaginosis after treatment with metronidazole: A double-blind, randomized study. *Am J Obstet Gynecol* 166:100, 1992

Livengood CH 3 et al: Pelvic inflammatory disease: Findings during inpatient treatment of clinically severe, laparoscopy-documented disease. *Am J Obstet Gynecol* 166:519, 1992

Mueller BA et al: Risk factors for tubal infertility. Influence of history of prior pelvic inflammatory disease. *Sex Transm Dis* 19:28, 1992

Peterson HB et al: Pelvic inflammatory disease: Key treatment issues and options. *JAMA* 266:2605, 1991

Rolfs RT et al: Pelvic inflammatory disease: Trends in hospitalizations and office visits, 1979 through 1988. *Am J Obstet Gynecol* 166:983, 1992

Safrin S et al: Long-term sequelae of acute pelvic inflammatory disease. A retrospective cohort study. *Am J Obstet Gynecol* 166:1300, 1992

Washington AE, Katz P: Cost of and payment source for pelvic inflammatory disease. Trends and projections, 1983 through 2000. *JAMA* 266:2565, 1991

Washington AE et al: Preventing pelvic inflammatory disease. *JAMA* 266:2574, 1991

Washington AE et al: Assessing risk for pelvic inflammatory disease and its sequelae. *JAMA* 266:2581, 1991

Wolner-Hanssen P et al: Decreased risk of symptomatic chlamydial pelvic inflammatory disease associated with oral contraceptive use. *JAMA* 263:54, 1990

Wolner-Hanssen P et al: Association between vaginal douching and acute pelvic inflammatory disease. *JAMA* 263:1936, 1990

For a more detailed discussion, see Weström L, Mårdh P-A: Acute Pelvic Inflammatory Disease (PID), Chap. 49, p. 593; Wølner-Hanssen P, Kiviat NB, Holmes KK: Atypical Pelvic Inflammatory Disease: Subacute, Chronic, or Subclinical Upper Genital Tract Infection in Women, Chap. 50, p. 615; and Eschenbach D, Wølner-Hanssen: Fitz-Hugh–Curtis Syndrome, Chap. 51, p. 621, in STD-2.

DEFINITIONS

Urethritis, manifested by urethral discharge, dysuria, or itching at the end of the urethra, is the response of the urethra to inflammation of any cause. The characteristic physical finding is urethral discharge, and the pathognomonic confirmatory laboratory finding is an increased number of polymorphonuclear leukocytes (PMNs) on Gram stain of a urethral smear or in the sediment of the first-voided urine.

ETIOLOGY

The causes are listed in Table 23-1.

Neisseria Gonorrhoeae

Neisseria gonorrhoeae is well recognized as a cause of male urethritis (see Chap. 3). Two points deserve reemphasis. First, penicillin and tetracycline resistance is now common. Second, although most new cases of gonococcal urethritis (GU) are symptomatic, up to one-half of men in the community with GU found through contact tracing have no symptoms at all. The incidence of asymptomatic GU is low, but the prevalence is high because the asymptomatic patient does not seek treatment; symptomatic patients do seek treatment, which removes them from the population of infected persons. Asymptomatic men are likely to remain sexually active and to spread gonorrhea.

Chlamydia Trachomatis

Multiple types of evidence suggest that *Chlamydia trachomatis* is a major cause of nongonococcal urethritis (NGU) and postgonococcal urethritis (PGU). Chlamydia can be isolated from about 30 to 40 percent of men who have NGU, approximately 15 to 25 percent of men with GU, and 0 to 7 percent of men without obvious urethritis. Chlamydia is isolated from asymptomatic men more frequently than *N. gonorrhoeae*. Antibiotics which selectively eradicate chlamydia treat urethritis more effectively in men with NGU and documented chlamydia than in those with NGU who have no evidence of chlamydia. Those with chlamydial urethritis who are treated with a 7-day course of antichlamydial therapy have a 17 percent relapse rate within 6 weeks, while patients without chlamydia have a 47 percent relapse rate.

Postgonococcal Urethritis

PGU frequently develops in men who have concurrent chlamydial infections because the incubation period of gonorrhea is shorter

TABLE 23-1. Etiology of Sexually Transmitted Urethritis in Males

Gonococcal:
  Neisseria gonorrhoeae
Nongonococcal:
  Chlamydia trachomatis, 30–50%
  Ureaplasma urealyticum, 10–40%
  Neither, 20–30%
    Trichomonas vaginalis, rare
    Yeasts, rare
    Herpes simplex virus, rare
    Adenoviruses, rare
    Haemophilus spp., rare
    Bacteroides ureolyticus?
    Mycoplasma genitalium?
    Other bacterial?
    Other???

than the incubation period of chlamydia, and because the antimicrobials used to treat gonococcal urethritis often have no effect on chlamydial infections. The incidence of PGU can be lowered by treatment with an antibiotic such as tetracycline which has activity against chlamydia.

Etiology of *Chlamydia*-negative NGU

Ureaplasma urealyticum

The most likely cause of many *C. trachomatis*–negative NGU cases is *U. urealyticum.* Ureaplasma has been isolated frequently from these patients; many have been cured with antibiotics such as spectinomycin or streptomycin that are directed specifically against ureaplasma. Nevertheless, the importance of this organism in the pathogenesis of urethritis remains controversial.

Miscellaneous Bacteria

In 20 to 30 percent of heterosexual men with NGU and most homosexual men with NGU, neither *C. trachomatis* nor *U. urealyticum* is isolated. These patients respond poorly to tetracycline therapy. Bacteria implicated as etiologic agents in such infections include *Bacteroides ureolyticus* and *Mycoplasma genitalium. Haemophilus influenzae* and *H. parainfluenzae* are rare causes of urethritis. Coliforms may infrequently cause urethritis in homosexual men.

Viruses

Viruses associated with NGU include primary genital herpes simplex virus (HSV). Approximately 30 percent of men with primary infection have urethritis. Attempts to identify other viruses as agents of NGU have been either unsuccessful or inconsistent.

Parasites and Yeasts

Trichomonas vaginalis has been associated with a high proportion of NGU cases in the Soviet Union, India, Africa, and South America but not in most European countries or North America. Although patients with yeast balanitis have symptoms of urethritis, yeasts are not a common cause of NGU.

Nonsexually Transmitted Causes of NGU

Nonsexually transmitted bacterial urethritis may occur in association with urinary tract infection, bacterial prostatitis, urethral stricture, or phimosis, or secondary to catheterization or other instrumentation of the urethra. Urethritis has also been described with congenital abnormalities, chemical irritation, and tumors. There is no evidence to support repeated stripping of the penis, masturbation, use of caffeine or alcohol, too little or too much sexual activity, or eating of certain foods as causes of urethritis.

EPIDEMIOLOGY

The incidence of NGU is greater than that of GU, but infection rates vary among different populations. The proportion of male urethritis cases that are nongonococcal varies from about 20 to 80 percent among different STD clinics; on college campuses more than 85 percent of urethritis is nongonococcal. For both NGU and GU, the peak age group affected is 20 to 24 years, followed by 15 to 19 years, and then by 25 to 29 years old.

Although the characteristics of men with NGU and GU vary somewhat, the differences are not usually adequate to distinguish one from another on clinical grounds. Men with NGU are more often white, better educated, more apt to be students, and less likely to be employed. Histories of previous gonorrhea are more frequent among men with gonorrhea, whereas histories of past episodes of NGU are more common among men with NGU. There are no distinguishing features, however, that reliably separate *C. trachomatis*–negative NGU patients.

CLINICAL MANIFESTATIONS

Comparison between GU and NGU

The signs and symptoms of NGU and GU differ quantitatively, but not qualitatively, so it is impossible to distinguish between the two infections with certainty on purely clinical grounds. Both may cause discharge, dysuria, or urethral itching. Frequency, hematuria, and urgency are infrequent in either infection. Mucoid discharge is more common in NGU; purulent discharge is suggestive of GU. Discharge may be very slight, especially with NGU, and thus may only be detected in the morning or noted as crusting on the meatus or staining on underwear. Men with GU describe more abrupt onset of symptoms and are more apt to seek medical care. More than three-fourths of men with GU but less than one-half with NGU seek treatment within 4 days of symptoms. Gonococcal urethritis has a shorter incubation period and often develops within 2 to 6 days of exposure. NGU develops between 1 to 5 weeks after exposure, with a peak around 2 to 3 weeks. However, longer incubation periods for both infections are seen, and a significant proportion of both groups of men remain asymptomatic.

Men with urethritis caused by HSV usually have severe dysuria, profuse mucoid discharge, and localized tenderness at the site of focal urethral ulceration. Regional lymphadenopathy and constitutional symptoms are common with primary HSV urethritis but uncommon in other forms of urethritis.

Other Manifestations of Urethritis

Some patients with NGU present with Reiter's syndrome (see Chap. 27), or they develop it soon after their initial presentation. A small proportion of patients with GU or chlamydial urethritis have conjunctivitis due to these organisms, probably as a result of autoinoculation. Inguinal lymphadenopathy is unusual and should suggest the possibility of HSV infection. Hematuria, chills, fevers, frequency, hesitancy, nocturia, urgency, perineal pain, scrotal masses, postvoid dribbling, or genital pain other than dysuria or urethral pain are not typical of urethritis. These signs and symptoms suggest the presence of other genitourinary abnormalities, such as classic urinary tract infection, prostatitis, or acute epididymitis or orchitis.

Asymptomatic Urethral Infection

Although rates vary widely, asymptomatic infections with NGU and GU appear to be very common. As many as 50 percent of male partners of women infected with *C. trachomatis* or *N. gonorrhoeae* may have no symptoms at all. Therefore, if a female index case has cervicitis or pelvic inflammatory disease, has delivered a baby with a sexually transmitted disease, or has had a positive test for *C. trachomatis* or *N. gonorrhoeae,* the possibility of asymptomatic infection in a male partner should be evaluated.

DIAGNOSIS

Algorithms for diagnosis and management of men with suspected urethritis are presented in Fig. 23-1 and Table 23-2. Diagnosis of gonorrhea requires demonstration of *N. gonorrhoeae* by Gram stain,

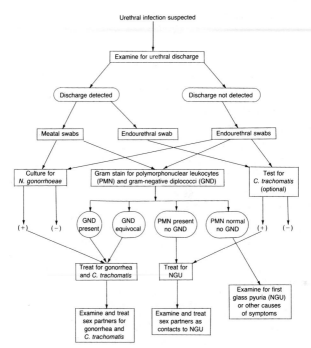

FIG. 23-1. Initial diagnosis and management in men with suspected urethritis.

culture, or a reliable nonculture technique. In contrast, the diagnosis of NGU requires not only exclusion of urethral infection with *N. gonorrhoeae* but also demonstration of urethritis. Distinction between *C. trachomatis* and *U. urealyticum* is difficult because there is no simple clinical or laboratory marker, and specific diagnostic tests are not always available.

Laboratory Differentiation between GU and NGU

Although clinical suspicion that a patient with urethritis has either GU or NGU may be strong, the final distinction requires laboratory examination to determine if *N. gonorrhoeae* is present. In the hands of an experienced microscopist, examination of Gram-stained urethral material for typical gram-negative intracellular diplococci is

TABLE 23-2. Management of Urethritis

1. Establish presence of urethritis
    a. Examine for urethral discharge
    b. Gram stain urethral discharge
    c. Examine first-voided urine if necessary
    d. Reexamine if necessary
2. Establish presence or absence of *N. gonorrhoeae*
    a. Gram stain
    b. Culture for *N. gonorrhoeae*
3. Diagnostic test for *C. trachomatis* (optional)
4. If gonorrhea, treat with
    a. Single-dose ceftriaxone 125 mg IM *plus*
    b. Doxycycline 100 mg p.o. twice daily for 7 days
5. If NGU, treat with 7 days of doxycycline 100 mg p.o. twice daily
6. Treat partner(s) appropriately
7. Follow-up examinations (optional)
    a. 3–5 days after completing therapy for gonorrhea
    b. 2–4 weeks after completing therapy for NGU

both sensitive and specific for the diagnosis of GU. The presence of greater than or equal to five polymorphonuclear leukocytes (PMNs) per oil-immersion field, with no evidence of gram-negative diplococci, is sufficient to diagnose NGU.

Cultures are necessary when inadequate expertise is available to immediately evaluate the Gram stain or when stains are interpreted as equivocal because only typical extracellular or atypical intracellular diplococci are present. Cultures should also be done when prior treatment has failed; when penicillinase-producing *N. gonorrhoeae*, tetracycline-resistant *N. gonorrhoeae*, or *N. gonorrhoeae* with chromosomally mediated resistance are suspected or prevalent in the community; or when one is testing for a cure. A strong argument can be made for performing a culture in all men with urethritis so that if *N. gonorrhoeae* is isolated, its susceptibility to tetracycline and penicillin can be evaluated. In current practice, however, cultures are performed infrequently in men because therapy with ceftriaxone or similar antimicrobial agents is so highly effective, even for penicillin-resistant strains.

Men who are symptomatic without objective evidence of urethritis should be examined in the morning without having voided overnight. The urethra should be stripped from the base to the meatus three to four times to detect urethral discharge. If the urethral Gram stain contains no PMNs or intracellular diplococci, 10 to 15 ml of the first-voided urine should be collected, centrifuged for 10 min, and examined for PMNs. Urinary PMNs are diagnostic of NGU when seen in men who have symptoms of urethritis but no evidence of *N. gonorrhoeae*.

THERAPY

Uncomplicated Gonococcal Urethritis

Chapter 3 describes recommended regimens, management of sex partners, and evaluation and management of treatment failures.

Treatment of NGU

Although there are many studies of NGU therapy, the optimal drug, dosage, and duration of therapy are unknown.

Recommended regimen: Doxycycline 100 mg orally 2 times a day for 7 days *or* azithromycin 1g orally, once.

Doxycycline is less expensive than azithromycin and has a long history of safety and efficacy. Azithromycin's major advantage is its simple dose administration, which may increase compliance with therapy.

Alternative regimen: Erythromycin base 500 mg orally 4 times a day or equivalent salt for 7 days *or* erythromycin ethylsuccinate 800 mg orally 4 times a day for 7 days.

If high-dose erythromycin regimens are not tolerated, the following regimen is recommended: erythromycin ethylsuccinate 400 mg orally 4 times a day for 14 days or erythromycin base 250 mg orally 4 times a day or equivalent salt for 14 days.

Erythromycin stearate 500 mg twice daily for 2 weeks is effective and probably also cures infection when given for only 7 days. The same medication given in a 250-mg dose for 7 days does not eradicate *C. trachomatis* in one-third of culture-positive men.

Trimethoprim-sulfamethoxazole is active but not synergistic against *C. trachomatis* and has no activity against *U. urealyticum.* Some of the new quinolones, especially ofloxacin, appear to be promising agents for the treatment of NGU. Ciprofloxacin, however, has been associated with relapse of infection.

After 1 week of doxycycline therapy, all but about 5 percent of compliant patients who are not reexposed to new or untreated partners will show definite and often total improvement by the end of therapy. However, if followed for 4 to 6 weeks, 30 to 35 percent of the initial responders will have recurrent or persistent pyuria, and about one-half of these men will have symptoms of urethritis. A positive follow-up culture in this situation may reflect either a false-positive result, a new infection, or noncompliance.

Treatment of Sexual Partners

As with other STDs, every effort should be made to evaluate and treat sexual partner(s). Although no one has demonstrated a decreased recurrence rate in male index cases through such therapy, female partners need treatment for their own benefit. *Chlamydia trachomatis* has been isolated from 30 to 60 percent of the female partners of men with GU or NGU. In general, the same regimens used to treat males with urethritis can be used to treat their female partners.

Management of Recurrent or Persistent NGU

Management of recurrent or persistent NGU is a difficult problem. The median time for recurrences is about 2 weeks after completion of therapy. Most are culture-negative for *C. trachomatis* and *U. urealyticum.* The first step in the evaluation is to ensure that the patient has complied with the course of therapy and not had any new genital contacts, and that the original sexual partner has been evaluated and treated. If an exudate is present, a drop should be mixed with saline to evaluate for *T. vaginalis,* and another drop should be mixed with 10% potassium hydroxide to look for yeast. Urethritis that has persisted and never resolved suggests HSV urethritis, which often lasts 2 weeks during the primary infection. Urethral foreign bodies and periurethral fistula or abscess should be excluded by palpation. Cultures for *N. gonorrhoeae* and *C. trachomatis* should be repeated at least once.

No standard guidelines for retreatment can be offered, since the cause of recurrent NGU is usually unknown and since repeated courses of antibiotics are often unsuccessful. Because tetracycline-resistant *U. urealyticum* is a cause of persistent urethritis, treatment with a 1- to 2-week course of erythromycin 500 mg four times daily is reasonable if no other cause is found.

About 30 percent of men will have recurrent symptoms after the second course of treatment. However, unless reinfection is a possibility or urethritis is severe, further antibiotics should be avoided. If the patient has florid urethral discharge or if symptomatic disease is prolonged and no cause is determined, treatment with a 4- to 6-week course with one of the following is often administered: tetracycline 500 mg four times daily, doxycycline 100 mg twice a day, or erythromycin 500 mg four times daily. It is not known whether a prolonged course of therapy improves ultimate outcome; most men will improve on this regimen, but some will have recurrent symptoms.

The patient should be given the following information:

1. Long-term sequelae such as infertility or cancer appear to be uncommon—even in men who have recurrent urethritis after both therapies.
2. The risk of transmission to women in the absence of *C. trachomatis* infection is low.
3. Even if no treatment were given, symptoms would probably disappear over time in most men with NGU.

4. In an ongoing monogamous sexual relationship, there is no need for further treatment of partners if both have completed initial therapy active against *C. trachomatis.*
5. Most recurrences arise independently of resumption of sexual activity, and these recurrences do not mean that the partner has been unfaithful.
6. Persistent urethritis is not a presentation of AIDS.
7. One episode of NGU does not provide immunity to future episodes.

Finally, the patient with atypical features, frequent recurrences, or persistent urethritis unresponsive to antibiotics should undergo microbiological studies to detect prostatic infection. If no pathogen is found, assessment of urine flow, urethrography and, if necessary, urethroscopy should be done to detect strictures, foreign bodies, or intraurethral lesions. Any patient with a history of concurrent or past genital warts should definitely undergo such evaluation.

PROGNOSIS

Complications of GU were frequent in the preantibiotic era and are now rare in developed countries. These include epididymitis, urethral strictures, seminal vesiculitis, prostatitis, prostatic abscess, disseminated gonococcal infection, and other less common complications.

NGU is usually a self-limited disease, and even without therapy physical consequences to the individual are usually slight. One to 2 percent of both *C. trachomatis*–positive and *C. trachomatis*–negative males develop epididymitis, and another 1 to 2 percent develop conjunctivitis. Urethritis is a manifestation of Reiter's syndrome, but it is unclear how frequently Reiter's syndrome develops as a consequence of NGU.

PREVENTION

Preventive measures are similar to those for other STDs. Patients and their partners must be identified and treated adequately. An individual should be advised to select his partner carefully and use a condom. Increased availability of adequate diagnostic facilities, especially for *C. trachomatis,* would also be useful.

ADDITIONAL READING

Handsfield HH, et al: A comparison of single-dose cefixime with ceftriaxone as treatment for uncomplicated gonorrhea. *N Engl J Med* 325:1337, 1991

Hay PE, et al: The value of urine samples from men with non-gonococcal urethritis for the detection of *Chlamydia trachomatis. Genitourin Med* 67:124, 1991

Hooton TM, et al: Ciprofloxacin compared with doxycycline for nongonococcal urethritis. Ineffectiveness against *Chlamydia trachomatis* due to relapsing infection. *JAMA* 264:1418, 1990

Hooton TM, et al: Erythromycin for persistent or recurrent nongonococcal urethritis. A randomized, placebo-controlled trial. *Ann Intern Med* 113:21, 1990

Kitchen VS, et al: Comparison of ofloxacin with doxycycline in the treatment of non-gonococcal urethritis and cervical chlamydial infection. *J Antimicrob Chemother* 26 Suppl D:99, 1990

Mclean KA, et al: Postgonococcal urethritis: A double-blind study of doxycycline vs placebo. *Genitourin Med* 66:20, 1990

Mitchell SA, et al: Aetiology of non-gonococcal urethritis: A possible relation to other infections. *Int J STD AIDS* 1:429, 1990

Mogabgab WJ: Single-dose oral temafloxacin versus parenteral ceftriaxone in the treatment of gonococcal urethritis/cervicitis. *Am J Med* 91:145S, 1991

Palmer HM, et al: Detection of *Chlamydia trachomatis* by the polymerase chain reaction in swabs and urine from men with non-gonococcal urethritis. *J Clin Pathol* 44:321, 1991

Segreti J: Fluoroquinolones for the treatment of nongonococcal urethritis/cervicitis. *Am J Med* 91:150S, 1991

Sellors J, et al: Rapid, on-site diagnosis of chlamydial urethritis in men by detection of antigens in urethral swabs and urine. *J Clin Microbiol* 29:407, 1991

Stamm WE: Azithromycin in the treatment of uncomplicated genital chlamydial infections. *Am J Med* 91:19S, 1991

Terry PM, et al: Diagnosing non-gonococcal urethritis: The gram–stained urethral smear in perspective. *Int J STD AIDS* 2:272, 1991

Whatley JD, et al: Azithromycin vs doxycycline in the treatment of non-gonococcal urethritis. *Int J STD AIDS* 2:248, 1991

Woolley PD, et al: Microbiological flora in men with non-gonococcal urethritis with particular reference to anaerobic bacteria. *Int J STD AIDS* 1:122, 1990

For a more detailed discussion, see Bowie WR: Urethritis in Males, Chap. 52, p 627, in STD 2.

The epididymis is a sausage-shaped organ on the posterior-inferior aspect of the testicle (Fig. 24-1). Inflammation of the epididymis causes pain and swelling which is almost always unilateral. Most cases of epididymitis are infectious, and sexually transmitted urethritis is often a precursor. Epididymitis can be a complication of gonococcal or chlamydial urethritis, or of genitourinary infection with enteric gram-negative rods or *Pseudomonas aeruginosa.* It occasionally occurs as a result of systemic infection such as tuberculosis. Because different pathogens require different therapies, every effort should be made to arrive at an accurate diagnosis. The term *nonspecific epididymitis* should be avoided; *idiopathic epididymitis* describes those cases for which no etiologic agent can be determined after a careful search.

EPIDEMIOLOGY AND ETIOLOGY

See Table 24-1 for a summary. In prepubertal boys with structural or neurologic abnormalities, epididymitis is frequently associated with coliform or *Pseudomonas* infection of the genitourinary tract. In adolescents with epididymitis, the level of sexual activity should be determined because sexually transmitted pathogens, especially *Neisseria gonorrhoeae* and *Chlamydia trachomatis,* may be important agents in these patients.

Among heterosexual males less than 35 years of age, epididymitis caused by coliforms or *P. aeruginosa* is unusual. The low prevalence of these organisms in this age group is probably due to low rates of structural abnormalities, such as prostatic hypertrophy, which predispose men to development of urinary tract infections. Coliform organisms cause epididymitis more often among homosexuals than heterosexuals; this may be related to exposure of the urethra to pathogenic enteric bacteria during anal-insertive intercourse.

Sexually transmitted organisms are the most common cause of epididymitis in heterosexual men under the age of 35. During the past 2 decades, studies in the United States and United Kingdom have revealed that *N. gonorrhoeae* caused about one-quarter, and *C. trachomatis* about one-half, of cases in this age group.

Characteristically, patients with epididymitis due to *N. gonorrhoeae* or *C. trachomatis* are young, are sexually active with multiple partners, and have no underlying urinary tract abnormalities. Symptoms of urethritis may be absent. Nonetheless, even in patients without symptoms of urethritis, it is sometimes possible to express a urethral discharge. Urinalysis may reveal pyuria, or a Gram-stained smear of an endourethral swab specimen may reveal greater than or equal to five polymorphonuclear cells per 1000× field.

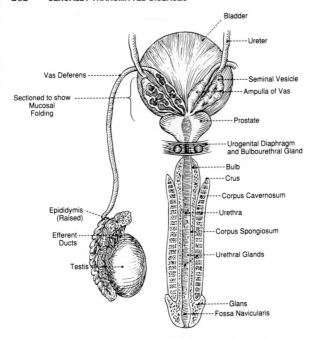

FIG. 24-1. Coronal section of male pelvis and urethra viewed posteriorly.

In contrast, up to 80 percent of epididymitis cases in men over 35 years of age are caused by coliform bacteria or *P. aeruginosa* urinary tract infections. This is probably due to the decreasing incidence of sexually transmitted diseases and an increased incidence of instrumentation or acquired genitourinary abnormalities, such as prostatic calculi, neurogenic bladder, benign prostatic hypertrophy, or chronic bacterial prostatitis.

Miscellaneous Causes of Epididymitis

Uncommon causes of epididymitis include systemic tuberculosis; nonenteric bacterial pathogens such as *Streptococcus pneumoniae*, *Brucella*, *N. meningitidis*, *Treponema pallidum*, and others that are believed to infect the organ by hematogenous spread; or fungi (as a manifestation of disseminated fungal infection). Interestingly, the antiarrhythmic drug amiodarone can cause epididymitis as a side effect.

TABLE 24-1. Microbial Etiology and Predisposing Factors in Acute Epididymitis

Prepubertal boys
Usual cause: Coliforms, *P. aeruginosa* *Unusual cause:* Hematogenous spread from primary infected site *Predisposing factors:* Underlying genitourinary abnormality

Men under 35
Usual cause: C. trachomatis, N. gonorrhoeae *Unusual cause:* Coliform or *P. aeruginosa*, *Mycobacterium tuberculosis* *Predisposing factors:* Sexually transmitted urethritis

Men over 35
Usual cause: Coliforms or *P. aeruginosa* *Unusual cause: N. gonorrhoeae, C. trachomatis, M. tuberculosis* *Predisposing factors:* Underlying structural abnormality or chronic bacterial prostatitis

CLINICAL MANIFESTATIONS AND DIAGNOSIS

In the patient with epididymitis secondary to coliform or *Pseudomonas* bacteriuria, the clinical history can suggest a urinary tract abnormality. The parents of infants whose presentation is suggestive of epididymitis should be asked whether any siblings have had similar problems, whether the quality of the urinary stream has changed, or whether hematuria is present. Adults may give a history of decreasing urinary stream, urinary tract surgery, or previous urinary tract infections. The patient with epididymitis secondary to a sexually transmitted disease often provides a history of urethral discharge or recent sexual exposure. Patients with tubercular epididymitis often have a history of tuberculosis or of exposure to TB.

Onset of scrotal pain is rapid in one-third of patients and more gradual in two-thirds. A history of lifting or straining prior to onset of pain is not helpful in differentiating epididymitis from other intrascrotal conditions. In addition to severe scrotal pain, the patient may complain of inguinal pain. A massively swollen spermatic cord can obstruct the ureter upon crossing it and cause flank pain.

On physical examination, the scrotum on the involved side is often red and edematous. The tail of the epididymis, which connects to the vas deferens near the lower pole of the testes, typically becomes swollen first, and swelling then spreads to the head of the epididymis near the upper pole of the testes. The groove between the epididymis and the testicle should be examined, as this can reveal whether swelling is greater in the testicle or the epididymis. However, progressive inflammation can obliterate this groove. The spermatic cord is often swollen and tender. Urethral discharge may be present in the patient who has not voided recently, but asymptomatic urethral infection without discharge is common. If no spontaneous discharge is noted, the urethra should be stripped and examined again. Digital rectal exam may reveal abnormalities suggesting prostatitis.

Gram stain of a urethral swab specimen can diagnose urethritis and establish with a high degree of certainty whether its cause is gonococcal or nongonococcal. Visualization of an average of at least five neutrophils per 1000× field in three areas of the slide containing the highest concentration of neutrophils suggests urethritis. First-voided and midstream urine specimens should be examined for bacteria and white cells. A Gram stain of one drop of unspun midstream urine may be helpful in diagnosis of bacteriuria: greater than or equal to one gram-negative rod per oil-immersion field correlates with the presence of greater than 100,000 bacteria per milliliter of urine. A quantitative midstream urine sample should be examined for urinary tract pathogens. Urethral swab specimens should be cultured for *N. gonorrhoeae* and tested for *C. trachomatis.*

Difficult cases may require needle aspiration of the epididymis to obtain cultures. This procedure, performed after regional anesthesia, can be useful in patients with indwelling urethral catheters, therapeutic failure, epididymitis found on surgical exploration for testicular torsion, or recurrent epididymitis of uncertain etiology.

Differential Diagnosis of Acute Epididymitis

See algorithm on Fig. 24-2. Acute epididymitis must always be differentiated from torsion of the testicle. In infants and prepubertal boys, torsion is far more common than acute epididymitis. Torsion is a surgical emergency; any acute swelling of the testes in a young male is due to this complication until proved otherwise. Among males over 18 years, however, epididymitis is more common.

Certain features can help distinguish torsion from infection. A history of previous scrotal pain suggests torsion, due to earlier intermittent torsion. History of trauma or exertion prior to the onset of pain may occur with either torsion or epididymitis. More patients with torsion exhibit swelling of the testes, whereas swelling of the epididymis alone is more common with infection. Nonetheless, scrotal swelling may be extensive in late epididymitis, and differences on physical exam are helpful but not completely reliable. If palpation of the uninvolved testicle reveals that the epididymis is anterior, torsion is likely because it suggests a congenital abnormality predisposing to this event. In torsion the testicle is often high in the scrotum, but the testicle rides in a normal position when infected. In epididymitis, the cord in the inguinal canal may be quite tender, whereas in torsion tenderness is often limited to the scrotal contents.

Examination of the urine and urethral smear is invaluable in distinguishing torsion from epididymitis. The first-voided specimen of urine should be examined. Pyuria occurs in patients with epididymitis but not with torsion; in the absence of pyuria, immediate surgical evaluation should proceed.

Diagnostic tools may distinguish torsion from epididymitis. The Doppler stethoscope shows decreased blood flow during torsion and increased blood flow in the presence of epididymal inflammation. Interpreting results requires skill; false positives and false negatives occur in the presence of hydroceles, late torsion, retracted scroti, and testicular tumor.

Unless torsion of the testicle can unequivocally be ruled out, the scrotum should be explored emergently. After 4 h of torsion there is a significant risk of irreversible testicular infarction. Finally, epididymitis and torsion can occur together; when any doubt exists, immediate surgery should be performed.

Testicular carcinoma is another condition which may be difficult to differentiate from epididymitis. The peak age of incidence for both is between the ages of 18 and 32, and approximately one-quarter of patients with carcinoma have pain as the presenting complaint. A testicular tumor can invade the epididymis and mimic physical findings of epididymitis. However, in testicular tumors, the urine and urethral smear should show no evidence of inflammation. When a man being treated for epididymitis fails to improve after a course of therapy, surgical exploration should be seriously considered to rule out carcinoma.

In summary, the differential diagnosis of epididymitis includes the "four t's": torsion, tumor, trauma, and tuberculosis or other chronic infections. Table 24-2 outlines other common conditions which should be considered in differential diagnosis.

COMPLICATIONS OF ACUTE EPIDIDYMITIS

The use of antibiotics to treat epididymitis has greatly reduced the incidence of surgical complications. Sequelae requiring surgery include abscess formation and testicular infarction. Infarction probably results from thrombosis of the spermatic vessels secondary to severe inflammation; gangrene of the testicle may result while the epididymis remains viable. Abscess formation is a complication requiring surgical drainage and often orchiectomy. Failure of the patient to improve with appropriate bed rest and antibiotic therapy suggests development of these complications. Hydrocele may also develop in as many as 8 percent of patients treated for epididymitis.

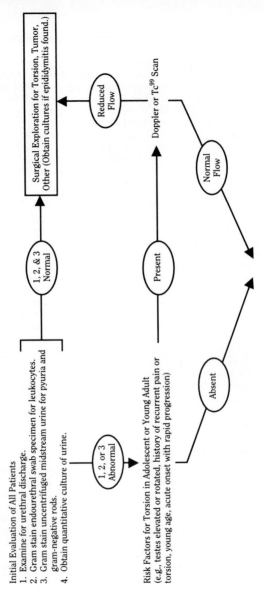

FIG. 24-2 Algorithm for the management of acute unilateral intrascrotal pain.

Initial Evaluation of All Patients
1. Examine for urethral discharge.
2. Gram stain endourethral swab specimen for leukocytes.
3. Gram stain uncentrifuged midstream urine for pyuria and gram-negative rods.
4. Obtain quantitative culture of urine.

Risk Factors for Torsion in Adolescent or Young Adult (e.g., testes elevated or rotated, history of recurrent pain or torsion, young age, acute onset with rapid progression)

1, 2, & 3 Normal

1, 2, or 3 Abnormal

Present

Absent

Doppler or Tc⁹⁹ Scan

Reduced Flow

Normal Flow

Surgical Exploration for Torsion, Tumor, Other (Obtain cultures if epididymitis found.)

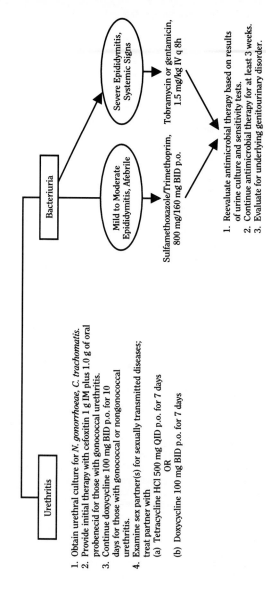

Urethritis

1. Obtain urethral culture for *N. gonorrhoeae, C. trachomatis.*
2. Provide initial therapy with cefoxitin 1 g IM plus 1.0 g of oral probenecid for those with gonococcal urethritis.
3. Continue doxycycline 100 mg BID p.o. for 10 days for those with gonococcal or nongonococcal urethritis.
4. Examine sex partner(s) for sexually transmitted diseases; treat partner with
   (a) Tetracycline HCl 500 mg QID p.o. for 7 days
   OR
   (b) Doxycycline 100 mg BID p.o. for 7 days

Bacteriuria

Mild to Moderate Epididymitis, Afebrile

Severe Epididymitis, Systemic Signs

Sulfamethoxazole/Trimethoprim, 800 mg/160 mg BID p.o.

Tobramycin or gentamicin, 1.5 mg/kg IV q 8h

1. Reevaluate antimicrobial therapy based on results of urine culture and sensitivity tests.
2. Continue antimicrobial therapy for at least 3 weeks.
3. Evaluate for underlying genitourinary disorder.

Bed rest and scrotal elevation are recommended for all patients with acute epididymitis.

287

TABLE 24-2. Common Differential Diagnosis of Acute Epididymitis in

	Usual age	Pain	Onset	Past history of pain	Spermatic cord tenderness	Scrotal tenderness
Epididymitis	Any	Mild–severe	Gradual to sudden	Infrequent	Frequent	Severe
Torsion of testes	< 30	Severe	Sudden	Frequent	Infrequent	Severe
Testes tumor	18–32	None–mild	Gradual	Infrequent	No	None–mild
Hydrocele	Any	None–mild	Gradual	Infrequent	No	None
Spermatocele	Any	None–mild	Gradual	Infrequent	No	None
Varicocele	Any	None–mild	Gradual	Infrequent	No	None
Hernia	Any	None–moderate	Gradual	Frequent	Frequent	None–mild

*In torsion of testicle, epididymis of normal testicle may be anterior.
†Spermatocele may feel like "third testicle."
‡Varicocele should disappear on lying down.

Recurrence of epididymitis often reflects inadequate or inappropriate treatment. Chronic epididymitis develops in approximately 15 percent of acute cases. It is generally idiopathic and poorly responsive to therapy.

Decreased fertility is another complication of acute epididymitis. Its incidence and pathophysiology are poorly understood.

TREATMENT

Symptomatic treatment of the patient with epididymitis is necessary. The patient should be placed at bed rest with the scrotum elevated on a towel between his legs to allow maximum lymphatic and venous drainage. He should remain at bed rest until the scrotal contents are nontender. If the pain returns on ambulation, he should again return to bed rest and scrotal elevation.

Because the vast majority of cases of epididymitis are infectious, antibiotics should never be withheld. Appropriate antibiotics must be chosen on the basis of culture and Gram stain as outlined in Fig. 24-2. Broad-spectrum parenteral antimicrobial therapy is recommended for patients with bacteriuria. If ambulatory therapy is chosen for afebrile patients with mildly or moderately severe

Adult Men

Trans-illu-min-ation	Decrease in swell-ing on lying down	Fever	Location of swelling	Ureth-ritis, pyuria, bacter-iuria	Activity on testic-ular scan	Blood flow on Doppler ultra-sonic
No	No	Frequent	Posterior to testes	Yes	↑	↑
No	No	Infrequent	Testes*	No	↓	↓
No	No	No	Testes	No	↑ or ↓	Normal
Yes	No	No	Entire hemi-scrotum	No	↓	Normal or ↓
Yes	No	No	Above testes†	No	↓	Normal or ↓
No	Yes‡	No	"Bag of worms"	No	Normal or ↑	Normal§
No	Yes¶	No	Above testes	No	Normal	Normal

§May get increased venous flow.
¶Hernia may be reducible on lying down.

epididymitis, trimethoprim-sulfamethoxazole or a quinolone anti-biotic provides activity against most Enterobacteriaceae. The organism recovered from the urine is also responsible for the epididymitis, and therapy can be modified on the basis of susceptibility tests. Prolonged antibiotic treatment may be needed to treat some cases.

In patients with epididymitis associated with urethritis, and young patients (even in the absence of urethritis), cultures should always be obtained for both *N. gonorrhoeae* and *C. trachomatis.* Chlamydia not only causes epididymitis in the absence of gonorrhea, but also is isolated in about 20 percent of patients with gonorrhea. Patients with epididymitis due to gonorrhea should therefore be treated with a regimen active against both chlamydia and penicillin-resistant *N. gonorrhoeae.*

Recommended regimen
Gonococcal epididymitis: ceftriaxone 250 mg IM and doxycycline 100 mg orally twice a day for 10 days.
Nongonococcal epididymitis and urethritis: doxycycline 100 mg orally twice a day for 10 days.
Alternative regimen
Ofloxacin 300 mg orally twice a day for 10 days.

When the etiologic agent is a sexually transmitted agent, treatment of the epididymitis is not complete without treatment of sexual contacts. This should prevent recurrences in the patient as well as prevent disease in the partner.

When treating a patient with acute epididymitis, the clinician must decide whether to evaluate for intrinsic genitourinary disease. Patients less than 50 years old do not usually require further workup unless a coliform agent or *P. aeruginosa* is isolated.

ADDITIONAL READING

Berger RE: Acute epididymitis: Etiology and therapy. *Semin Urol* 9:28, 1991

Eisner DJ, et al: Bilateral testicular infarction caused by epididymitis. *Am J Roentgenol* 157:517, 1991

Fenner MN, et al: Testicular scanning: Evaluating the acute scrotum in the clinical setting. *Urology* 38:237, 1991

Krishnan R, Heal MR: Study of the seminal vesicles in acute epididymitis. *Br J Urol* 67:632, 1991

Middleton WD, et al: Acute scrotal disorders: Prospective comparison of color Doppler US and testicular scintigraphy. *Radiology* 177:177, 1990

Robinson AJ, et al: Acute epididymitis: Why patient and consort must be investigated. *Br J Urol* 66:642, 1990

Thind P, et al: Is micturition disorder a pathogenic factor in acute epididymitis? An evaluation of simultaneous bladder pressure and urine flow in men with previous acute epididymitis. *J Urol* 143:323, 1990

Trambert MA, et al: Subacute scrotal pain: Evaluation of torsion versus epididymitis with MR imaging. *Radiology* 175:53, 1990

Vordermark JS, et al: Role of surgery in management of acute bacterial epididymitis. *Urology* 35:283, 1990

For a more detailed discussion, see Berger RE: Acute Epididymitis, Chap. 53, p. 641, in STD 2.

| Sexually Transmitted Proctitis
and Diarrheal Disease

Five categories of intestinal infection are related to STD. First, receptive anorectal intercourse causes localized anal or rectal infection with usual sexually transmitted pathogens, such as *Chlamydia trachomatis, Neisseria gonorrhoeae, Haemophilus ducreyi, Treponema pallidum,* herpes simplex virus (HSV), and human papilloma virus. In women, contiguous spread from the genitalia can also result in rectal gonorrhea or chlamydial infection. Second, receptive anorectal intercourse represents the most efficient way of sexually acquiring certain systemic STDs, such as HIV and hepatitis B virus infection. Third, systemic manifestations of certain STDs, such as secondary syphilis, may have prominent effects on the gastrointestinal tract. Fourth, oral–anal sexual contact, fellatio after rectal intercourse, or insertion of a penis contaminated with feces into the rectum can result in any of the usual intestinal infections caused by ingestion of pathogens shed in feces. A fifth category— intestinal infections due to HIV-induced immunosuppression—has begun to replace the first four categories as modification of sexual practices reduces the first four categories, while the incidence of AIDS continues to rise. Finally, certain types of opportunistic intestinal infection in AIDS may themselves be sexually transmitted in gay men. Thus, while the clinical and etiologic spectrum of STD-related intestinal infections is rather complex, careful epidemiologic risk assessment is needed to direct the diagnostic evaluation. Furthermore, in the patient without AIDS, clinical manifestations of sexually transmitted intestinal infection can often be differentiated into three syndromes—proctitis, proctocolitis, and enteritis—each with distinctive etiologies. This chapter concerns the approach to these three syndromes in sexually active patients without AIDS.

DEFINITIONS

Symptoms and clinical manifestations of sexually transmitted proctitis, proctocolitis, and enteritis vary widely, depending on the location of the infection and character of the mucosa at the site of infection. The presence of fecal leukocytes on Gram's stain or methylene blue stain of stool or rectal swabs indicates inflammation but does not provide information as to the site of infection.

Figure 25-1 illustrates normal anorectal anatomy. The distal rectum terminates in the anus and anal verge. The anal canal, which extends 2 cm from the anal verge internally to the anorectal line, is supplied with one of the richest networks of sensory nerve endings in the body. Anal infection is therefore very painful and results in

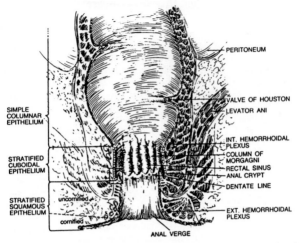

FIG. 25-1. Diagram of the rectum and anal canal, showing normal anal and rectal structures with the types of epithelium lining the anus and rectum.

constipation and tenesmus (ineffectual straining to defecate) due to spasm of the anal sphincter muscle.

The term *proctitis* refers to inflammation of the rectum, which begins at the anorectal line. Symptoms include constipation, tenesmus, rectal discomfort or pain, hematochezia (passage of bloody stools), and a mucopurulent rectal discharge. The combination of tenesmus with frequent attempts to defecate plus rectal discharge is occasionally misinterpreted as diarrhea. Although stretching of rectal tissue causes pain, the area is insensitive to other direct stimuli. Hence, infections which involve the rectum but spare the anus are relatively painless. Sigmoidoscopic findings may range from normal mucosa with only mucopus present to diffuse inflammation of the mucosa, which bleeds easily or forms petechiae after swabbing, or discrete ulcers. When these findings are limited to the rectum, and the mucosa is normal above 15 cm, the condition is called proctitis. If the mucosa is abnormal above this point, the term *proctocolitis* is used. Proctocolitis causes all of the above symptoms of proctitis, together with those caused by colitis, such as diarrhea, abdominal cramping, and fever.

Enteritis is inflammation of the duodenum, jejunum, and/or ileum. Sigmoidoscopy shows no abnormalities. Symptoms typically include diarrhea, abdominal pain, bloating, cramps, and nausea and can also include flatulence, urgency, mucous rectal discharge, and, in severe cases, melena. Systemic symptoms, such as fever, dehydration, acidosis, hypokalemia, malabsorption, weight loss, and myalgias may also be present.

ETIOLOGY AND EPIDEMIOLOGY

Enteric organisms that do not require an intermediate host can be transmitted by the oral–anal or genital–anal routes. Sexual transmission of enteric pathogens that are shed in feces may occur through ingestion of feces during anilingus, during fellatio of a fecally contaminated penis, or through direct intrarectal inoculation of organisms by a fecally contaminated penis. Heterosexuals can acquire enteric infections by anilingus, and women can become infected through anal intercourse. Sexually transmitted intestinal or anal infections are most common, however, among homosexually active men. Table 25-1 lists enteric pathogens which have been proved to be or have the potential to be sexually transmitted.

Prominent pathogens in patients with proctitis include *N. gonorrhoeae,* HSV, *C. trachomatis,* and *T. pallidum. Campylobacter, Shigella,* and lymphogranuloma venereum (LGV) strains of *C. trachomatis* are associated with proctocolitis, while *Giardia lamblia* is associated with enteritis. Patients frequently have multiple enteric pathogens.

RECTAL GONORRHEA

Rectal gonococcal infection occurs in 30 to 50 percent of women with gonorrhea. Most cases in women are probably caused by contiguous spread of infected vaginal secretions, although some are due to rectal intercourse. The clinical manifestations of rectal gonococcal infection in women have not been well defined.

In contrast, rectal gonorrhea in men occurs almost exclusively as a result of receptive anorectal intercourse. Although infection is usually symptomatic, asymptomatic infection of the rectum constitutes the main reservoir of gonococcal infection in homosexual men.

Symptoms are usually mild and include constipation, anorectal discomfort, tenesmus, and a mucopurulent rectal discharge. Occasionally, the patient may only notice strands of mucus on his stool or small amounts of blood commonly mistaken for hemorrhoidal bleeding.

Findings during proctoscopy are also nonspecific and are limited to the distal rectum. Mucopus in the rectum is the most frequent finding. The rectal mucosa may appear completely normal or demonstrate generalized erythema with localized areas of easily induced bleeding.

Diagnosis is made by Gram stain and culture of material obtained

TABLE 25-1. Sexually Transmissible Causes of Intestinal or Anal
Infections in Homosexual Men

Bacterial pathogens
  Neisseria gonorrhoeae
  Neisseria meningitidis
  Chlamydia trachomatis
  Haemophilus ducreyi
  Calymmatobacterium granulomatis
  Treponema pallidum
Enteric bacterial pathogens
  Shigella spp.
  Salmonella spp.
  Campylobacter spp.
Fungus
  Candida spp.*
Protozoa
  Giardia lamblia
  Entamoeba histolytica
  Dientamoeba fragilis
  Cryptosporidium spp.*
  Isospora belli *
  "Nonpathogenic" protozoans
Helminths
  Enterobius vermicularis
  Strongyloides stercoralis
Viruses
  Herpes simplex virus
  Cytomegalovirus*
  Human papilloma virus
  Human immunodeficiency virus
  Hepatitis A and B viruses

*Most commonly seen in HIV-infected men; not necessarily sexually
transmitted.

by swabbing the epithelial mucosa of the distal rectum. Use of an
anoscope to examine the rectum and obtain specimens may increase
the yield of Gram stain. A positive smear, showing intracellular
gram-negative diplococci, is usually reliable when the smear has
been taken and analyzed properly, and therapy can be instituted
while awaiting culture results. In men without symptoms, a sterile
cotton swab can be inserted blindly 2 to 3 cm into the rectum for
specimen collection.

   **Recommended treatment: Ceftriaxone 125 mg IM once (or another
agent effective against anal and genital gonorrhea)** *plus* **doxycycline
100 mg orally 2 times a day for 7 days.**

   Doxycycline or tetracycline alone is no longer considered adequate therapy for gonococcal infections but is added for treatment
of coexisting chlamydial infections.

ANORECTAL HSV INFECTION

Anorectal herpes is usually acquired by anal intercourse, although oral–anal contact with an individual who has herpes simplex virus type 1 (HSV-1) infection of the mouth or lips presumably could lead to anorectal infection with HSV-1. Herpes infection may involve the perianal areas, the anal canal, and/or the rectum. Some individuals are totally asymptomatic, but symptoms are quite prominent in most cases. Patients with AIDS sometimes develop progressive mucocutaneous herpes involving the anorectal area.

Anorectal HSV infections are typically characterized by severe, often debilitating anal pain. Constipation, a nonspecific manifestation of proctitis, is usually also present. Urinary retention is not uncommon. The occurrence of constipation, anorectal pain, and urinary retention in a homosexual man strongly suggests herpetic proctitis. Other symptoms include tenesmus, hematochezia, and rectal discharge. Constitutional symptoms such as fever, chills, malaise, and headache are common with primary anorectal HSV infection. Tender inguinal lymphadenopathy occurs in nearly one-half of men with primary anorectal herpes. Anal lesions drain to inguinal lymph nodes, while rectal lesions drain to perirectal nodes. However, recurrent anorectal attacks are often mild and rarely associated with constitutional symptoms.

Many infected persons have no perianal lesions but instead present with ulcerative findings deep in the anal canal or rectal mucosa. With HSV infection of the rectum, the lower 10 cm of the rectum may appear edematous, and discrete focal vesicular or ulcerative lesions may occasionally be present. The rectal mucosa is usually normal above this level. A clinical diagnosis can often be made. Cultures of external lesions, of rectal swabs, or of rectal biopsy are confirmatory.

Recommended therapy for first clinical episode: Acyclovir 400 mg orally 5 times a day for 10 days or until clinical resolution occurs. Analgesics and sitz baths may also be effective in ameliorating symptoms. Recurrent anorectal infections occur, but the temporal pattern and clinical manifestations of anorectal recurrences have not been well studied.

ANORECTAL SYPHILIS

Anorectal chancres usually appear within 2 to 6 weeks after exposure by rectal intercourse. Symptoms are commonly absent in the primary stage of anorectal syphilis, but when symptoms are present, they include mild anal pain or discomfort, constipation, rectal bleeding, and occasionally a rectal discharge. Primary anorectal syphilis may appear as single or multiple ulcers in the perianal region or within the anal canal or rectum. Within the rectum, secondary syphilis may cause discrete polyps, smooth lobulated masses, and mucosal ulcerations, as well as nonspecific mucosal erythema or bleeding. Similar lesions occur in the gastric and intestinal mucosae. Condylomata lata lesions of secondary syphilis may be found near or inside the anal canal.

Diagnosis of anorectal syphilis is based on serologic examination, perirectal and digital rectal examination, and anoscopy. Detection of motile treponemes by dark field examination is useful for evaluation of perianal and anal lesions but may be less specific for rectal lesions, since nonpathogenic treponemes can be found in the intestine. Biopsies of rectal lesions or masses should be processed for silver staining or immunofluorescence staining, as well as routine histologic examination.

Differential diagnosis of anorectal syphilis includes ulcers due to HSV infection, chancroid, granuloma inguinale, and LGV. They may be commonly misdiagnosed as anal fissures, fistulas, hemorrhoiditis, traumatic lesions, rectal polyps, condylomata acuminata, and even rectal carcinoma. Treatment of early syphilis is discussed in Chap. 6.

Chlamydia trachomatis PROCTITIS

Both LGV and non-LGV immunotypes of *C. trachomatis* cause proctitis. Anorectal LGV, described in Chap. 5, is characterized by severe anorectal pain, a bloody mucopurulent discharge, and tenesmus. Inguinal or perirectal adenopathy is also often present. Sigmoidoscopy reveals diffuse bleeding, or easily induced bleeding with discrete ulcerations in the rectum that occasionally extend to the descending colon. Strictures and fistulas may become prominent and can be easily misdiagnosed clinically as Crohn's disease or carcinoma. Histopathologic examination of biopsy material may show granulomata that are easily confused with Crohn's disease, leading to inappropriate therapy.

The non-LGV immunotypes of *C. trachomatis* are less invasive than LGV and cause a mild proctitis associated with rectal discharge, tenesmus, and anorectal pain. Anal lesions have not been described. Many infected individuals may be asymptomatic and are diagnosed only by routine culturing. Sigmoidoscopy may be normal or may reveal mild inflammatory changes in the lower 10 cm of the rectum.

Diagnosis of chlamydial proctitis is best made by isolation of *C. trachomatis* from the rectum, together with response to appropriate therapy. Direct fluorescent antibody staining of rectal secretions using monoclonal antibodies can also be used to make the diagnosis. Serotyping by microimmunofluorescence can differentiate LGV from non-LGV isolates. Serologic examination is also useful for the diagnosis of LGV, particularly with the microimmunofluorescent (micro-IF) technique.

Treatment

Anorectal LGV
   Recommended regimen: Doxycycline 100 mg orally 2 times a day for 21 days.
   Alternative regimens:
   Erythromycin, in a dosage equivalent to 500 mg orally of erythromycin base, 4 times a day for 21 days *or*
   Sulfisoxazole 500 mg orally 4 times a day for 21 days *or* **equivalent sulfonamide course.**
Non-LGV C. trachomatis rectal infections
   Recommended regimen: As above for LGV, but duration of therapy for all regimens other than sulfisoxazole is only 7 days. Sulfisoxazole requires a 10-day course.

PROCTOCOLITIS AND ENTERITIS DUE TO ENTERIC PATHOGENS

Bacterial Agents

Shigella, Salmonella, and *Campylobacter* are the bacteria most commonly associated with sexually transmitted diarrhea. These pathogens produce similar illnesses and can cause clinically severe bacteremia or persistent enteric infection. Fluoroquinolones are generally effective against all three of these organisms. *Campylobacter* is also susceptible to erythromycin. *Shigella* and *Salmonella* are sensitive to third-generation cephalosporins, such as cefotaxime and ceftriaxone, but sensitivity to trimethoprim-sulfamethoxazole varies with geographic location.

Shigella

Although several species of *Shigella* are responsible for human disease, *Shigella sonnei* and *S. flexneri* account for most of the *Shigella* infections in the United States. The sexual transmission of *Shigella* was recognized in 1972 when reports from San Francisco, and later from Seattle and New York, documented that 30 to 70 percent of patients with *Shigella* were homosexual men. Contact tracing demonstrated recovery of the same serotype from sexual partners, and no contaminated food or water source was common to any of the cases. Whereas *S. sonnei* is the most common cause of shigellosis in the United States, and most often associated with mild to moderate watery diarrhea, the most common species found in homosexual men has been *S. flexneri,* which causes more severe disease. Shigellosis produces colitis, with most severe disease in the distal colon, suggesting tropism for the rectum.

Clinically, shigellosis presents with an abrupt onset of diarrhea, fever, nausea, and cramps. The diarrhea is usually watery but, in classic bacillary dysentery caused by *Shigella*, also contains mucus and blood. Sigmoidoscopy usually reveals inflamed mucosa with easily induced bleeding not limited to the distal rectum. Diagnosis is made by culturing the organisms from the stool on selective media. Treatment is usually supportive, but antibiotics are of benefit in selected cases. Due to widespread development of resistance, selection of antibiotics should be based on regional antibiotic sensitivities.

Campylobacter

Campylobacter jejuni is a curved gram-negative rod that causes Shigella-like illness, ranging from self-limited watery diarrhea to febrile bloody mucoid diarrhea with abdominal pain. It generally produces an acute diarrhea of several days' duration with fever, chills, myalgias, and abdominal pain. Although the infection usually involves the small intestine, involvement of the colon and rectum also is seen, with sigmoidoscopic findings similar to those described for shigellosis. Fecal leukocytes are uniformly present, and diagnosis is confirmed by isolating the organisms from the stool by culture on selective media in a microaerophilic atmosphere.

Salmonella

Salmonellae cause four clinical types of infection: acute enterocolitis, enteric (typhoid) fever, septicemia with or without focal systemic lesions, and an asymptomatic carrier state. Enteric fever has become uncommon in the United States (and will not be discussed here) as the number of human host reservoirs has decreased with improved sanitation. The number of cases of *Salmonella* enterocolitis, however, has increased. Clinical manifestations of *Salmonella* enterocolitis, including fever, headache, vomiting, abdominal pain, and diarrhea, usually begin 24 to 36 h after exposure. Bacteremia is frequently detected if blood cultures are obtained early in the infection, and this may become clinically significant in a few patients; generally, bacteremia is transient and self-limited without therapy. The diarrhea is watery, and it often contains mucus and, on occasion, blood. Microscopic examination of the stool reveals a few erythrocytes but usually shows large numbers of leukocytes. The ileum is the major site of infection with *Salmonella*. Although *Salmonella* enterocolitis is thus associated with dysentery less often than shigellosis and *Campylobacter* infection are, a few patients do develop dysenteric symptoms, with frankly bloody stools, tenderness over the sigmoid colon, and tenesmus. Endoscopic examination in these cases reveals colonic mucosal edema, hyperemia, and easily induced bleeding or petechial hemorrhages, as seen in shigellosis and *Campylobacter* infection.

Parasitic Infections

The major protozoan causes of diarrhea in normal hosts are *G. lamblia* and *Entamoeba histolytica.*

Giardia lamblia

Giardia lamblia is a flagellated protozoon that is widely distributed throughout the world (Fig. 25-2). Food- and waterborne transmission and person-to-person contact are the most common means of transmission, but sexual transmission of *Giardia* by oral–anal or other sexual practices has also been reported in recent years.

Giardia is typically an infection of the small intestine. Symptoms of giardiasis include diarrhea, abdominal cramps, bloating, and nausea. Multiple stool examinations are sometimes necessary to document infection. Often, when stool examination has been negative, sampling of jejunal mucus by the Enterotest or small bowel biopsy is necessary to confirm the diagnosis.

Quinacrine hydrochloride, 100 mg, or metronidazole, 250 mg three times a day for 7 days, is presently recommended in the United States, but both drugs are associated with a 10 to 15 percent failure rate.

Entamoeba histolytica

Entamoeba histolytica infects 10 percent of the world's population; although the vast majority of infected persons are asymptomatic, invasive amebiasis is the third leading parasitic cause of death worldwide. The infection is usually acquired by person-to-person transmission, but sexual transmission also occurs. Some investigators classify *E. histolytica* strains into pathogenic and nonpathogenic types, termed *zymodemes,* based upon protozoal isoenzyme analysis; *E. histolytica* strains from homosexual men have belonged to supposedly nonpathogenic zymodemes. However, the validity of this method, and the existence of nonpathogenic variants of *E. histolytica,* are debated. Nonetheless, because homosexual men found to have *E. histolytica* in stools have often been asymptomatic, therapy is probably unnecessary in such cases.

When symptoms of amebiasis are present in infected homosexual men, they may vary from mild diarrhea to fulminant bloody dysentery. Amebic proctocolitis in general causes diffuse inflammation and ulceration of the distal colon, often clinically indistinguishable from inflammatory bowel disease, shigellosis, *Yersinia* enterocolitis, and *C. jejuni* infection.

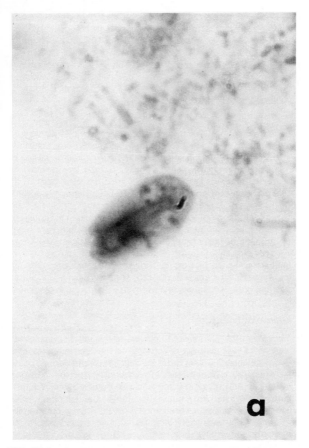

FIG. 25-2. *Giardia lamblia (a)* cyst and *(b)* trophozoite from fecal specimens of a patient with active giardiasis. Gomori-Wheatley trichrome stain, oil immersion × 640 magnification. *(Courtesy of GR Healy.)*

Diagnosis is based on the demonstration of *E. histolytica* in the stool or in a wet mount of a swab or a biopsy of rectal mucosal lesions (Fig. 25-3). Occasionally, multiple fresh stool examinations are necessary to demonstrate the cysts or trophozoites. Serologic examination (indirect hemagglutination) is useful in acute amebic

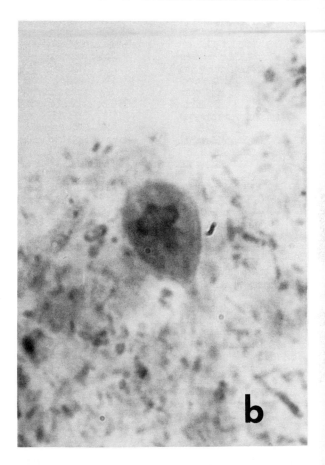

colitis because it is positive in about 90 percent of infected patients. Recommended treatment for symptomatic disease is with metronidazole (750 mg orally 3 times daily for 10 days), followed by diiodohydroxyquin (650 mg orally 3 times daily for 20 days).

Other Parasites

Sexual transmission among homosexual men has been suspected for other parasites, such as *Iodamoeba butschlii, Dientamoeba fragilis,*

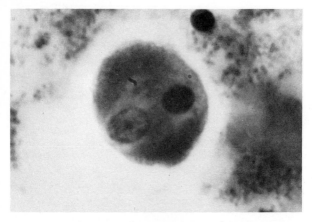

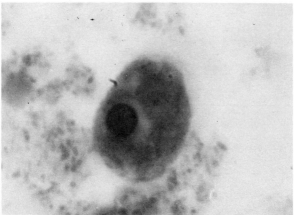

FIG. 25-3. *Entamoeba histolytica* trophozoites from fecal specimens of a patient with amebic colitis. Gomori-Wheatley trichrome stain, oil immersion. *(Facing page)* × 320 magnification. *(This page)* × 640 magnification. Note single nuclei with central, punctate karyosome, with delicate peripheral nuclear chromatin. The top two trophozoites also have an ingested red blood cell. *(Courtesy of GR Healy.)*

inflammatory disease. Cultures for *N. gonorrhoeae* should be obtained from the rectum, urethra, and pharynx, and a rectal culture for *C. trachomatis* should be performed. A serologic test for syphilis should be performed in all cases. If external ulcers, rectal mucosal lesions, or suspected condylomata lata are seen, dark field examinations of these lesions and a rapid plasma reagin (RPR) test should be performed. HSV cultures should be performed if vesiculopustular or ulcerative lesions are present, as HSV has become increasingly common as a cause of proctitis in the AIDS era and is not always associated with typical symptoms in HIV-infected patients. If proctocolitis is likely on the basis of either symptoms or sigmoidoscopic examination, then additional cultures for *Campylobacter, Salmonella,* and *Shigella,* and stool examination for *E. histolytica* are indicated. Attempts to demonstrate *Clostridium difficile* toxin may also be indicated.

If symptoms and signs suggest enteritis rather than proctitis or proctocolitis, then stool should be cultured for *Campylobacter* and other enteric pathogens and examined for *G. lamblia.*

If a diagnosis of gonorrhea is initially made by a positive Gram stain or if syphilis is confirmed by dark field examination or RPR, appropriate treatment should be given promptly. Similarly, anyone who has sexual contact with a person with known gonorrhea, syphilis, or chlamydial urethritis should be treated appropriately on an epidemiologic basis after complete physical examination, while results of gonorrhea cultures and syphilis serologic tests are pending. A presumptive diagnosis of HSV can often be made initially on clinical appearance alone or by history, but laboratory confirmation of suspected herpetic lesions is always desirable unless the clinical appearance of vesicular lesions is diagnostic.

If the patient remains symptomatic and a careful search reveals no pathogen, or if the patient remains symptomatic despite appropriate therapy for any pathogen found or after empirical therapy, then the patient should be evaluated for the possibility of inflammatory bowel disease or other diseases which are not sexually transmitted.

Identification of any of the enteric pathogens should result in specific therapeutic regimens. Failure to respond to specific antimicrobial regimens may represent drug resistance or, more commonly, the presence of additional pathogens, necessitating more comprehensive microbiological and immunologic evaluation. If symptoms persist after eradication of infection or if no pathogens are identified, one must consider idiopathic inflammatory bowel disease, neoplastic lesions, or antibiotic-resistant opportunistic infections and begin diagnostic and therapeutic approaches to these diseases.

Because of the complexity of diagnosis and treatment of enteritis and proctitis in an STD population and the different levels of laboratory support at STD clinics and in office practice, we have outlined two algorithms. Algorithm A (Fig. 25-4) represents a systematic approach to diagnosis and treatment that is comprehensive and employs treatment only for identified pathogens. It represents a stepwise progression toward specific diagnosis and treatment of patient and exposed contacts. The major problem with this algorithm is that the microbiological evaluation is expensive and time-consuming, factors that may indirectly allow continued discomfort of the patient and transmission of the pathogen before final diagnosis and treatment.

Algorithm B (Fig. 25-5) is based on empirical therapy, which has the advantage of decreasing the cost of laboratory tests and provides

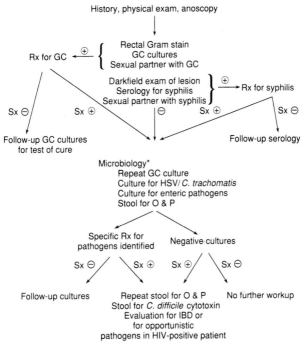

FIG. 25-4. Algorithm A: Evaluation and treatment of anorectal and/or intestinal symptoms in homosexual men. This algorithm emphasizes a full diagnostic evaluation and treatment for specific pathogens identified. Ideally, microbiological evaluation should be based on presenting symptoms and sigmoidoscopy findings. Rx = treatment, Sx = symptoms, GC = *N. gonorrhoeae,* O & P = ova and parasites, IBD = inflammatory bowel disease.

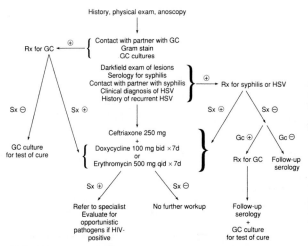

FIG. 25-5. Algorithm B: Evaluation and treatment of anorectal and/or intestinal symptoms in homosexual men. This algorithm emphasizes empirical therapy after an initial evaluation for gonorrhea and syphilis. Empirical therapy consists of intramuscular aqueous procaine penicillin, 4.8 million units, with 1.0 g of oral probenecid, followed by either doxycycline or erythromycin. If the patient remains symptomatic, he is referred for more complete evaluation. GC = *N. gonorrhoeae,* APPG = aqueous procaine penicillin G, Rx = treatment, Sx = symptoms.

immediate therapy to patients who may not return for follow-up visits. In a controlled trial, syndromic treatment of proctitis in homosexual men with drugs active against gonorrhea and chlamydial infection was found to be more effective than treatment of documented infections. This approach has the disadvantage, however, of interfering with the public health efforts to trace contacts of the patient who may harbor a specific pathogen. Such public health efforts are possible only if a specific diagnosis is made.

Selection between these two methods of approach must be based on clinic and public health priorities, budget, laboratory support, and patient population.

PREVENTION

Examination and treatment of the sexual contacts of homosexual men with sexually transmitted enteric infection should be considered. When a specific pathogen is identified in a symptomatic homosexually active male patient, epidemiologic investigation of all sexual contacts should be performed and appropriate diagnostic tests for the pathogen(s) involved should be obtained from the contacts. This is especially important for those agents that can be eliminated by treatment, such as *N. gonorrhoeae, C. trachomatis, T. pallidum,* and the enteric pathogens. Most of the pathogens we have discussed should be reported to local public health workers, whose assistance in coordinating efforts to identify and examine culture contacts is helpful. Household as well as sexual contacts should be screened for infection when investigating the spread of enteric pathogens. After the acute infection subsides or following therapy, repeat laboratory tests should be performed to detect possible development of a carrier state. Infected individuals should abstain from sexual practices that might spread infection and should be educated regarding safer sex practices in the AIDS era.

ADDITIONAL READING

Law C: Sexually transmitted diseases and enteric infections in the male homosexual population. *Semin Dermatol* 9:178, 1990

Law CL et al: Factors associated with the detection of *Entamoeba histolytica* in homosexual men. *Int J STD AIDS* 2:346, 1991

Law CL et al: Nonspecific proctitis: Association with human immunodeficiency virus infection in homosexual men. *J Infect Dis* 165:150, 1992

For a more detailed discussion, see Keusch GT: Enteric Bacterial Pathogens: *Shigella, Salmonella, Campylobacter,* Chap. 27, p 295; Guerrant RL, Weikel CS, Ravdin JI: Intestinal Protozoa: *Giardia lamblia, Entamoeba histolytica,* and *Cryptosporidium,* Chap. 44, p 493; Quinn TC, Stamm WE: Proctitis, Proctocolitis, Enteritis, and Esophagitis in Homosexual Men, Chap. 55, p 663, in STD-2.

DEFINITION

Genital ulcer adenopathy syndrome is an epithelial defect in the skin or mucosa of the genitalia, often accompanied by lymphadenopathy in the genital region. Many sexually transmitted pathogens cause the genital ulcer adenopathy syndrome. The importance of genital ulcer disease has increased enormously with growing evidence that genital ulceration is a major risk factor for transmission of human immunodeficiency virus (HIV).

EPIDEMIOLOGY

Genital ulcer adenopathy syndrome is rarely reported as such. Among the many different causative agents, only syphilis has a widely available diagnostic test. A specific diagnosis is made in only 50 to 85 percent of genital ulcer cases. Thus, epidemiologic data on the syndrome are incomplete.

Genital ulcers are more common in developing countries than in the industrialized world. From 1 to 5 percent of STD patients in the United States and Europe present with genital ulceration, but 20 to 70 percent of such patients in Asia and Africa present in this manner. The etiology of genital ulcer disease also shows striking geographic variability. Genital herpes is by far the most common diagnosis in North America and Europe, whereas chancroid is more common in Africa, Asia, and Latin America. Lymphogranuloma venereum (LGV) and donovanosis occur mainly in certain tropical areas.

Risk factors for genital ulcer disease also vary by population and etiologic agents. Homosexual men used to account for the majority of syphilis cases in the industrialized world, but the incidence in this population has declined as a result of behavioral change during the AIDS epidemic. In most countries, chancroid patients belong to lower socioeconomic strata, and prostitutes are usually the source of the disease. Uncircumcised men are at higher risk for acquiring chancroid than those who are circumcised. LGV is usually an imported disease in North America and Europe, but it occasionally causes anorectal ulcers in homosexual men in the United States.

Many types of genital ulcers have serious sequelae. In addition, genital ulcers enhance susceptibility and transmission of HIV infection during sexual intercourse. Therefore, genital ulcer disease should be considered a very high priority in STD control programs.

ETIOLOGY

Major pathogens of the genital ulcer adenopathy syndrome include *Treponema pallidum;* herpes simplex virus; *Haemophilus ducreyi; Chlamydia trachomatis* serovars L1, L2, and L3; and *Calymmato-*

bacterium granulomatis (the agent of donovanosis). Other causes include fixed drug eruption, Behçet's and Reiter's syndromes, trauma, and malignancy. Rare or uncertain causes include *Phthirus pubis, Entamoeba histolytica, Sarcoptes scabiei, Trichomonas vaginalis,* and nonsyphilis spirochetes. HIV has also been reported as a cause.

CLINICAL MANIFESTATIONS

Clinical features of the major causes of genital ulcer adenopathy syndrome are shown in Table 26-1. Diagnosis is complicated because clinical presentations are often atypical, and mixed infections are common. The use of antibiotics or corticosteroids, systemically or topically, or the presence of immunodeficiency can alter the classic manifestations. When clinical findings alone are used, even experienced clinicians incorrectly diagnose the different agents of genital ulcers in 20 to 50 percent of cases.

Genital Ulcers

Most genital ulcers in the male are located on the coronal sulcus, glans, prepuce, and shaft of the penis. Herpes and chancroid often involve the frenulum. If a condom has been used, lesions may be located only at the root of the penis. Perianal and rectal lesions should be sought in women and homosexual males. Lesions can also occur on the scrotum and on extragenital sites such as the lips and oropharynx. In women, lesions may occur on the labia, vagina, cervix, fourchette, and perianal area.

The number and size of lesions can be a clue to the diagnosis. Herpes and chancroid may appear as a single serpiginous ulcer which is actually composed of multiple coalesced lesions. Because morphology often suggests a specific pathogen, the examiner should note whether the lesion is vesicular, papular, or pustular; round, oval, or irregular; and whether the edges are elevated, undermined, or erythematous. Itching is often reported with herpes simplex in the prodromal phase.

Lymphadenopathy

In both men and women the lymphatic system of the external genitalia drains into the inguinal nodes and sometimes the femoral nodes. The sacral nodes drain the inner two-thirds of the vagina and cervix. Genital lymphadenopathy is usually associated with genital ulcers, with the latter usually appearing first.

Features of lymphadenopathy that may be helpful in diagnosis include whether the nodes are bilateral or unilateral, fluctuance, pain or tenderness, and the consistency of the nodes and overlying

TABLE 26-1. Clinical Features of Genital Ulcers

	Syphilis	Herpes	Chancroid	Lymphogranuloma venereum	Donovanosis
Incubation period	2–4 weeks (1–12 weeks)	2–7 days	1–14 days	3 days–6 weeks	1–4 weeks (up to 6 months)
Primary lesion	Papule	Vesicle	Papule or pustule	Papule, pustule, or vesicle	Papule
Number of lesions	Usually one	Multiple, may coalesce	Usually multiple, may coalesce	Usually one	Variable
Diameter, mm	5–15	1–2	2–20	2–10	Variable
Edges	Sharply demarcated, elevated, round or oval	Erythematous	Undermined, ragged, irregular	Elevated, round or oval	Elevated, irregular
Depth	Superficial or deep	Superficial	Excavated	Superficial or deep	Elevated
Base	Smooth, nonpurulent	Serous, erythematous	Purulent	Variable	Red and rough ("beefy")
Induration	Firm	None	Soft	Occasionally firm	Firm
Pain	Unusual	Common	Usually very tender	Variable	Uncommon
Lymphadenopathy	Firm, nontender, bilateral	Firm, tender, often bilateral	Tender, may suppurate, usually unilateral	Tender, may suppurate, loculated, usually unilateral	Pseudoadenopathy

skin. LGV usually involves several nodes, and when inguinal and femoral nodes are both swollen and divided by the inguinal ligament, this creates a *groove sign.* This finding is considered pathognomonic for LGV, but it occasionally occurs in chancroid. If a genital ulcer becomes secondarily infected, the adenopathy may reflect the secondary process rather than the primary infection. The pseudobuboes which occur in donovanosis are granulomatous nodules in the skin and subcutaneous tissue of the inguinal region, not the lymph nodes. Inguinal lymphadenopathy that is chronic, nontender, and not associated with an ulcer or other infection suggests a cutaneous genital or lymphatic malignancy. However, in the tropics many adults have inguinal adenopathy as a result of recurrent lower extremity trauma and infection.

COMPLICATIONS AND SEQUELAE

Many of the agents of genital ulcer adenopathy syndrome have debilitating, deforming, and even lethal complications. Individual chapters on these agents detail the syndromes.

The presence of the ulcer creates an opportunity for secondary infection, which may result in phagedenic ulceration, massive edema, necrotic balanitis, paraphimosis, and phimosis. The glans penis can be destroyed by untreated chancroid or donovanosis. These infections can also cause satellite ulcers in adjacent gluteal or groin folds or ruptured inguinal lymph nodes.

Lymphatic obstruction and fistulas can result from LGV. Stenosis of urethral, vaginal, and anal orifices, and massive swelling and deformity of the genitalia can result from donovanosis. If untreated, syphilis can progress to secondary and tertiary stages, though the primary lesion usually heals without event.

DIAGNOSIS (Table 26-2)

Genital ulcers are difficult to correctly diagnose clinically; clinicians are wrong at least 20 percent of the time. History and examination can provide clues, but laboratory evaluation should be performed to the extent possible. A dark field examination for *T. pallidum,* a viral culture for herpes, and serologic tests for syphilis are essential. In developing countries where laboratory facilities are limited, priority should be given to diagnosis of syphilis, since this is potentially the most debilitating disease.

Collection of Specimens

To collect specimens, the lesions should be washed with saline and dried with a swab or gauze, then squeezed between thumb and index finger until an exudate appears. This exudate should be collected

TABLE 26-2. Laboratory Tests for the Diagnosis of Genital Ulcer Adenopathy Syndrome

	Syphilis	Herpes	Chancroid	Lymphogranuloma venereum	Donovanosis
Microscopy	Dark field examination	Antigen detection	Gram stain has low sensitivity and specificity	Not available	Giemsa- or Wright-stained tissue smears and sections
Culture	Not available	Cell culture	Sensitive, selective media available	Cell culture	Not available
Serology	RPR/VDRL, FTA-ABS, MHA-TP*	Rarely useful (primary herpes)	Experimental	Complement fixation and immunofluorescent antibody tests	Not available

*RPR = rapid plasma reagin; VDRL = Veneral Disease Research Laboratory; FTA-ABS = fluorescent antibody absorption; MHA-TP = microhemagglutination assay for antibodies to *T. pallidum*.

313

for dark field microscopy using a spatula, loop, or coverslip. Specimens for culture of herpes simplex virus, *H. ducreyi,* and *C. trachomatis* should be collected after vigorous swabbing. Aspiration of lymph nodes, particularly fluctuant nodes, can demonstrate an organism in some cases. To avoid fistula formation, aspiration should always be performed through intact skin.

Microscopy

Dark field examination requires skill and a suitable microscope but remains the gold standard for diagnosis of primary syphilis. If the initial result is negative, the examination should be repeated the following day.

Smears and scrapings can be examined for herpes simplex virus by immunofluorescent or immunoperoxidase techniques, or by a Tzanck preparation (presence of giant multinucleated cells in scrapings from the floor of the lesion). These tests are sensitive when vesicles are present, but the yield is lower for ulcers.

Gram stain does not diagnose chancroid reliably and is therefore not recommended. Donovanosis can be diagnosed by Giemsa- or Wright-stained tissue; a positive slide reveals encapsulated, intracytoplasmic Donovan bodies in macrophages.

Isolation of Causative Agent

Viral isolation is the method of choice for the diagnosis of genital herpes, but sensitivity decreases after vesicles have ulcerated.

The diagnosis of chancroid should be confirmed by isolation of *H. ducreyi* from an ulcer or bubo. In experienced hands sensitivity of a single culture can be 80 percent on selective media.

Isolation of *C. trachomatis* LGV serovars L1, L2, or L3 confirms the diagnosis of LGV. Although bubo aspirate is the best culture material, the fluid may be toxic to cell cultures and yield an inconclusive test result. Chlamydia can occasionally be isolated from the ulcer base or rectal lesions.

Serology

A serologic test for syphilis should be part of every evaluation for genital ulcer adenopathy syndrome. A cardiolipin test (RPR, VDRL) may be negative when a patient presents with a chancre but will usually become positive during primary syphilis. Although the fluorescent treponemal antibody absorption test (FTA-ABS) is more sensitive than a cardiolipin test, a positive FTA-ABS may reflect prior, treated syphilis. Serologic tests should not replace dark field examination for diagnosis of primary syphilis but should be used to further evaluate genital ulcers and to quantitatively document response to therapy.

Serum antibody to herpes simplex can be detected by many methods, but serologic testing diagnoses primary herpes simplex virus infection only when a seroconversion or a fourfold or greater rise in antibody titer is noted.

LGV is most commonly diagnosed with the complement-fixation test, which becomes positive within 1 to 3 weeks after infection. Antibody titers are greater than or equal to 1:64 in over half of the patients. Because many patients present late in the disease, rising antibody titers are rarely observed.

DIFFERENTIAL DIAGNOSIS

See Fig. 26-1 for an algorithm outlining the major aspects of differential diagnosis. Ulcers not restricted to the genital area may indicate a systemic disease of nonvenereal origin, such as Behçet's disease, erythema multiforme, or dermatitis herpetiformis. A medication history should always be obtained to assess the possibility of a drug reaction.

TREATMENT

No single antimicrobial has activity against all the agents causing genital ulcer adenopathy syndrome, and treatment is best initiated after proper diagnosis. See individual chapters for therapy for specific organisms. Until syphilis is excluded by a dark field examination, it is preferable to use an antibiotic without activity against *T. pallidum,* such as trimethoprim-sulfamethoxazole or ciprofloxacin. With the exception of *H. ducreyi,* antibiotic resistance is not yet a problem in genital ulcer adenopathy syndrome.

Virtually all ulcers contain abundant bacterial flora, and in severe cases of secondary infection, a broad-spectrum antibiotic should be given. Topical antimicrobial therapy is not recommended. Frequent application of warm-water compresses should be used to remove necrotic material and purulent exudate. A dorsal slit incision of the prepuce may be needed to relieve the urinary retention caused by severe phimosis.

The fluctuant buboes of chancroid and LGV should be aspirated since they often do not respond to antimicrobial therapy and may even become larger after successful treatment of the associated ulcer. Aspiration should be performed through adjacent normal skin to avoid fistula formation; repeated aspirations may be necessary. Incision and drainage should be avoided because the procedure increases healing time and makes scarring more likely.

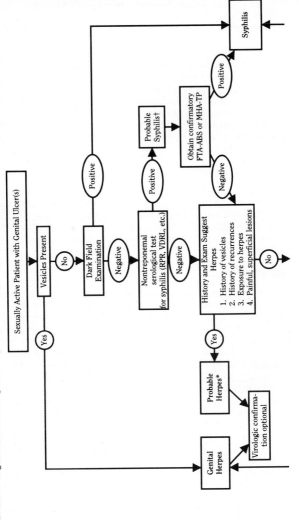

FIG. 26-1 Algorithm for the diagnosis of genital ulcer–inguinal adenopathy syndromes in sexually active patients.

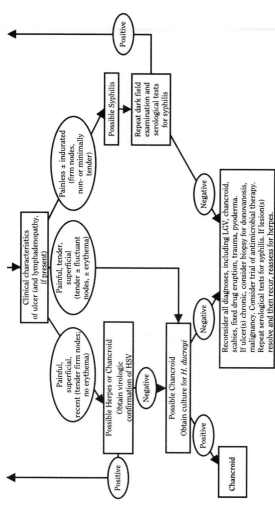

*Confirmation of probable herpes is desirable. If the confirmation test for herpes is negative, or if the course is atypical, reevaluate the diagnosis, repeat serological test for syphilis in 3 to 4 weeks, consider fixed drug eruption if there is history of recurrent lesions at the same time, and rule out herpes at the next recurrence.

†While awaiting the FTA-ABS test results, most clinicians would initiate syphilis therapy for patients having dark-field-negative, RPR-positive ulcers which resemble chancres.

ADDITIONAL READING

Chirgwin K, et al: HIV infection, genital ulcer disease, and crack cocaine use among patients attending a clinic for sexually transmitted diseases. *Am J Public Health* 81:1576, 1991

Jessamine PG, Ronald AR: Chancroid and the role of genital ulcer disease in the spread of human retroviruses. *Med Clin North Am* 74:1417, 1990

Jessamine PG, et al: Human immunodeficiency virus, genital ulcers and the male foreskin: Synergism in HIV-1 transmission. *Scand J Infect Dis* 69 (suppl):181, 1990

Kraus SJ: Diagnosis and management of acute genital ulcers in sexually active patients. *Semin Dermatol* 9:160, 1990

Schmid GP: Approach to the patient with genital ulcer disease. *Med Clin North Am* 74:1559, 1990

Zenilman JM: Update on bacterial sexually transmitted disease. *Urol Clin North Am* 19:25, 1992

For a more detailed discussion, see Piot P, Plummer FA: Genital Ulcer Adenopathy Syndrome, Chap. 59, p 711, in STD-2.

DEFINITION

Reactive arthritis is the general term for inflammatory arthritis that follows a localized infection, which usually involves a mucosal surface. Reiter's syndrome is a reactive arthritis associated with various combinations of urogenital, ocular, and mucocutaneous inflammation. It typically follows a primary genital or lower gastrointestinal infection. The term *Reiter's syndrome* includes the disorders referred to as reactive spondyloarthropathy, reactive uroarthritis, postgonococcal arthritis, and postdysenteric arthropathy.

Other sexually transmitted diseases associated with acute arthritis include hepatitis B virus (HBV) and human immunodeficiency virus (HIV) infections, and rarely syphilis, lymphogranuloma venereum (LGV), genital herpes, cytomegalovirus (CMV), and genital mycoplasma infections. Arthritis may also result from allergic reactions to drugs used in the treatment of sexually transmitted infections.

REITER'S SYNDROME

Etiology and Pathogenesis

The pathogenesis of reactive arthritis is not well understood. It appears that certain infections trigger the syndrome in a genetically predisposed host and that the disease may persist despite eradication of the initial infection. The infectious agents implicated include *Chlamydia trachomatis, Shigella flexneri, Salmonella* spp., *Yersinia enterocolitica, Campylobacter* spp., and perhaps *Neisseria gonorrhoeae.*

C. trachomatis appears to be the most common etiologic agent of sexually transmitted Reiter's syndrome. Genital chlamydial infection has been documented in about 50 percent of men with the syndrome. Antichlamydial antibody titer is even more common in these patients and is usually present in a higher titer than in patients with uncomplicated chlamydial infection.

However, not all cases of sexually acquired Reiter's syndrome can be associated with prior chlamydial infection. Twenty-five percent of patients have no immune response to *C. trachomatis,* and no sexually transmitted organisms can be isolated from the urethra in one-third to one-half of men with sexually transmitted reactive arthritis. *N. gonorrhoeae* itself may initiate some cases; Reiter's syndrome has been documented after gonococcal urethritis in the absence of cultural and serologic evidence of *Chlamydia.* Other infectious agents such as *Ureaplasma urealyticum* may be involved.

In some cases of Reiter's syndrome the urethritis may be noninfective. Urethritis occurs in patients with the postdysenteric form of reactive arthritis and also may recur during late exacerbations of the syndrome despite absence of recent sexual contact.

The HLA-B27 haplotype is strongly associated with Reiter's syndrome and may predispose persons with this haplotype to develop the disease. The prevalence not only of HLA-B27 but also of haplotypes that cross-react with HLA-B27 is much greater in both black and white patients with Reiter's syndrome than in their respective general populations. Nonetheless, no more than 25 percent of patients with HLA-B27 haplotype who contract nongonococcal urethritis (NGU) or shigellosis subsequently develop Reiter's syndrome. The initial manifestations and clinical course of Reiter's syndrome in patients with the HLA-B27 haplotype tend to be more severe and aggressive than in those without it.

Chlamydia trachomatis and *Y. entercolitica* have been found in the synovium or synovial fluid of patients with Reiter's syndrome. Nevertheless, the role of direct synovial infection in pathogenesis is unclear, in part because antimicrobial therapy has no clinical benefit.

Epidemiology

Reiter's syndrome appears to have two forms: a more common, endemic form that is usually sexually acquired, and a less common, epidemic form most often associated with enteric infection. Although sexually acquired Reiter's syndrome commonly follows a new sexual contact, documentation of sexual transmission of individual cases is rare.

The incidence and prevalence of Reiter's syndrome are unknown but probably vary geographically. One series from Seattle described Reiter's syndrome as constituting 11 percent of acute nontraumatic arthritis in adults; the syndrome was second only to disseminated gonococcal infections as a cause of arthritis (Fig. 27-1). The overall risk of acquiring Reiter's syndrome in a man with NGU or acute shigellosis was estimated at 1 to 3 percent, but may be as high as 20 to 25 percent in those who have the HLA-B27 haplotype.

Most patients with Reiter's syndrome present between the ages of 30 and 40, and 80 to 90 percent of patients are white. Differences in racial susceptibility remain poorly defined, but it is likely that blacks are less susceptible than whites, at least to the extent that the prevalence of the HLA-B-27 haplotype is lower in blacks.

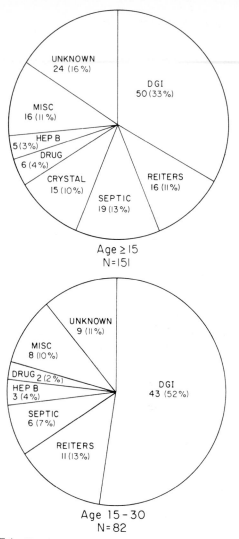

FIG. 27-1. Diagnoses in 151 consecutive adults (age ≥ 15 years) hospitalized in Seattle because of acute, nontraumatic arthritis of ≤ 14 days' duration. REITERS includes postgonococcal arthritis; DRUG denotes drug-induced arthritis; HEP B denotes hepatitis B infection. *(From HH Handsfield.[1])*

Traditionally, males were believed to develop Reiter's syndrome more often than females. Recent series, however, report that women constitute from 3.6 to 52 percent of sexually acquired Reiter's syndrome. Some investigators have found associations between histories of salpingitis, gonorrhea, bacterial urinary tract infection, trichomoniasis, and nonspecific rheumatic complaints and overt Reiter's syndrome in women. The sexual partners of men with Reiter's syndrome have been described as having a high prevalence of musculoskeletal disorders. In addition, other investigators have reported an association between salpingitis and radiologic evidence of sacroiliitis. Prospective studies with complete microbiological and immunologic evaluations and careful clinical examinations will be required to define the true sex distribution and other epidemiologic features of this disease.

Clinical and Laboratory Manifestations

The clinical manifestations of Reiter's syndrome include acute arthritis, lower urogenital tract inflammation, conjunctivitis, and mucocutaneous inflammatory lesions. It is uncommon for all these findings to be observed at presentation, but many patients, especially those who are HLA-B27 positive, will eventually develop all features. Table 27-1 outlines the frequencies of each finding at presentation and follow-up. The articular, mucocutaneous, and ocular manifestations usually follow the onset of urethritis or diarrhea by 1 to 4 days, but delays of several months can be seen.

Urogenital Inflammation

Patients with Reiter's syndrome frequently give histories of contact with a new sexual partner, followed by the development of urethritis that is clinically indistinguishable from uncomplicated NGU. The spectrum of urogenital inflammation in women with Reiter's syndrome is unknown, but cervicitis, urethritis, cystitis, and salpingitis all may be important.

Arthritis

A wide range of articular disease occurs. Asymmetrical polyarticular synovitis-tendinitis is often seen initially, followed by persistence in one or two joints. Tendon insertion sites, such as those of the Achilles tendon and plantar fascia, are commonly involved. Eighty-six percent of patients have involvement of more than one joint, and many have involvement of four or more. The arthritis characteristically begins in the distal weight-bearing joints such as knees, ankles, and feet. Knee effusions and fusiform dactylitis ("sausage digits") are common (Fig. 27-2). Sacroiliitis occurs in up to 10 percent of acute cases and is even more common among persons

TABLE 27-1. Frequencies of Clinical Manifestations in Patients with
Reiter's Syndrome

	Initial attack, percent*	Entire course, percent†
Urogenital inflammation:		
Urethritis (criteria not specified)	85	87
Cervicitis (criteria not specified)	71	NA
Arthritis:		
Monoarticular	14	3
Polyarticular	81	86
Arthralgia only	0	9
Sacroiliitis back pain	49	21
Heel pain	40	Not recorded
Tendinitis	25	25
Fusiform dactylitis ("sausage" digits)	17	Not recorded
Ocular involvement:		
Conjunctivitis	57	50
Uveitis	0	12
Mucocutaneous involvement:		
Balanitis/vulvovaginitis	39	69
Stomatitis	31	17
Keratodermia blennorrhagica	21	18
Nail changes	9	16
Other:		
Cardiac	0	9
Neurologic	1	2
Diarrhea	14	12

*Data from Wilkens et al (N = 83).[2]
†Data from Kousa (N = 173).[3]

with chronic disease. In contrast to ankylosing spondylitis and other
spondyloarthropathies, spinal involvement is uncommon in Reiter's
disease.

Mucocutaneous Manifestations

Painless mucocutaneous lesions are common in Reiter's syndrome
that is sexually acquired or associated with shigellosis, but uncommon in reactive arthritis following infection with *Campylobacter,
Salmonella,* and *Yersinia.*

Circinate balanitis, the most common skin manifestation, occurs
in about 20 to 40 percent of men with sexually acquired Reiter's
syndrome and is the most common skin finding (Fig. 27-3). This
lesion is a painless, serpiginous, "geographic" dermatitis of the glans
penis in uncircumcised men and is diagnostic of the syndrome. In
circumcised men, circinate balanitis often consists of hyperkeratotic
papules that closely resemble the other lesion typical of Reiter's

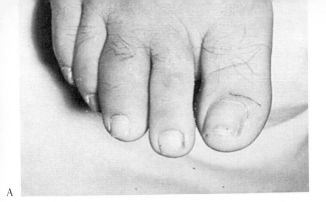

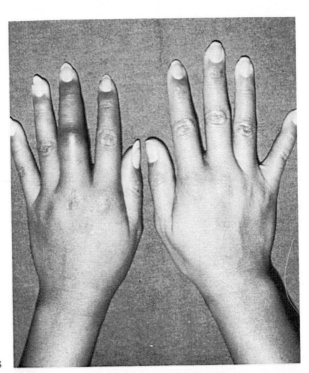

FIG. 27-2. Acute fusiform dactylitis in patients with Reiter's syndrome: *(A)* "sausage toe" involving middle toe; *(B)* "sausage finger" involving middle finger. *(Courtesy of RF Willkens.)*

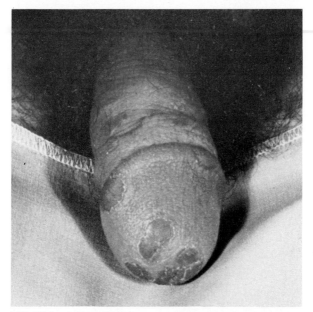

FIG. 27-3. Circinate balanitis in a circumcised man with Reiter's syndrome (see also Plate 67, STD-2e). *(Courtesy of RF Willkens.)*

syndrome, keratodermia blennorrhagica. Erosive vulvitis, perhaps the female equivalent of circinate balanitis, has been documented in some women with Reiter's syndrome.

Lesions of keratodermia blennorrhagica begin as erythematous macules that gradually enlarge to form hyperkeratotic papules, sometimes with red halos and central clearing (Fig. 27-4). The lesion resembles psoriasis, and well-documented cases of Reiter's syndrome have progressed to become clinically indistinguishable from psoriatic arthritis. Though keratodermia blennorrhagica can occur anywhere, it most commonly involves the plantar surfaces of the feet.

Painless, shallow ulcers on the palate, tongue, buccal mucosa, lips, tonsillar pillars, and pharynx occur in up to 20 percent of patients with Reiter's syndrome. Nail involvement consists of thickening and brown-yellow discoloration due to subungual accumulation of hyperkeratotic material and occurs in up to 10 percent of patients.

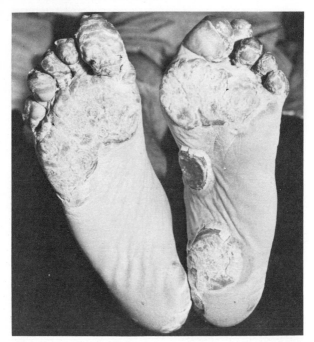

FIG. 27-4. Lesions of keratodermia blennorrhagica involving *(A)* the soles of the feet and *(B)* the palms (see also Plate 68). *(Courtesy of RF Willkens.)*

Ocular Inflammation

Ocular manifestations are common and occur in up to half of patients with acute sexually acquired Reiter's syndrome. Conjunctivitis is the most common finding but is often mild enough to be overlooked. Iritis and extensive uveitis develop in up to 10 percent of patients.

Other Systemic Manifestations

Systemic manifestations are common in acute Reiter's syndrome and include fever, malaise, anorexia, and weight loss. From 9 to 30 percent of patients with acute reactive arthritis develop transient and usually benign electrocardiogram abnormalities, including atrioventricular conduction disturbances, ST-segment elevation or depression, and nonspecific T-wave changes. Rare but potentially

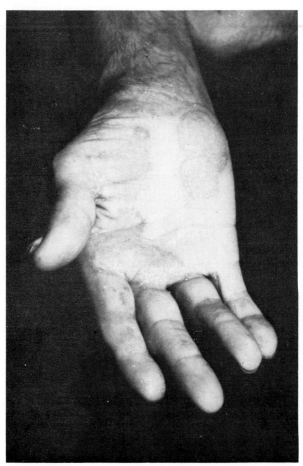

B

serious complications include complete heart block, myocarditis, pericarditis, and acute aortitis with aortic valve incompetence and congestive heart failure. Less than 1 percent of patients experience peripheral neuropathy, hemiplegia, meningoencephalitis, generalized lymphadenopathy, pleuritis, pneumonitis, thrombophlebitis, or amyloidosis.

Laboratory Features

There are no diagnostic laboratory features, but nondiagnostic laboratory features that may be helpful include the erythrocyte sedimentation rate (ESR). The ESR exceeds 20 mm/h in about 60 percent of patients and 50 mm/h in 40 percent, but does not correlate with disease activity. Mild anemia and leukocytosis with up to 20,000 WBC per cubic millimeter are common. Other findings, which are occasionally present, include antinuclear antibodies, rheumatoid factor, cryoglobulins, C-reactive protein, and circulating immune complexes.

Synovial fluid analysis is nonspecific and resembles that of septic arthritis. Leukocyte counts range from 500 to >50,000 per cubic millimeter and are greater than or equal to 20,000 in about 50 percent of patients. Differential counts usually reveal at least 90 percent neutrophils. Other common findings include decreased viscosity, normal or elevated complement levels, decreased ratio of synovial fluid to serum complement concentration, and elevated protein levels. Synovial fluid glucose levels are usually normal.

Clinical Course

Most initial episodes of acute Reiter's syndrome resolve completely within 2 to 6 months, but one-third of patients have symptoms for more than a year, and a few have symptoms indefinitely. The annual risk of recurrent episodes is believed to be about 15 percent. Recurrences may be manifested by any of the clinical features, alone or in combination. The most persistent symptoms are arthritis (83 percent), urethritis or cervicitis (42 percent), ocular disease (31 percent), circinate balanitis (29 percent), and other mucocutaneous lesions (25 percent). The severity of functional impairment caused by chronic Reiter's syndrome is controversial.

OTHER ARTHRITIS SYNDROMES

Disseminated Gonococcal Infection (DGI)

See Chap. 3 for a discussion of *N. gonorrhoeae,* the most common sexually transmitted pathogen that causes infective arthritis.

Evidence suggests that pathogenesis of DGI may involve immunologic mechanisms as well as direct synovial infection. The overall risk of DGI after local gonococcal infection is estimated to be 0.5 to 3 percent. Local infection with serum-resistant gonococcal strains is associated with increased likelihood of dissemination.

Table 27-2 outlines the major clinical manifestations in patients with DGI. The primary genital, rectal, or pharyngeal gonococcal infection is usually asymptomatic. Signs of articular or periarticular inflammation occur in approximately 80 percent of patients; an

TABLE 27-2. Major Presenting
Clinical Manifestations in 102 Patients
with Bacteriologically Confirmed DGI

	Number
Arthritis and dermatitis	71
Arthritis alone	23
Dermatitis alone	7
Endocarditis*	1

*Without arthritis or dermatitis.
SOURCE: Handsfield,[1] Handsfield et al.[4]

additional 10 to 15 percent complain of arthralgias but lack
objective findings. About 30 to 40 percent of patients present with
monoarthritis, usually with frank synovial effusions; the remainder
have involvement of two to three joints. Any joint can be affected,
but the most commonly involved are the wrists, knees, small joints
of the hands, and the ankles. Tenosynovitis is common, but not
pathognomonic, since it also is found in Reiter's syndrome and
other arthritides.

From 50 to 75 percent of patients have characteristic skin
findings. These lesions usually occur on the extremities and consist
of petechiae, pustules, papules, and necrotic lesions in various stages
of development. Over 90 percent of patients with dermatitis have 5
to 30 skin lesions, but the number of lesions can vary from 1 to
over 100. Chemical hepatitis that is usually not clinically apparent
occurs in up to 50 percent of patients. Fever and leukocytosis each
occur in only about 50 to 70 percent of patients with DGI.

Hepatitis B Virus Infection

Generalized arthralgias occur in up to 50 percent of patients during
the prodrome of hepatitis B. Acute arthritis is due to immune-complex deposition and is associated with low serum and synovial fluid
complement levels, which return to normal as the arthritis abates.

The clinical manifestations are similar to those of serum sickness.
Ten to 20 percent of hepatitis B patients have overt polyarthritis,
with symmetrical involvement of the hands, knees, ankles, shoul-
ders, wrists, and feet. About 25 percent of patients with arthralgias
and 50 percent of those with arthritis develop an urticarial rash
which often involves the lower extremities. The arthritic symptoms
usually resolve when the patient develops frank hepatitis. Because
many people never develop jaundice or hepatomegaly, performance
of assay for hepatitis B surface antigens and liver function tests
should be seriously considered in the evaluation of all patients with
acute polyarthritis.

Syphilis

Less than 1 percent of patients with secondary syphilis develop osseous or synovial involvement. Acute periostitis, sometimes mimicking acute arthritis, is a more common finding, but at least some cases of true arthritis result from direct synovial invasion by *Treponema pallidum.* Acute or chronic arthritis can develop in late syphilis due to spread from adjacent osteomyelitis or periostitis. Charcot joints are believed to be traumatic in origin, the indirect result of syphilitic neuropathy and, perhaps, of microvascular disease.

Lymphogranuloma Venereum

Acute and chronic LGV is occasionally associated with a serum sickness–like syndrome that involves polyarthritis, rash, cryoglobulinemia, and circulating rheumatoid factor. The pathogenesis is unclear.

Human Immunodeficiency Virus

Patients infected with HIV can develop any number of rheumatic manifestations at any stage of the disease. Sjögren's syndrome with arthritis and Reiter's syndrome have been described among patients with HIV disease, although the relationship of these arthritides to HIV infection is uncertain. Nonspecific, generalized arthralgias and unexplained oligo- or polyarthritis are relatively common.

Other Diseases with Arthritic Complications

Other sexually transmitted organisms that rarely cause arthritis include *Mycoplasma hominis, Ureaplasma urealyticum,* herpes simplex virus, Epstein-Barr virus, and CMV. Finally, therapy of sexually transmitted diseases with penicillins or other drugs occasionally causes allergic reactions manifested by a serum sickness–like syndrome with skin eruptions, arthralgias, or arthritis, and is associated with high concentrations of circulating immune complexes.

Differential Diagnosis

The differential diagnosis of acute arthritis is broad, but sexually transmitted agents are common causes among young adults. DGI and Reiter's syndrome are the two most common causes of sexually acquired arthritis. Both commonly present with a combination of arthropathy, dermatitis, and genitourinary inflammation, but it is usually possible to distinguish between these two diseases on clinical grounds. The characteristic mucocutaneous lesions, the presence of NGU, conjunctivitis, and radiographically confirmed sacroiliitis are almost always a feature of Reiter's syndrome rather than DGI. Sacroiliitis, typical fusiform dactylitis, or calcaneal tendon insertion site inflammation also support the diagnosis of Reiter's syndrome. Tenosynovitis is a nonspecific finding.

Genital, anorectal, or pharyngeal gonococcal infection occurs in at least 70 to 80 percent of patients with DGI. Therefore, all mucosal sites should be cultured, regardless of the presence or absence of local symptoms. All sexual partners should also be examined; *N. gonorrhoeae* and *C. trachomatis* infection in patients with reactive arthritis can sometimes be confirmed only in a sexual contact.

Synovial fluid analysis and culture or specific antigen detection tests are important in distinguishing patients with crystal-induced arthritis and gonococcal or nongonococcal septic arthritis. Radiographs of peripheral joints, tests for serum uric acid levels, erythrocyte sedimentation rate, rheumatoid factor, antinuclear antibodies, complement levels, and circulating immune complexes may be helpful or diagnostic in the appropriate setting but should not be part of the routine initial workup of all patients with acute arthritis. Likewise, HLA typing may be useful in an equivocal case of Reiter's syndrome, but it is not a primary diagnostic tool.

The diagnosis of DGI is unequivocal if *N. gonorrhoeae* is identified in a nonmucosal site such as blood or synovial fluid, and is probable when a mucosal gonococcal infection is documented in the presence of a typical syndrome that responds promptly to appropriate antibiotic therapy. A typical clinical syndrome that responds rapidly to antibiotics or documentation of gonorrhea in a sexual partner supports the diagnosis.

The American Rheumatism Association defines Reiter's syndrome as an episode of peripheral arthritis of more than 30 days' duration occurring in association with urethritis or cervicitis. These criteria accurately classify most patients with Reiter's syndrome. The occurrence of conjunctivitis or the typical mucocutaneous inflammatory lesions, documentation of the HLA-B27 haplotype, and clinical or radiographic evidence of sacroiliitis help to confirm the diagnosis. The pattern of joint involvement and other clinical and laboratory features distinguish the reactive arthritides from rheumatoid arthritis and arthropathies due to immune-complex deposition.

Neither of the above sets of criteria allows immediate diagnosis of Reiter's syndrome or DGI. The algorithm in Fig. 27-5 illustrates an approach that may be used after performance of a careful history

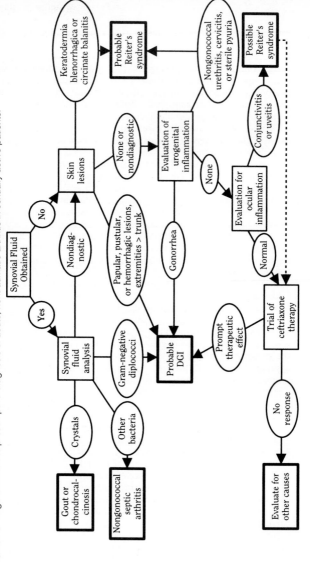

FIG. 27-5 Algorithm for the presumptive diagnosis of acute, nontraumatic arthritis in sexually active patients.

and physical examination to reach a tentative diagnosis when a sexually active patient presents with acute arthritis. If synovial fluid is obtained, examination for crystals by wet preparation and for bacteria by Gram stain should be performed. If synovial fluid is either unobtainable or nondiagnostic, a careful skin exam should be performed. The patient should always undergo examination for either cervicitis or urethritis. It is essential to obtain cultures or antigen-detection tests for *C. trachomatis* and cultures for *N. gonorrhoeae* from the cervix, urethra, and rectum. Pharyngeal, blood, and synovial fluid gonococcal cultures should be obtained as well.

A trial of antibiotic therapy often is warranted. Failure of the arthritis to respond to antibiotics necessitates further evaluation for other causes of arthritis, such as rheumatoid arthritis, Lyme arthritis, systemic lupus erythematosus, and infective endocarditis.

Management

Ceftriaxone is now the treatment of choice for DGI (see Chap. 3). For treatment of NGU or cervicitis in Reiter's syndrome, see Chaps. 20 and 23. Similarly, specific antibiotic therapy should be administered if infectious enteritis is documented. Treatment of the triggering infection, however, does not affect the course of the arthritis or the mucocutaneous manifestations. The mainstay of treatment for Reiter's syndrome is anti-inflammatory drugs, especially indomethacin 25 to 50 mg orally 3 times daily. Several other nonsteroidal anti-inflammatory drugs have been effective for symptomatic relief. Salicylates and corticosteroids are of little benefit for most patients. In fulminant, nonresponsive cases, methotrexate or immunosuppressive agents (e.g., azathioprine) have been reported to be successful.

Arthritis due to hepatitis B is self-limited; when therapy is required, symptoms can be palliated by use of aspirin or other nonsteroidal anti-inflammatory drugs. Patients with arthritis secondary to syphilis, LGV, or other sexually transmitted infections should be treated with standard antibiotic regimens.

REFERENCES

1. Handsfield HH: Disseminated gonococcal infection. *Clin Obstet Gynecol* 18:131, 1975
2. Wilkens RF et al: Reiter's syndrome: Evaluation of preliminary criteria for definite disease. *Arthritis Rheum* 24:844, 1981
3. Kousa M: Clinical observations on Reiter's disease with special reference to the venereal and nonvenereal aetiology: A follow-up study. *Acta Derm Venereol* (Stockh) 58(suppl 81):1, 1978
4. Handsfield HH et al: Unpublished data.

ADDITIONAL READING

Keat A: Sexually transmitted arthritis syndromes. *Med Clin North Am* 74:1617, 1990

For a more detailed discussion, see Handsfield HH, Pollock PS: Arthritis Associated with Sexually Transmitted Diseases, Chap. 61, p 753, in STD-2.

Pregnancy modifies the manifestations of many sexually transmitted diseases (STDs) and presents unique problems for diagnosis and management. As the spectrum of STDs has broadened, the medical and social consequences of STD in pregnancy have become more apparent. Ectopic pregnancy, spontaneous abortion and stillbirth, prematurity, congenital and perinatal infection, and puerperal maternal infections represent outcomes of pregnancy in which sexually transmitted infectious agents play important etiologic roles. The incidence of many STDs has increased during the last three decades, and the number of pregnancies per year is also again increasing. These two factors have further amplified the effects of STD on pregnancy and neonatal morbidity.

ALTERATIONS OF HOST–PARASITE RELATIONSHIPS DURING PREGNANCY

Immunologic rejection of the fetus does not normally occur during pregnancy, perhaps partly because of suppression of maternal immunocompetence. Maternal immunosuppression may in turn affect the natural history of many infectious diseases. Attack rates or severe morbidity have been greater in the pregnant host than in the nonpregnant host for pneumococcal pneumonia, influenza, candidiasis, malaria, viral hepatitis, and a variety of other infections.

The bases for alterations in host immune response are probably multifactorial. Substantial decreases have been found in the CD4+ subset of the T-lymphocyte population of pregnant women. Studies have also revealed impairment of the in vitro lymphocyte transformation response to a number of microbial antigens and to phytohemagglutinin.

The anatomy of the genital tract changes dramatically during pregnancy and may also contribute to the observed alterations in host–parasite relationships. Figure 28-1 illustrates the relationship of the cervix and mucus plug, chorioamnion, and placental bed in late pregnancy. Vaginal walls become hypertrophic and engorged with blood. The glycogen content of the vaginal epithelium increases, and the intravaginal pH significantly decreases during pregnancy. These changes probably influence vaginal microbial flora. The cervix hypertrophies, and a larger area of ectopic columnar epithelium appears on the exocervix, where it is exposed to microorganisms. The increased area of cervical ectopy during pregnancy may predispose the cervix to infection, but this has not been studied. The cervix secretes highly viscid mucus during

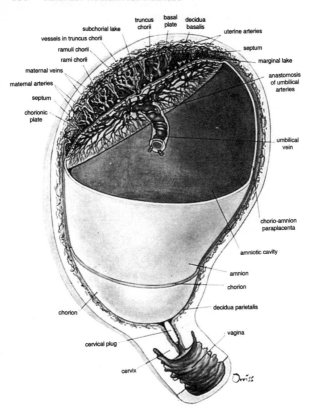

FIG. 28-1. The relationship within the gravid uterus of the mucus plug, fetal membranes (chorion and amnion), decidua, and placenta. *(From JD Boyd and WJ Hamilton,* The Human Placenta.*)*

pregnancy, forming the *mucus plug*. This mucus is generally believed to limit the access of microorganisms into the uterus, but little research has been done to study the actual effectiveness of cervical mucus as a physical or antimicrobial barrier.

ECTOPIC PREGNANCY

Histologic evidence of salpingitis has been identified in about 50 percent of surgically removed ectopic pregnancies. Two sexually transmitted organisms, *Neisseria gonorrhoeae* and *Chlamydia trachomatis,* produce the majority of primary salpingitis cases. The risk of ectopic pregnancy increases about ten-fold after an initial episode of salpingitis. The incidence of ectopic pregnancy has tripled since 1970 in the United States; this trend has also been observed in Sweden, Canada, and England. It is likely that this rising incidence of ectopic pregnancy is partly due to an increasing incidence of gonococcal and chlamydial infections, and of resulting tubal infections, and partly to increased detection of subclinical ectopic pregnancy with improved diagnostic tests.

INTRAUTERINE INFECTION

Intrauterine infection can result from either hematogenous or ascending microbial spread. Hematogenous origin appears to be the major route of spread for organisms present in maternal blood, such as *Treponema pallidum.* Ascending infection by microorganisms present in the cervix or vagina can occur, producing inflammation of the fetal membranes (chorioamnionitis) and the syndrome of amniotic fluid infection.

Chorioamnionitis

Chorioamnionitis is strongly associated with prematurity and neonatal sepsis. It is defined histologically by the presence of polymorphonuclear leukocytes in the membranes—usually within the chorion. Chorioamnionitis probably occurs by transcervical infection of amniotic fluid rather than primary hematogenous spread. The role of coitus in causing ascending infection is controversial. However, the weight of evidence suggests that coitus in pregnancy can be harmful—especially if the sexual partner harbors genital pathogens.

The risk of chorioamnionitis is highest among patients of low socioeconomic status who have not received prenatal care. Although frequently asymptomatic, many women with chorioamnionitis have intrapartum fever, prolonged rupture of membranes, and/or premature labor. Most cases, however, probably occur in the setting of intact membranes. Indeed, it is likely that chorioamnionitis can cause premature rupture of membranes, with delayed delivery after rupture as a result, rather than a cause of the chorioamnionitis.

The cause of acute chorioamnionitis is in many cases unknown. However, bacterial vaginosis is associated with increased risk of chorioamnionitis, and organisms isolated from the chorioamnion more often from patients with chorioamnionitis than from normal patients include some of those found in the vagina of women with bacterial vaginosis. Such organisms include *Ureaplasma urealyticum* and vaginal anaerobes such as *Bacteroides* spp., *Fusobacterium,* and *Peptostreptococcus,* as well as organisms not associated with bacterial vaginosis, such as group B *streptococcus* (GBS) and *Escherichia coli.*

Bacterial vaginosis is also associated with increased risk of amniotic fluid infection, and bacteria recovered from amniotic fluid of patients with chorioamnionitis include anaerobic organisms such as *Peptostreptococcus, Fusobacterium,* and *Bacteroides* spp., as well as facultative organisms such as GBS, enteric gram-negative rods, and, rarely, *Haemophilus influenzae.* These infections are often polymicrobial, resembling the spectrum of organisms found in the upper genital tract of women with salpingitis or postpartum endometritis.

It is unclear whether these organisms are the primary cause of chorioamnionitis or whether chorioamnionitis is primarily attributable to necrosis or mechanical rupture of the membranes. Alternatively, chorioamnionitis may be due to other pathogens which infect and compromise the integrity of the fetal membranes, with secondary infection by vaginal bacteria.

MATERNAL PUERPERAL INFECTION AS A COMPLICATION OF ANTENATAL STDs

Epidemiology and Pathogenesis

Puerperal endometritis, the most common maternal postpartum infection, can be divided into early infections occurring within the first 48 h after delivery and late infections occurring from 2 days to 6 weeks after delivery. Cesarean section greatly increases the risk of early postpartum infection, which is probably due to direct myometrial and peritoneal contamination by organisms present within the amniotic cavity at the time of surgery.

In developed countries, most postpartum infections are related to cesarean section. In developing countries where cesarean sections are less frequently performed and maternal STDs may be more prevalent, postpartum upper genital tract infections after vaginal delivery are approximately 10 times more common than in developed countries.

Microbial Etiology

N. gonorrhoeae and *C. trachomatis* are important causes of post-partum pelvic infection. An important study in Kenya during the 1980s confirmed that undetected antepartum infection with either of those organisms often led to postpartum endometritis. Other microorganisms, such as anaerobic bacteria and *Mycoplasma hominis,* also cause postpartum infection and puerperal sepsis and may be relatively more important causes in areas of low prevalence of maternal gonococcal and chlamydial infection, or where antepartum screening leads to early treatment of these infections.

Bacterial vaginosis per se has recently been implicated as a risk factor for post–cesarean section endometritis and is a suspected risk factor for endometritis following vaginal delivery as well. This is consistent with the association of vaginal anaerobes and *M. hominis* with postpartum pelvic infection after both vaginal and cesarean section delivery, and with the fact that early postpartum bacteremia among women following cesarean delivery is usually due to the anaerobic and facultative bacteria of the cervicovaginal flora, which are predominantly but not exclusively those associated with bacterial vaginosis.

In contrast, in the United States, late postpartum endometritis has been correlated with *C. trachomatis* infection. Clinical manifestations of puerperal chlamydial endometritis, like those of nonpuerperal chlamydial endometritis and salpingitis, are generally mild. Patients are often afebrile, with mild uterine tenderness, and usually with no adnexal tenderness. Such minimally symptomatic postpartum chlamydial infections may contribute to the high rate of chlamydial antibody among women with secondary infertility due to distal tubal obstruction.

NEONATAL CONSEQUENCE OF STDs

Systemic perinatal bacterial infection is acquired in utero or during delivery in 1 to 5 per 1000 live births. About half of all neonatal bacterial infections in the United States are due to GBS, although marked regional variations occur. Table 28-1 summarizes the clinical manifestations of congenital or neonatal infection with STD agents.

CONSEQUENCES, RECOGNITION, AND MANAGEMENT OF SPECIFIC STDs DURING PREGNANCY

Syphilis

Epidemiology

When untreated primary or secondary syphilis occurs during pregnancy, it affects virtually 100 percent of fetuses, with 50 percent of

TABLE 28-1. Clinical Manifestations of Neonatal Infection with Sexually Transmitted Agents Acquired in Utero or at Delivery

Clinical sign	Microorganism*					
	Cytomegalovirus	Herpes simplex virus	Treponema pallidum	Group B streptococci	Chlamydia trachomatis	Neisseria gonorrhoeae
Hepatosplenomegaly	+	+	+	+	−	−
Jaundice	+	+	+	+	−	−
Adenopathy	−	−	+	−	−	−
Pneumonitis	+	+	+	+	++	−
Lesions of skin or mucous membranes						
Petechiae or purpura	+	+	+	+	−	+
Vesicles, ulcers	?	++	+	−	−	−
Maculopapular exanthem	−	+	++	−	−	−
Lesions of nervous system						
Meningoencephalitis	+	+	+	+	−	+
Microcephaly	++	+	−	−	−	−
Intracranial calcifications	++	+	−	−	−	−
Bone lesions	+	+	++	−	−	−
Joint lesions	−	−	+	−	−	+
Eye lesions						
Chorioretinitis	+	+	+	−	−	−
Conjunctivitis	−	+	−	−	++	++

*− Indicates finding rare or not present.
+ Indicates finding occurs in neonates during infection.
++ Indicates finding has special diagnostic significance for this infection.
SOURCE: Modified from AJ Nahmias and AM Visintine from Brown ZA et al. in Remington JS, Klein JO (eds): *Infectious Diseases of the Fetus and Newborn Infant.* Philadelphia, Saunders, 1976.

such pregnancies resulting in premature delivery or perinatal death. Untreated early latent syphilis during pregnancy results in a 40 percent rate of prematurity or perinatal death. Ten percent of infants born to mothers with untreated latent syphilis show signs of congenital infection. While syphilis is rarely sexually transmissible longer than 2 years after acquisition, women with untreated syphilis apparently may remain infectious for their fetuses for many years. However, the proportion of affected fetuses and the severity of fetal disease decrease with longer duration of untreated maternal infection. Chapter 31 discusses the manifestations and pathogenesis of congenital syphilis.

Case Detection

Congenital syphilis can be prevented by early prenatal diagnosis and treatment. Serologic testing remains the most useful diagnostic test for syphilis in women. Signs or symptoms are confirmatory but often are not demonstrable; almost half of women with early syphilis have no manifestations and are detected only by serologic examination. The U.S. Centers for Disease Control (CDC) recommends serologic testing at the first prenatal visit and at delivery, with intermediate testing at the beginning of the third trimester (28 weeks) for high-risk women. In addition, other practical measures may improve early detection of syphilis in pregnant women. These strategies include on-site pregnancy testing of women whose menstrual periods are late in STD clinics and drug-addiction programs; routine rapid plasma reagin (RPR) testing whenever a positive pregnancy test is obtained in all pregnancy-testing programs; and early testing by prenatal programs, before the regularly scheduled prenatal visit when the waiting time for the first scheduled visit is long.

Treatment

A positive screening test should be further evaluated with a quantitative nontreponemal test, such as the Venereal Disease Research Laboratory (VDRL) test and a confirmatory treponemal test, such as the fluorescent treponemal antibody absorption (FTA-ABS) or the microhemagglutination *T. pallidum* (MHA-TP) tests.

Seropositive pregnant women should be considered infected unless treatment history and sequential serologic antibody titers are clearly documented.

Patients should be treated with the penicillin regimen appropriate for the woman's stage of syphilis (see Chap. 6 for recommended treatment of syphilis). Tetracycline and doxycycline are contraindicated in pregnancy. Erythromycin should not be used because of the high risk of failure to cure fetal infection. Pregnant women with histories of penicillin allergy should first be carefully questioned regarding the validity of the history. They should then be skin-tested and either treated with penicillin or referred for desensitization. Women who are treated in the second half of pregnancy are at risk for premature labor and/or fetal distress if their treatment precipitates a Jarisch-Herxheimer reaction. They should be advised to seek medical attention if they notice a change in fetal movements or have any contractions. Stillbirth is a rare complication of treatment; however, since therapy is necessary to prevent further fetal damage, this concern should not delay treatment.

Monthly follow-up of quantitative serologic tests is mandatory so that retreatment can be given if needed. The fall in VDRL titer should be appropriate for the stage of disease.

Gonorrhea

Epidemiology

The reported prevalence of gonococcal infection among pregnant women varies widely by population studied. Generally, prenatal gonorrhea prevalence rates are higher in the United States than in other industrialized countries, and rates in most of the developing world are higher than rates in industrialized countries. In North America, gonorrhea rates are highest in young, nonwhite, unmarried, urban mothers of low socioeconomic status. In addition, history of a new sex partner or multiple partners within the past 3 months, and illegal drug use, are associated with increased risk of gonorrhea and other STDs.

Manifestations and Pathogenesis

The manifestations and pathogenesis of gonococcal infection in the pregnant host have some unique features. Pharyngeal infection is often the sole site of infection. In some studies, 15 to 35 percent of infected pregnant women have had *N. gonorrhoeae* isolated only from the throat and not from the endocervix or anal canal.

Disseminated gonococcal infection may be more common in pregnant women than in nonpregnant women. However, acute gonococcal pelvic inflammatory disease (PID) appears to be a rare event during pregnancy, perhaps because of hormonal and anatomic changes.

Nonetheless, maternal gonococcal infection is detrimental to pregnancy. Intrapartum gonococcal infection is associated with premature rupture of membranes, prolonged rupture of membranes, chorioamnionitis, and prematurity. The effect of gonococcal infection on early pregnancy is less well studied than its effect on late pregnancy, but early infection may cause septic abortion.

Case Detection and Treatment

Pregnant women should have samples cultured for *N. gonorrhoeae* at the first prenatal care visit. In women at high risk for STD, a second culture for gonorrhea should be obtained late in the third trimester. Nearly 40 percent of pregnant women with gonorrhea give a past history of the disease; therefore, past history of gonorrhea is a strong indicator for repeated screening cultures. In patients with premature rupture of membranes, intrapartum fever, or septic abortion, an endocervical swab for Gram stain and culture for *N. gonorrhoeae* should also be obtained.

Recommended regimen

Ceftriaxone 250 mg IM once *plus*

Erythromycin base 500 mg orally 4 times a day for 7 days. (Erythromycin stearate 500 mg or erythromycin ethylsuccinate 800 mg or equivalent may be substituted for erythromycin base.)

Pregnant women allergic to β-lactams should be treated with spectinomycin 2.0 g once (followed by erythromycin). Follow-up cervical and rectal cultures for *N. gonorrhoeae* should be obtained 3 to 7 days after completion of treatment.

Ideally, pregnant women with gonorrhea should be tested for chlamydial infection and treated if infected. If chlamydial diagnostic testing is not available, then treatment for chlamydia with erythromycin should be given together with gonorrhea treatment (as indicated above) because of the high likelihood of coinfection with both *N. gonorrhoeae* and *C. trachomatis.* Tetracyclines (including doxycycline) are contraindicated in pregnancy because of the possibility of adverse effects on the fetus. Quinolones (for example, ciprofloxacin and ofloxacin) are also contraindicated during pregnancy.

For complicated gonococcal infection in pregnancy (e.g., septic abortion, chorioamnionitis), we recommend treatment for several days with ceftriaxone or cefoxitin plus erythromycin for possible coexisting chlamydial infections.

Neonatal Gonococcal Infection

Neonates born to mothers with untreated antepartum or intrapartum gonococcal infection are at high risk for gonococcal ophthalmia neonatorum as well as infection at other body sites. These infants should receive parenteral antibiotics in standard curative dosage (see Chap. 29), in addition to topical ocular prophylaxis.

Chlamydia trachomatis Infections

The reported prevalence of *C. trachomatis* infection among pregnant women has ranged widely from 2 to 30 percent. In addition to the usual demographic correlates of STD in pregnancy (described above for gonorrhea), young age, especially adolescence, is a very strong predictor of chlamydial infection in pregnancy.

Antepartum chlamydial infection appears to play a role in amnionitis, postpartum endometritis, and postabortal salpingitis. We recommend that women undergoing therapeutic abortion be screened for chlamydial infection to prevent postabortal ascending infection.

Pregnant women should undergo diagnostic testing for *C. trachomatis* at their first prenatal visit. Women at high risk should be tested again during the third trimester.

Recommended regimen

Erythromycin base 500 mg 4 times a day for 7 days.

If the above therapy is not tolerated, the following regimens are recommended:

Alternative regimen

Erythromycin base 250 mg 4 times a day for 14 days *or*
Erythromycin ethylsuccinate 800 mg 4 times a day for 7 days *or*
Erythromycin ethylsuccinate 400 mg 4 times a day for 14 days.

Alternative if erythromycin cannot be tolerated

Amoxicillin 500 mg orally 3 times a day for 7 days. (Although penicillins are not generally recommended for chlamydial infection, one large study suggested that this regimen may be effective in pregnant women.)

Erythromycin estolate is contraindicated during pregnancy because of frequent hepatotoxicity. As previously noted, tetracyclines, the drugs of choice for *C. trachomatis* infection in nonpregnant adults, cannot be recommended for pregnant or nursing women. Quinolones are also contraindicated for pregnant of nursing women.

Group B Streptococcus

GBS *(Streptococcus agalactiae)* is part of the vaginal flora of 5 to 25 percent of women. Although 65 to 75 percent of exposed neonates become colonized, only 1 in 50 to 1 in 100 neonates born to women with GBS vaginal colonization develop invasive GBS disease. The mortality rate of neonatal GBS sepsis is 50 percent. Vertical transmission accounts for most early-onset disease, and early infection is significantly associated with premature birth, prolonged rupture of membranes, and maternal intra- and postpartum fever. With late-onset disease, infection occurs after the first week of life; it is not associated with vertical transmission or with maternal obstetric complications. Although the importance of GBS is greatest in neonatal infections, GBS has also been implicated in obstetric and puerperal complications, such as amnionitis and postpartum endometritis.

Strategies for prevention of perinatal or neonatal GBS disease are being evaluated. Proposals under evaluation include antenatal culture screening and treatment of maternal carriers (especially those with higher concentrations of GBS in the vagina), identification and immunization of mothers who are seronegative for GBS antibodies, and prophylactic treatment of exposed neonates.

Genital Mycoplasmas

Many reproductive disorders have been ascribed to infection with the genital mycoplasmas. However, the ubiquity of these organisms and the high frequency of coinfection with other STD agents make it difficult to assess their etiologic roles in these disorders. In general, *M. hominis* has been associated with endometritis and postpartum fever while *U. urealyticum* has been correlated with amniotic fluid infection, chorioamnionitis, low birth weight, and prematurity. The etiologic role of these agents, however, remains to be elucidated.

At present, antenatal serologic studies or vaginal culture for either *U. urealyticum* or *M. hominis* are not recommended.

Bacterial Vaginosis

Bacterial vaginosis (BV) is characterized by a nonpurulent, homogeneous, malodorous vaginal discharge; increase in vaginal pH; the presence of characteristic amines and organic acids in vaginal fluid; and polymicrobial changes in vaginal flora, including a decrease in H_2O_2-producing facultative lactobacilli, and an increase in *Gardnerella vaginalis* and several anaerobic species (see Chap. 21). BV and BV-associated microorganisms have been found to be correlated with amniotic-fluid-infection syndrome, prematurity, and puerperal infections.

BV is not generally treated during pregnancy since (1) the symptoms, if any, are well tolerated, (2) although a relationship of BV to pregnancy morbidity has been confirmed in a large multicenter study, it has not yet been shown in a randomized clinical trial that treatment of BV during pregnancy reduces pregnancy or puerperal morbidity, and (3) the use of any drugs should be minimized in the pregnant woman. In a pregnant woman who wants treatment for BV because of symptoms, use of intravaginal clindamycin cream can be considered.

Cytomegalovirus Infection

Cytomegalovirus infection (CMV) is the commonest cause of congenital viral infection of the fetus and is the most common infectious cause of mental retardation. The role of sexual transmission in the epidemiology of CMV is discussed in Chap. 12.

No clinical illness is recognized in most pregnant women who develop primary CMV infection. Women with recurrent (nonprimary) CMV infections almost always have no recognizable clinical abnormality.

Congenital infection is most common and most often associated with early clinical manifestations among neonates born to mothers who develop primary CMV infection during pregnancy. About 40 percent of infants born to such women develop congenital infection, and nearly one-third of infected infants have clinical manifestations of CMV infection at birth or shortly thereafter.

Congenital infection is less common and much less often clinically apparent among neonates born to mothers with preexisting persistent or recurrent CMV infection.

Symptomatic congenital CMV infection is characterized by hepatomegaly, splenomegaly, microcephaly, mental retardation, motor retardation, motor disability, jaundice, and petechiae. Often CMV-infected neonates are born prematurely and are of low birth weight. The mortality and long-term morbidity for such children are exceedingly high.

Case Detection

Women who develop a viral-like illness during pregnancy should probably have serologic studies performed to exclude primary CMV, although most primary CMV infections in pregnancy are asymptomatic. Primary CMV infection, if recognized in early pregnancy, may be an indication for offering abortion since severe fetal involvement occurs in at least 30 percent of infants.

Congenitally or perinatally infected infants often shed large amounts of the virus in saliva, respiratory secretions, and urine. Pregnant women should not be exposed to infants recognized to be shedding CMV.

Herpes Simplex Virus Infection

Herpes simplex virus (HSV) infection in pregnancy is of concern for two reasons: (1) primary HSV infection during pregnancy has been associated with an increased risk of spontaneous abortion and prematurity, and (2) maternal HSV shedding at term is associated with life-threatening neonatal infection. Most neonatal HSV infection is presumed to be due to intrapartum exposure to HSV-2 in the birth canal; up to 86 percent of HSV isolates from neonates are type 2.

Primary adult infection with HSV, unlike recurrent disease, is characterized by prolonged clinical illness, frequent systemic involvement (indicating viremia), frequent cervical infection, and high-titered viral shedding. Transplacental infection with HSV is a rare complication of viremia, and congenital infection with HSV occurs only rarely. The syndrome of disseminated HSV infection, with potentially fatal hepatotoxicity and nephrotoxicity, may occur with increased frequency in pregnant women but is nonetheless extremely rare even in pregnancy.

Primary HSV infection during pregnancy is a major risk factor for neonatal HSV infection and is also associated with spontaneous abortion, preterm delivery, and intrauterine growth retardation. Primary genital HSV infection is much more strongly associated with neonatal infection and disease than recurrent herpes is. This is probably because women with primary infection have a large inoculum of virus present in the birth canal, extensive cervical involvement, absence of HSV antibodies, and frequent viremia. The risk of neonatal transmission from a mother with primary infection ranges from 20 to 50 percent. Up to one-half of neonates who acquire HSV infection have been exposed to mothers with primary infection occurring late in pregnancy.

In contrast, recurrent genital herpes during pregnancy is associated with a much lower risk of neonatal infection and disease. Most studies estimate the risk of neonatal transmission through vaginal delivery in women with recurrent HSV cervicitis at 3 to 5 percent. Recurrence rates of herpes during pregnancy are high; 70 percent of women with a history of recurrent disease have at least one positive HSV culture while pregnant. However, recurrences during pregnancy are not clinically worse than recurrences in nonpregnant women, and recurrent disease is not associated with prematurity.

The route of delivery and duration of rupture of membranes correlate with risk of neonatal infection among mothers who have genital herpes at term. Approximately 50 percent of neonates exposed to HSV during vaginal delivery acquire the disease. Cesarean section appears to significantly reduce this risk if performed within 4 h of rupture of membranes. When membranes have been ruptured for greater than 4 h, nearly all exposed neonates acquire the disease, irrespective of the route of delivery.

Management

Clinicians should solicit and record in the prenatal record a history of genital herpes in the patient or her partner(s). Women with a positive history should be observed carefully for recurrences near the end of pregnancy.

At the onset of labor, all women should be carefully questioned about symptoms and examined. Women without symptoms or signs of genital herpes infection or prodrome may be delivered vaginally. If herpetic lesions are in the genital tract when membranes rupture or during labor, cesarean section should be performed if it can be done within 4 h of rupture of membranes. In women who have a history of genital herpes, or have a sex partner with genital herpes, cultures of samples from the birth canal at delivery may be helpful in decisions about neonatal management, though the cost-benefit ratio of perinatal HSV screening in this way is doubtful. Infants delivered through an infected birth canal (proved by culture or by observation of presumptively herpetic lesions) should have samples cultured and should be followed carefully. Although existing data are not sufficient to recommend the use of acyclovir in asymptomatic infants, some clinicians presumptively treat infants who were exposed to HSV at delivery. Herpes cultures should be obtained from infants before therapy; positive cultures obtained 24 to 48 h or more after birth indicate active viral infection.

Human Papillomavirus

Genital human papillomaviruses (HPVs), the causative agents of genital warts and most cases of cervical intraepithelial neoplasia (CIN), are of concern in pregnancy because (1) warts may rapidly enlarge with advancing gestation and mechanically obstruct labor, (2) the most common form of therapy, topical application of podophyllin, is contraindicated during pregnancy, and (3) perinatal exposure may result in development of laryngeal or genital papillomatosis in infancy or childhood. It is not certain whether intrapartum exposure of the infant to an infected mother also commonly leads to genital HPV infection of the infant. The worsening of CIN frequently observed during pregnancy may also be due to accelerated HPV replication.

A history of current or past genital warts may be useful in monitoring pregnant patients for recurrent or excessive growth of wart lesions. Pregnant women should have Pap smears to detect evidence of CIN.

Genital warts should be removed before delivery by electrocoagulation, cryotherapy, or electrodesiccation. Laser therapy has also been successful. Podophyllin should not be used during pregnancy because both maternal and neonatal deaths have resulted from excessive use of this agent.

Cesarean section is not currently recommended to prevent neonatal exposure to HPV. However, it may be necessary if extensive lesions obstruct the vaginal outlet.

Human Immunodeficiency Virus (HIV)

Whether pregnancy alters the natural history of HIV infection is still unknown. However, HIV infection has been associated with preterm delivery or low-birth-weight infants in some, but not all, studies. Prospective studies suggest that perhaps 20 to 30 percent of infants exposed to a seropositive mother in the United States will acquire HIV infection. However, the risk of perinatal transmission has varied widely and may be greater from symptomatic, immuno-suppressed pregnant women than from asymptomatic, immunologically normal pregnant women with HIV infection.

Confirmation of infection in exposed infants can be difficult since infants passively acquire maternal IgG antibodies against HIV. IgM and IgA antibody testing of cord blood has not yet proved reliable for predicting future serologic status of the exposed neonate. The detection of HIV-1 by culture or by the polymerase chain reaction can be insensitive early in life. In general, infants may have to be followed for 15 months to correctly determine whether they have been infected. Multiple antibody, antigen, and viral isolation studies may therefore be necessary to determine whether infection has occurred.

The relative frequency of in utero, intrapartum, and postpartum transmission from the mother is still uncertain. At least some infants are infected prenatally. Cesarean section has not yet been found to prevent HIV transmission, and the proportion of infants infected during birth is not known. Postnatal transmission via breastfeeding is well documented, although the efficiency of transmission by this route requires further study.

There is no clear scientific or political consensus on many of the various potential interventions in HIV-positive pregnant women. However, pregnant women with high-risk behaviors should certainly be counseled and offered HIV testing, and the American Academy of Pediatrics recommends routine HIV testing of all pregnant women on a voluntary basis.

Trichomonas vaginalis Vaginitis

Trichomonas vaginalis presents two problems unique to the pregnant host: (1) an association with puerperal maternal morbidity (postpartum fever) has been noted, and (2) a recent multicenter study of vaginal and cervical infections in pregnancy found that vaginal trichomoniasis was one of the infections that was associated with a small but statistically significant increased risk of preterm delivery.

Therapy for trichomoniasis during pregnancy has been problematic, especially in view of the evidence associating trichomoniasis with preterm delivery. Metronidazole and other nitroimidazoles are the only highly effective forms of therapy for trichomoniasis. They have not been approved in the United States for use during pregnancy. Although not yet associated with pregnancy morbidity or birth defects, metronidazole has generally been withheld early in pregnancy and reserved for use (single 2-g dose) in later pregnancy in very symptomatic women. This policy now requires careful review.

SUMMARY: APPROACH TO MANAGEMENT OF STDs IN PREGNANCY AND THE PERINATAL PERIOD

A standard history concerning sexual and drug-using behavior and past STDs should be obtained from all pregnant patients. Information on age, socioeconomic status, marital status, and health care behavior may also help identify those at highest risk of having STD.

Pregnant women in most populations should routinely undergo cervical screening culture for gonorrhea and serologic testing for syphilis. Those with a history of past gonococccal infection or who have more than one current sex partner should be screened again in late pregnancy with both tests. A routine screening test for *C. trachomatis* is indicated in pregnant women who have risk factors for chlamydial infection.

The occurrence of a number of clinical situations during pregnancy should prompt evaluation of the patient for selected STDs. Dysuria, a common complaint in pregnancy, should not be automatically attributed to urinary tract infection without excluding vaginitis, cervicitis, or urethritis as a possible cause. Endocervical cultures for *N. gonorrhoeae* and *C. trachomatis* should be obtained from women at any stage of gestation who have signs of mucuopurulent cervicitis or history of exposure to a sex partner with urethritis. Women with otherwise unexplained complications such as septic abortion, premature labor, premature rupture of membranes, and intrapartum fever should be evaluated for sexually transmitted infection. Treatable infections (e.g., with *N. gonorrhoeae* and *C. trachomatis*) should always be excluded in women with these complications. Women who have a syndrome consistent with CMV infection during pregnancy should have serologic tests performed to exclude primary CMV infection. Women who have a history of genital herpes should be examined closely for recurrent clinical evidence of herpetic lesions late in pregnancy and during labor, as described above. Screening for HIV infection, on a voluntary basis and with appropriate counseling, is being advocated by many in the United States, to permit counseling of infected parents and early management of HIV infection in the infant.

Finally, it must be emphasized that in the setting of neonatal STD, both parents must be interviewed, examined, and treated where appropriate. Special surveillance of the neonate may be necessary when the mother is at high risk for STDs or develops puerperal infection or intrapartum fever.

ADDITIONAL READING

Arvin AM: Relationships between maternal immunity to herpes simplex virus and the risk of neonatal herpesvirus infection. *Rev Infect Dis* 13:S953, 1991

Brown ZA et al: Neonatal herpes simplex virus infection in relation to asymptomatic maternal infection at the time of labor [see comments]. *N Engl J Med* 324:1247, 1991

Catalano PM et al: Incidence of genital herpes simplex virus at the time of delivery in women with known risk factors. *Am J Obstet Gynecol* 164:1303, 1991

Elliott B et al: Maternal gonococcal infection as a preventable risk factor for low birth weight. *J Infect Dis* 161:531, 1990

Fowler KB, Pass RF: Sexually transmitted diseases in mothers of neonates with congenital cytomegalovirus infection. *J Infect Dis* 164:259, 1991

Gibbs RS, Mead PB: Preventing neonatal herpes—Current strategies, editorial; comment. *N Engl J Med* 326:946, 1992

Hillier SL et al: Microbiologic causes and neonatal outcomes associated with chorioamnion infection. *Am J Obstet Gynecol* 165:955, 1991

Hillier SL et al: The relationship of hydrogen peroxide–producing lactobacilli to bacterial vaginosis and genital microflora in pregnant women. *Obstet Gynecol* 79:369, 1992

Hillier SL et al: Characteristics of three vaginal flora patterns assessed by Gram stain among pregnant women. Vaginal Infections and Prematurity Study Group. *Am J Obstet Gynecol* 166:938, 1992

Larsson PG et al: Incidence of pelvic inflammatory disease after first-trimester legal abortion in women with bacterial vaginosis after treatment with metronidazole: A double-blind, randomized study. *Am J Obstet Gynecol* 166:100, 1992

Libman MD et al: Strategies for the prevention of neonatal infection with herpes simplex virus: A decision analysis. *Rev Infect Dis* 13:1093, 1991

Minkoff HL: Preventing fetal damage from sexually transmitted diseases. *Clin Obstet Gynecol* 34:336, 1991

Minkoff HL et al: Pregnancy outcomes among mothers infected with human immunodeficiency virus and uninfected control subjects. *Am J Obstet Gynecol* 163:1598, 1990

Much DH, Yeh SY: Prevalence of *Chlamydia trachomatis* infection in pregnant patients. *Public Health Rep* 106:490, 1991

Silver HM et al: Evidence relating bacterial vaginosis to intraamniotic infection. *Am J Obstet Gynecol* 161:808, 1989

Temmerman M et al: Infection with HIV as a risk factor for adverse obstetrical outcome. *AIDS* 4:1087, 1990

Watts DH et al: Bacterial vaginosis as a risk factor post-Cesarean endometritis. *Obstet Gynecol* 75:52, 1990

Watts DH et al: Upper genital tract isolates at delivery as predictors of post-cesarean infections among women receiving antibiotic prophylaxis. *Obstet Gynecol* 77:287, 1991

For a more detailed discussion, see Brunham RC, Holmes KK, and Embree JE: Sexually Transmitted Diseases in Pregnancy, Chap. 64, p 771, in STD-2.

The worldwide epidemic of *Neisseria gonorrhoeae* infections has been widely publicized, but the increasing risk of infection in children has gained public recognition relatively slowly. Retrospective reviews and case reports based on detection of symptomatic cases provide us with the estimates of infection in preadolescent children and early adolescent youths. Presenting complaints of children who are subsequently determined to have *N. gonorrhoeae* infection are primarily vaginal or urethral discharge, but some present for evaluation of sexual assault, and a number of children have complaints not related to the genitalia. Gonococcal infection in prepubertal children is particularly important because it may be an indicator of child abuse. Identification of infection in children should lead to a search for adult contacts.

Gonococcal infections in children produce different clinical syndromes which are age-related. In addition, the means of acquisition of infection varies by age; thus, newborn gonococcal infection will be considered separately from *N. gonorrhoeae* in prepubertal children.

MATERNAL AND PERINATAL *N. GONORRHOEAE* INFECTION

Untreated maternal gonococcal disease can have substantial effects on the health of the fetus and infant. A number of studies have demonstrated associations between maternal gonococcal infection and prematurity, perinatal distress, premature rupture of membranes, and spontaneous abortion (see Chap. 28).

Neonatal Gonococcal Ophthalmia

In earlier times, gonococcal conjunctivitis of the newborn was common and a leading cause of blindness. This is no longer true in industrialized countries. The causes of neonatal ophthalmic disease include chemical conjunctivitis due to silver nitrate, *Chlamydia trachomatis, Staphylococcus aureus, Hemophilus spp.,* other respiratory tract bacteria such as pneumococci, herpes simplex, and *N. gonorrhoeae.*

Conjunctival infection caused by *N. gonorrhoeae* in the newborn usually produces an acute purulent conjunctivitis that appears from 2 to 5 days after birth. However, the initial course is occasionally indolent, and onset can occur later than 5 days after birth, perhaps because of partial suppression of infection by ophthalmic prophylaxis, because of small inoculum size, or because of strain-to-strain variations in gonococcal virulence. Prolonged incubation after perinatal acquisition is hard to distinguish from delayed onset due to postnatal acquisition. Therefore, gonococcal infection must be ruled out in every case of conjunctivitis in infants, regardless of severity or time of onset.

Although gonococcal conjunctivitis is usually less severe and less rapidly progressive in the newborn than in the adult, permanent corneal damage was usual in the preantibiotic era. The infant typically develops tense edema of both lids, followed by chemosis and a progressively purulent and profuse conjunctival exudate, which pours or squirts from the lids when they are separated. If treatment is delayed, the infection extends beyond the superficial epithelial layers, reaching the subconjunctival connective tissue of the palpebral conjunctivae and, more significantly, the cornea. Corneal complications include ulcerations that may leave permanent nebulae or cause perforation and lead to anterior synechiae, anterior staphyloma, panophthalmitis (rarely), and loss of the eye.

In addition to ocular complications of neonatal gonococcal ophthalmia, the disease may spread locally, cause primary disease at other mucous membrane sites, or cause systemic disease. About 35 percent of infants with gonococcal ophthalmia also yield *N. gonorrhoeae* from pharyngeal culture. The ocular disease serves as a signal that the infant has been infected.

Exposed infants who receive ocular silver nitrate prophylaxis have a less than 5 percent incidence of gonococcal ophthalmia, while exposed infants who have not had prophylaxis have an incidence of 2 to 30 percent.

Gonococcal Arthritis in the Neonate

Septic arthritis is the most commonly recognized manifestation of gonococcemia in the neonatal period. The source of bacteremia is often not apparent.

Clinical evidence of gonococcal arthritis in the newborn usually appears from 1 to 4 weeks after delivery. In most cases it is impossible to distinguish between perinatal and postnatal acquisition of infection. Multiple joints are usually involved; the characteristic presentation is the infant's unwillingness to move the involved limb(s). Conjunctivitis is absent in most cases of neonatal gonococcal arthritis; its absence may partially be explained by ophthalmic prophylaxis and prompt recognition and treatment of gonococcal ophthalmia neonatorum when it occurs despite prophylaxis. The pustular and necrotic skin lesions that characteristically appear during gonococcemia in the adult have not been described in the newborn. The natural history of gonococcal arthritis in the infant is uncertain. Fatality rates varied markedly among series in the preantibiotic era.

Other Manifestations of Neonatal Gonococcal Infection

In addition to gonococcal ophthalmia and septic arthritis, the spectrum of neonatal disease attributable to *N. gonorrhoeae* includes sepsis without arthritis and local infections such as vaginitis, rhinitis, anorectal infection, funisitis, urethritis, and, recently, scalp abscesses at the site of intrauterine fetal monitoring electrodes.

Diagnosis of Neonatal Gonococcal Disease

Direct culture is the method of choice for diagnosis of all forms of childhood gonorrhea. When gonococcal arthritis is suspected, Gram stain of aspirated joint fluid should be performed, and blood and joint fluid should be cultured for *N. gonorrhoeae.*

In infants with suspected gonococcal ophthalmia, conjunctival exudate should be examined by Gram stain; detection of typical gram-negative intracellular bean-shaped diplococci supports the presumptive diagnosis of gonococcal conjunctivitis, although other *Neisseria* species, such as *N. meningitidis,* have also been associated with purulent ophthalmia neonatorum. Conjunctival exudate should be plated directly onto blood agar, MacConkey agar, and either chocolate agar or Thayer-Martin medium (containing no more 3 µg/ml of vancomycin) for recovery of *N. gonorrhoeae.* If gonococcal conjunctivitis is suspected on the basis of a positive Gram stain, cultures for *N. gonorrhoeae* should also be obtained from the oropharynx and anal canal, since concomitant infection of these sites has been demonstrated in association with gonococcal ophthalmia neonatorum. Because of the social implications of gonorrhea in a child, all presumptive *N. gonorrhoeae* isolates should be confirmed by at least two tests that use different principles (e.g., biochemical, enzyme substrate, or serologic).

GONOCOCCAL DISEASE BEYOND INFANCY

Vaginitis

Beyond the neonatal period, gonococcal vaginitis is the most common form of gonorrhea in childhood. In contrast to adults, in prepubertal girls the nonestrogenized alkaline vaginal mucosa can be colonized and infected with *N. gonorrhoeae.* Gonococcal vaginitis is usually a mild disease, perhaps because it is restricted to the superficial mucosa. Asymptomatic disease is probably common among infected children and is usually recognized when a child is undergoing evaluation for suspected sexual abuse. The majority of symptomatic girls have vaginal itching and minor crusting discharge, which may discolor the underwear. Signs of systemic infection are minimal or absent. Dysuria and pyuria may be present. A Gram stain of the vaginal secretions may lead to diagnosis.

Although gonococcal vaginitis occasionally results in salpingitis or peritonitis, ascending infection is uncommon, probably because of the lack of patency of the endocervix until age 9 or 10 years.

Other causes of vaginitis in girls include irritative and infectious agents such as pinworms, foreign bodies, streptococci, *Trichomonas vaginalis,* diphtheroids, and other bacteria.

Pelvic Inflammatory Disease and Salpingitis

Vaginal infection, especially in adolescents, may progress to involve the fallopian tubes or disseminate to the pelvis, resulting in perihepatitis and pelvic inflammatory disease (PID). PID in adolescents is particularly likely to result in ectopic pregnancy and infertility, and PID is the single most common cause of infertility in young women.

Identification of the cause of PID is complicated by the difficulty of obtaining fallopian tube specimens prior to therapy. Gonococcal infections are a common cause of acute PID in adolescents, but not the only one. Other causes include *Chlamydia trachomatis, Mycoplasma hominis,* and mixed aerobic flora, especially *Peptostreptococcus* and *Peptococcus* species.

Risk factors for PID and acute salpingitis include a history of previous PID, multiple sexual partners, and use of an IUD for contraception. Approximately 15 percent of teenagers who develop gonorrhea progress to PID.

Diagnosis of PID may be difficult. Differential diagnosis in the adolescent includes numerous other causes of abdominal pain, such as appendicitis, ectopic pregnancy, mesenteric adenitis, pyelonephritis, and septic abortion. Clinical diagnosis of PID is supported by the presence of lower abdominal pain and adnexal and cervical motion tenderness. Fever, leukocytosis, elevated sedimentation rate, and adnexal mass on abdominal ultrasonography support the diagnosis but may be absent. Culdocentesis, if performed, may reveal evidence of purulent reaction in the peritoneal cavity.

The outcome for fertility presumably improves with prompt and vigorous therapy. All adolescents with PID probably should be hospitalized. Other indications for hospitalization are listed in Table 29-1.

Urethritis

Gonococcal urethritis in prepubertal males is less common than vaginitis is in females. The disease is usually symptomatic and resembles gonococcal urethritis in adults, but it can also cause asymptomatic pyuria. Gonococcal infection of the genital urinary

TABLE 29-1. Indications for Hospitalization of Children with Suspected Salpingitis

---

All adolescents
Diagnostic uncertainty
Failure to respond to prior regimen
Pregnancy
Fever, peritoneal signs
Adnexal mass
IUD use
Noncompliance with medical regimen

---

tract is often accompanied by anorectal or oropharyngeal infection which may be either symptomatic or asymptomatic.

Disseminated Disease

Gonococcal arthritis in older children resembles that of adults and may be accompanied by cutaneous lesions. Involvement of multiple joints is not as common as in the newborn period, although some patients have a migratory polyarthritis.

Cultures of nasopharynx, rectum, vagina or endocervix, blood, and involved joint(s) should be obtained. The need for drainage of an affected joint must be assessed in each patient. Complete response to medical therapy may not occur for several days, even with drainage of affected joints. Open drainage procedures should be avoided if possible; needle aspirations are adequate to drain most joints (knees, ankles, wrists, elbows). Purulent arthritis of the hips, however, usually requires early open (surgical) drainage to prevent necrosis of the femoral head.

Gonorrhea as an Indicator of Sexual Abuse in Children

Gonorrhea in children other than newborns should be assumed to be sexually transmitted and is thus often an indicator of sexual abuse. Among all STDs diagnosed in children evaluated for suspected abuse, gonorrhea is the single most common diagnosis (see Chap. 32).

TREATMENT

Treatment of Infants Born to Mothers with Gonococcal Infection

Infants born to mothers with untreated gonorrhea are at high risk of infection [e.g., ophthalmia and disseminated gonococcal infection (DGI)] and should be treated with a single injection of **ceftriaxone (50 mg/kg IV or IM, not to exceed 125 mg)**. Ceftriaxone should be given cautiously to hyperbilirubinemic infants, especially premature infants. Topical prophylaxis for neonatal ophthalmia is not adequate treatment for documented infections of the eye or other sites.

Treatment of Infants with Gonococcal Infection

Infants with documented gonococcal infections at any site (e.g., eye) should be evaluated for DGI. This evaluation should include a careful physical examination, especially of the joints, as well as blood and CSF cultures. Infants with ophthalmia neonatorum may be treated with **ceftriaxone 25–50 mg/kg IV or IM once, not to exceed 125 mg.** Infants with DGI should be treated for 10 to 14 days with one of the following regimens:

Ceftriaxone 25 to 50 mg/kg per day in a single daily dose *or* **cefotaxime 25 mg/kg 2 times a day.**

Infants with no signs of gonococcal infection should be treated with **single injection of ceftriaxone (50 mg/kg up to 125 mg)** if their mothers have gonococcal infection.

If the gonococcal isolate is proved to be susceptible to penicillin, **crystalline pencillin G may be given. The dose is 100,000 units/kg per day given in 2 equal doses (4 equal doses per day for infants more than 1 week old). The dose should be increased to 150,000 units/kg per day for meningitis.**

Infants with gonococcal ophthalmia should receive eye irrigation with buffered saline solutions until discharge has cleared. Topical antibiotic therapy alone is inadequate. Simultaneous infection with *C. trachomatis* has been reported and should be considered in patients who do not respond satisfactorily. The mother and infant should be tested for chlamydial infection.

Gonococcal Infections of Children

Children who weigh 45 kg or more should be treated with adult regimens. Children who weigh less than 45 kg should be treated as follows:

Recommended regimen:

For uncomplicated vulvovaginitis, cervicitis, urethritis, pharyngitis, and proctitis: **ceftriaxone 125 mg IM once.**

Patients who cannot tolerate ceftriaxone may be treated with **spectinomycin 40 mg/kg IM once.**

Children 8 years of age or older should also be treated presumptively for concomitant chlamydial infection with **doxycyline 100 mg 2 times a day for 7 days.** All patients should be evaluated for coinfection with syphilis and *C. trachomatis.* Follow-up cultures are necessary to ensure that treatment has been effective.

Bacteremia or arthritis should be treated with **ceftriaxone 50 mg/kg (maximum 1 g) once daily for 7 days. For meningitis, the** duration of treatment is increased to 10 to 14 days, and the maximum daily dose is 2 g.

PREVENTION OF OPHTHALMIA NEONATORUM

Instillation of a prophylactic agent into the eyes of all newborn infants is recommended to prevent gonococcal ophthalmia neonatorum and is required by law in most states. While all regimens proposed below effectively prevent gonococcal eye disease, their efficacy in preventing chlamydial eye disease is not clear. Furthermore, they do not eliminate nasopharyngeal colonization with *C. trachomatis.*

Recommended regimens:
Erythromycin (0.5%) ophthalmic ointment, *or*
Tetracycline (1%) ointment, *or*
Silver nitrate (1%).

One of these should be instilled into the eyes of every neonate as soon as possible after delivery, and definitely within 1 h after birth.

The efficacy of tetracycline and erythromycin in the prevention of ophthalmia caused by tetracycline-resistant and penicillinase-producing organisms is unknown. Because of the high concentrations of drug in these preparations, both are probably effective. Bacitracin is not a recommended regimen.

Treatment of gonococcal and chlamydial infections in pregnant women is the best method for preventing neonatal gonococcal and chlamydial disease. Pregnant women should have specimens cultured for *N. gonorrhoeae* at the first prenatal care visit. Those at high risk for STD should have specimens cultured again late in the third trimester.

ADDITIONAL READING

Ahmed HJ, et al: An epidemic of *Neisseria gonorrhoeae* in a Somali orphanage. *Int J STD AIDS* 3:52, 1992

Desenclos JC, et al: Pediatric gonococcal infection, Florida, 1984 to 1988. *Am J Public Health* 82:426, 1992

Lepage P, et al: Treatment of gonococcal conjunctivitis with a single intramuscular injection of cefotaxime. *J Antimicrob Chemother* 26 Suppl A:23, 1990

Lewis LS, et al: Gonococcal conjunctivitis in prepubertal children. *Am J Dis Child* 144:546, 1990

Vermund SH, et al: History of sexual abuse in incarcerated adolescents with gonorrhea or syphilis. *J Adolesc Health Care* 11:449, 1990

For a more detailed discussion, see Gutman LT, Wilfert CM: Gonococcal Diseases in Infants and Children, Chap. 65, p 803, in STD-2.

The biology and the spectrum of adult infection by *Chlamydia trachomatis* are discussed in Chap. 4. The infections considered in this chapter include neonatal inclusion conjunctivitis and infant pneumonitis.

EPIDEMIOLOGY

As with gonorrhea, the link between adult and infant chlamydial infections is vertical transmission from a cervically infected pregnant woman. About 5 to 10 percent of pregnant women have *C. trachomatis* infection. Infected women tend to be younger, of lower socioeconomic status and gravidity, and more often unmarried and nonwhite. Several studies indicate that infants born to women with chlamydial infection have an 18 to 50 percent risk of developing conjunctivitis and 11 to 20 percent risk for pneumonia.

PATHOGENESIS

Infants are probably inoculated with *C. trachomatis* during passage through an infected endocervical canal. The pathogenesis of infection has not been completely elucidated. One hypothesis is that individual sites (eye, nasopharynx, lung, vagina) are inoculated independently. Alternatively, infection may progress by direct extension of infected secretions from eye to nasopharynx to lung.

Once transmitted to the infant, *C. trachomatis* infects and disrupts epithelial surfaces but does not invade or destroy deep tissue or produce exotoxins. Disease manifestations appear to be a consequence of the host response to infection rather than the inherent destructiveness of the organism.

CLINICAL MANIFESTATIONS

Inclusion Conjunctivitis

Clinical findings generally appear between the fifth and twelfth postnatal days. In many cases, determination of the day of onset is difficult because early conjunctivitis due to silver nitrate is often present. Clinical manifestations range widely from asymptomatic infection to severe purulent conjunctivitis. Disease usually begins as a mucoid discharge that becomes progressively more purulent. The eyelids then become edematous, the palpebral conjunctivae become diffusely erythematous, and the normal vascular pattern is obliterated. The bulbar conjunctivae become inflamed, and papillary hypertrophy, primarily of the upper tarsal plate, is present. If the disease is prolonged, lymphoid follicles usually develop between 3 and 6 weeks of age. When untreated, active disease can persist for 3 to 12 months. Inclusion conjunctivitis can be complicated by conjunctival scarring and superficial corneal vascularization.

Differential diagnosis of neonatal conjunctivitis is wide. Silver nitrate prophylaxis can cause conjunctival inflammation with marked lid swelling but little discharge; the reaction usually resolves within 3 days. Gonococcal ophthalmia most often presents at 2 to 5 days of life with a copious purulent exudate and marked lid edema. Other causes of infant conjunctivitis include *Staphylococcus aureus, Streptococcus pneumoniae, Haemophilus influenzae, H. aegyptius,* other gram-negative organisms such as *Klebsiella* and *Neisseria meningitidis,* and streptococci. All of these organisms produce similar clinical findings: purulent discharge, edema, and erythema of the conjunctiva. Gram stain and bacterial culture of the discharge are necessary for diagnosis.

Viral infection is another important consideration. Herpes simplex virus, acquired by passage through the mother's infected genital secretions, may cause neonatal ophthalmia. Signs of meningitis, disseminated infection, or skin vesicles help to distinguish this infection from bacterial conjunctivitis.

Infant Pneumonitis

Infants typically present at 3 to 11 weeks of age with a history of prolonged cough and congestion. They are usually afebrile and without significant systemic illness; conjunctivitis is sometimes present. Cough, congestion, tachypnea, and rales dominate respiratory findings, although in some infants, the clinical picture is more suggestive of bronchiolitis than pneumonitis. A pertussoid staccato cough, although not always present, should suggest the possibility of chlamydial pneumonia. Radiographs reveal hyperinflation with infiltrates (Fig. 30-1), and blood examination reveals eosinophilia and hyperimmunoglobulinemia. When untreated, the course may be protracted.

Differential diagnosis includes cytomegalovirus and adenovirus, which can cause afebrile pneumonia in infants. Pertussis can cause a similar cough (often subacute), may be afebrile, and may show hyperaeration on chest radiograph. Other agents that must be considered, particularly in the presence of fever and systemic findings, are the influenza viruses and the bacterial pathogens of infancy: group A and B β-hemolytic streptococci, *S. aureus, Escherichia coli, Klebsiella* spp., *H. influenzae, S. pneumoniae,* and *N. meningitidis.* Tuberculosis and coccidioidomycosis also must be considered in infant respiratory diseases, given appropriate exposures or residence in endemic areas.

DIAGNOSIS

Inclusion Conjunctivitis

There are several methods of diagnosing inclusion conjunctivitis. The Giemsa-stained conjunctival smear is the most widely used technique. The eyelid is everted, and conjunctival scrapings are taken, usually with a platinum spatula (not with a swab). The scrapings are spread thinly on a microscope slide and stained with Giemsa stain. *Chlamydia trachomatis* inclusions are seen in the cytoplasm of conjunctival cells as a circumscribed group of blue or purple granules. The inclusions are frequently adjacent to the nucleus and may replace much of the cell cytoplasm.

Newer and more sensitive methods for diagnosis include in vitro cell culture and antigen detection using either direct fluorescent antibody smears or enzyme immunoassay.

A culture for the Neisseria gonorrhoeae should be obtained in every case of neonatal conjunctivitis.

Infant Pneumonitis

Diagnosis of chlamydial pneumonitis has been made by isolation of the organism in cell culture of specimens from the nasopharynx, tracheal aspirates, and lung biopsy material. More recently, antigen detection methods, by direct fluorescent antibody smear or enzyme immunoassay, have been used. In addition, serum antichlamydial antibody titers have been useful in diagnosing acute infection, especially in patients with prior antibiotic therapy, in whom cultures may be negative.

Both culture and serologic techniques require experienced laboratories. In the absence of readily available facilities, the diagnosis of chlamydial pneumonitis should be suspected in an infant with the clinical syndrome described earlier in this chapter. The chest radiograph, the eosinophil count, and the serum IgG and IgM levels may be used as corroborative information. The concurrent presence of Giemsa-positive inclusion conjunctivitis also suggests a chlamydial cause in an infant with pneumonitis. Bacterial cultures and nasopharyngeal fluorescent antibody for pertussis should rule out other treatable pathogens.

MANAGEMENT

Inclusion Conjunctivitis

Recommended regimen: erythromycin, 30 to 50 mg/kg of body weight per day in 4 divided doses for 2 weeks.

Topical treatment of inclusion conjunctivitis with sulfonamide, tetracycline, or erythromycin ophthalmic preparations is no longer

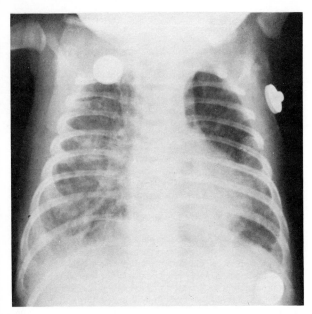

A

FIG. 30-1. *(A)* Anteroposterior and *(B)* lateral chest radiographs of a severely ill 1-month-old male infant with chlamydial pneumonitis. Diffuse interstitial infiltrates and hyperaeration with flattened diaphragms are prominent.

recommended because they are often not applied correctly and therefore do not decrease the risk of recurrent conjunctivitis or pneumonia.

Infant Pneumonitis

Recommended regimen: erythromycin, 30 to 50 mg/kg of body weight per day in 4 divided doses for 2 weeks.

Other regimens which have been used with success include sulfisoxazole 150 mg/kg per day or erythromycin ethyl succinate 40 mg/kg per day for approximately 2 weeks.

PREVENTION

Most neonatal chlamydial infections appear to be vertically transmitted from mother to infant at birth. Pregnant women should

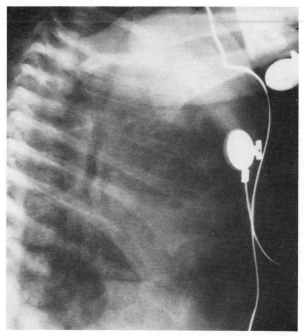

B

undergo diagnostic testing for *C. trachomatis* at their first prenatal visit and, if at high risk, during the last trimester. Studies suggest that erythromycin therapy given to the infected mother and her sexual partner(s) is effective in preventing disease in the newborn.

Studies of eye prophylaxis regimens for prevention of inclusion conjunctivitis have yielded contradictory results. Erythromycin and tetracycline appear to be more efficacious than silver nitrate in preventing chlamydial ophthalmic disease. None of the eye prophylaxis regimens, however, are adequate for prevention of nasopharyngitis or pneumonia.

ADDITIONAL READING

Bell TA, et al: Chronic *Chlamydia trachomatis* infections in infants. *JAMA* 267:400, 1992

Centers for Disease Control: False-positive results with the use of chlamydia tests in the evaluation of suspected sexual abuse—Ohio, 1990. *MMWR* 39:932, 1991

Phillips G, et al: Diagnosis of neonatal chlamydial conjunctivitis. *Arch Dis Child* 65:894, 1990

For a more detailed discussion, see Alexander ER, Harrison HR: Chlamydial Infections in Infants and Children, Chap. 66, p 811, in STD-2.

The cause of congenital syphilis is not *Treponema pallidum* alone. The web of social and economic factors that permit syphilis in pregnancy to occur and to remain untreated must be considered a part of the etiology. Rates of congenital syphilis in the United States declined dramatically following the introduction of penicillin, but incidence is once more rising ominously.

EPIDEMIOLOGY

While only 688 cases were reported among infants younger than 1 year of age in 1988, 2841 cases were reported for 1990. The new surveillance case definition recently approved by the Centers for Disease Control partly accounts for the increase in observed incidence. This definition requires reporting all infants whose mothers had untreated or inadequately treated syphilis at delivery, regardless of clinical signs in the infant. However, escalating syphilis rates among women indicate that the skyrocketing incidence of congenital syphilis reflects a true increase in maternal disease and not simply a reporting artifact.

The congenital syphilis statistic that reflects recent transmission best is the number of cases under 1 year of age per 100,000 live births. The incidence of infantile congenital syphilis closely follows that of primary and secondary syphilis in women in the peak childbearing age group (15 to 29 years); this is also the peak age group in which early syphilis occurs. However, the relationship between the two incidence figures is not constant. The incidence curve for congenital syphilis lags behind the curve for infectious syphilis in 15- to 29-year-old females by approximately 1 year. The vertical transmission index (VTI) for syphilis is the number of cases of congenital syphilis under 1 year of age per 1000 cases of primary and secondary syphilis *for the preceding year* and reflects this relationship. It can be used as an index of the effectiveness of prevention of syphilitic births among pregnant women who have or acquire syphilis in the year prior to delivery. The substantial increases in the VTI and rising rates of congenital syphilis that have been observed in the United States in recent years suggest that prenatal care is becoming less adequate.

The demographic profile of women in the United States who deliver syphilitic babies resembles that of women with other STDs, as well as those who fail to obtain adequate prenatal care; they are more likely than the general population to be adolescent, unmarried, and black. The greatest risk factor for congenital syphilis is lack of prenatal care. Likelihood of obtaining prenatal care is strongly associated with age, marital and socioeconomic status, rural residence, and low educational attainment.

PATHOLOGY AND PATHOGENESIS

The fundamental histologic lesions of congenital and acquired syphilis are vasculitis and resulting necrosis and fibrosis. Histopathologic patterns depend on the gestational age at the time of infection and examination. Three tissue reactions are usually attributed to syphilitic vasculitis: (1) focal ischemic necrosis, (2) fibrosis, and (3) gummas.

Structures most affected include the placenta, dentition, and bony skeleton. Striking inflammatory and fibrotic changes are noted in the placenta.

Teeth are abnormal in form, structure, and size. Syphilis affects morphodifferentiation and apposition, primarily of the permanent incisors and first molars. Whether deciduous teeth are affected probably depends upon whether infection occurs prior to 18 weeks' gestation, when deciduous teeth are fully formed.

Characteristic bony lesions are found in 97 percent of infants autopsied by 6 months of age. Endochondrial (long) bones are commonly affected at the metaphyseal-epiphyseal junction. When membranous bone is involved, the result is a focal periostitis causing exostosis and osteoporosis at the site. A perivascular inflammatory infiltrate erodes the trabeculae in both types of bone and eventually gives way to fibrosis. In surviving infants these lesions heal over the first 6 months, usually without residual lesions, and seem little influenced by penicillin. This suggests that much of the pathogenesis of these lesions may be trophic rather than directly infectious.

CLINICAL MANIFESTATIONS

Congenital syphilis is divided into two clinical syndromes. Those features that typically appear within the first 2 years of life constitute early congenital syphilis. Those that occur later than 2 years, most often near puberty, are considered late congenital syphilis.

Early Congenital Syphilis

Virtually any organ in the body can be involved by the widespread inflammatory changes that result from generalized spirochetemia.

Most syphilitic infants lack signs of infection at birth, but two-thirds of such infants demonstrate clinical signs of early congenital syphilis within the third to eighth week of life, and nearly all present within 3 months. Infants born with manifest syphilis are usually severely infected and have a worse prognosis.

Liver, Spleen, and Lymph Nodes

Hepatosplenomegaly occurs in approximately half of all patients with early manifest congenital syphilis. Both hepatic and splenic enlargement are caused by subacute inflammation and compensatory extramedullary hematopoiesis. Serum transaminase levels may be elevated, and up to 30 percent of patients exhibit jaundice due to either indirect or direct and indirect bilirubin, depending on whether hemolysis or hepatitis is predominant. Hepatosplenomegaly may persist for more than a year despite treatment and progress to cirrhosis with a fatal outcome.

Generalized lymphadenopathy occurs in 20 to 50 percent of patients. Nodes are firm, rubbery, and nontender. Epitrochlear adenopathy is found in 20 percent of those with adenopathy and is considered especially characteristic of syphilis.

Mucocutaneous Lesions

Mucocutaneous lesions are many and varied. Nasal discharge is often the earliest sign of congenital syphilis (Fig. 31-1). The discharge is initially watery but becomes thicker, more purulent, and finally hemorrhagic. Ulceration can progress to chondritis and necrosis, resulting in septal perforation or saddle nose deformity of late congenital syphilis.

Various cutaneous lesions occur in 30 to 60 percent of patients and often resemble those of acquired secondary syphilis. The most common lesion is a large round pink macule that fades to a dusky or coppery hue, develops slowly over a period of weeks, and lasts 1 to 3 months without treatment, leaving a residual pigmentation. Typical distribution includes the back, perineum, extremities, palms, and soles, sparing the anterior trunk.

A variety of papular and maculopapular eruptions may also be seen. Purpura and petechiae may appear when thrombocytopenia is severe; as a response to anemia, cutaneous extramedullary hematopoiesis produces the "blueberry muffin" rash.

A vesiculobullous eruption occurs and is most prominent on the palms and soles. Dark field examination of the blister fluid reveals spirochetes. Even without bulla formation, desquamation is common (Fig. 31-2). Paronychia can cause narrow atrophic nails, producing a claw-nail deformity, particularly of the fourth and fifth digits. The hair may be brittle and sparse; infantile alopecia, especially of the eyebrows, is suggestive of syphilis.

Eczematoid, impetiginous, or even gangrenous lesions may occur, particularly on the face, perineum, or intertrigenous areas. The facial eruption preferentially affects the middle third of the face, from the medial portions of the supraorbital ridge to the chin.

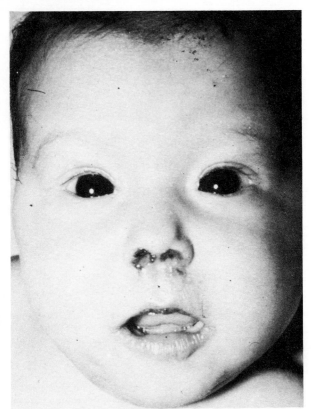

FIG. 31-1. Snuffles: a persistent, often sanguinous, nasal discharge. Treponemes abound in the discharge, providing a definitive means of diagnosis. *(Courtesy of C Ginsburg.)*

Mucous patches are found on the tongue and palate. Condyloma lata are raised, flat, moist verrucae in mucocutaneous and intertriginous areas that are seen in recurrences of untreated congenital syphilis, usually toward the end of the first year of life.

Skeletal Involvement

Over 30 percent of syphilitic infants less than 1 year of age have physical signs of skeletal defects, and approximately 80 percent have

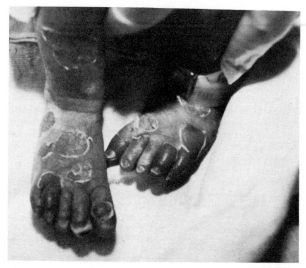

FIG. 31-2. Typical bullae and desquamation of congenital syphilis. *(Courtesy of C Ginsburg.)*

radiographic evidence. Generalized osteochondritis is the cardinal finding. Periostitis is seen as well. The long bones (radius, femur, humerus, and fibula) are preferentially involved, but other sites may be affected. Therefore, a skeletal survey is mandatory when a diagnosis of congenital syphilis is considered.

Hematologic Manifestations

Hematologic abnormalities are common. Anemia has been noted in more than 90 percent of infants and is Coombs' test–negative, normochromic and normocytic, or macrocytic. Autoimmune hemolysis is a common mechanism. Neutrophilic leukocytosis occurs in over 70 percent of cases; congenital syphilis is one of the classic causes of leukemoid reactions in infancy. Monocytosis is also frequently seen. Significant thrombocytopenia occurs in 30 percent of babies with syphilis and is associated with a high incidence of bleeding complications.

Other Manifestations

A variety of other complications can occur. Glomerulonephritis has been noted. Chorioretinitis, glaucoma, and uveitis are also associated with congenital syphilis. Pneumonitis is usually present in fatal cases but is otherwise uncommon.

Late Congenital Syphilis

Eighty percent of children ultimately diagnosed as having congenital syphilis pass through the early stage undetected. Inadvertent partial treatment associated with management of other intercurrent infections seems to have so greatly modified the expression of the disease that classic syndromes of late congenital syphilis are now rare, in spite of a persistent incidence of infant syphilis. Late congenital syphilis particularly affects the bones, soft tissues, eyes, ears, and central nervous system, but spares the cardiovascular system. The distinctive lesions of late disease are the stigmata. These are malformations that occur because of prior infection at a critical period of growth and development and, presumably, at a relatively immature stage of immunologic development.

Malformations (Stigmata)

Chondritis and focal osteitis in infancy can lead to craniofacial malformations. The most common is frontal bossing, which occurs in 30 to 87 percent of symptomatic cases. Deep necrotizing chondritis in infancy causes a saddle nose deformity in 10 to 30 percent of syphilitic children. Anterior bowing of the tibia (saber shin) is also seen.

Dental malformations are highly characteristic. Hutchinson's teeth are widely spaced and peg- or screwdriver-shaped canines and incisors which taper from the gingival bases toward a notched biting edge (Fig. 31-3). In the first year of life, the diagnosis can be made by radiographs of unerupted central incisors.

Inflammatory Lesions

Keratitis is the most common late manifestation. Its onset is between the ages of 5 and 16 years, and when accompanied by neural deafness and typical teeth, forms Hutchinson's triad. Symmetrical, painless swelling of the knees or elbows occurs between the ages of 8 and 15 in 1 to 3 percent of children. Gummata of the palate, throat, and nasal septum begin in late childhood or adulthood and may lead to perforation of the septum and soft palate. Asymptomatic neurosyphilis is common, but symptomatic disease is quite rare. When present, it is usually delayed until adolescence and fits the adult patterns of tabes dorsalis, general paresis, and local gummata. Attacks of paroxysmal cold hemoglobinuria occur, but cease following penicillin therapy.

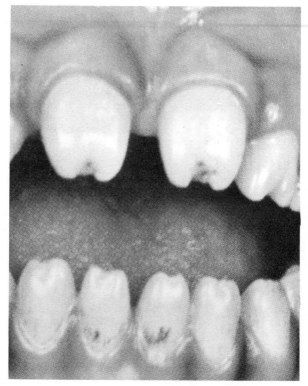

FIG. 31-3. Hutchinson's teeth: the upper and lower incisors are conical, tapered toward the apex, and notched; the canine teeth are hypoplastic and poorly enamelized. *(From RA Colby et al.[1])*

DIAGNOSIS

Diagnosis of congenital syphilis is complicated by the occasional biological false-positive nontreponemal test due to pregnancy. False-positive fluorescent treponemal antibody-absorption (FTA-ABS) tests can occur during pregnancy, but the probability of two such false-positive tests is exceedingly low. After therapy, some patients will be VDRL "serofast"; the only way to distinguish serofast, treated women and the reinfected patient is by re-treatment and serologic follow-up. All pregnant women with a positive nontreponemal and confirmatory treponemal test should be treated.

Criteria for Diagnosis in the Infant

Definite Congenital Syphilis: Visualization of T. pallidum

The diagnosis of congenital syphilis may be classified as definite, compatible, or unlikely. A definite diagnosis requires demonstration of *T. pallidum* in a lesion by dark field examination, immunofluorescence, or histologic examination. One of these tests should be performed whenever nasal discharge, mucous patches, vesiculobullous lesions, or condylomata are present, as treponemes abound in such lesions.

Compatible Congenital Syphilis: Serodiagnosis

When treponemes cannot be demonstrated, the diagnosis rests mainly on serology. A positive nontreponemal test confirmed by a treponemal test (FTA-ABS or MHA-TP) should be regarded as due to syphilis until proven otherwise. Three clinical circumstances sometimes cause diagnostic confusion, however: the recently treated mother, the apparently "serofast" mother (who remains seropositive following adequate treatment in the absence of active infection), and the seronegative infant or mother. In the first two situations, the difficulty is in distinguishing between passively transferred maternal IgG and fetal antibody produced in response to continuing active infection. In this setting it is sometimes useful to determine umbilical cord blood IgM levels. An elevated infant IgM level in combination with positive nontreponemal and treponemal tests strongly suggests congenital syphilis.

One strategy for distinguishing maternal from infant antibody in the asymptomatic infant is to follow the baby's titer. An infant titer due to maternal antibody should fall fourfold within 2 months and disappear by 6 months of life; a stable or rising titer indicates active infection. This approach should be reserved for babies whose mothers have been treated *during* pregnancy and in whom reinfection during pregnancy can be reasonably excluded by an appropriate serologic response and prompt treatment of sexual partners. For asymptomatic seropositive infants who do not meet these criteria, an alternative is to treat at birth or upon discovery and to retest by treponemal serology at 3 to 6 months. If the treponemal test is still positive, the baby may be reported as a case; if the nontreponemal test also remains positive, the baby should be re-treated.

Thorough clinical evaluation can identify additional cases. CSF pleiocytosis and characteristic bony abnormalities on radiographic tests are particularly helpful in establishing a diagnosis. Table 31-1 outlines clinical criteria for infant syphilis. Tables 31-2 and 31-3 list

TABLE 31-1. Clinical Criteria for Infant Syphilis

Major	Minor
Condylomata lata Osteochondritis or periostitis (symmetric metaphyseal lesions) Snuffles or hemorrhagic rhinitis Vesiculobullous eruption, other causes excluded	Perioral fissures Characteristic rash, especially vesiculobullous eruption Mucous patches Hepatomegaly or splenomegaly Generalized lymphadenopathy CNS signs or CSF pleocytosis Hematologic signs (hemolysis or thrombocytopenia) Nonimmunologic hydrops Pseudoparalysis Nephrotic syndrome or glomerulonephritis

SOURCE: After Kaufman et al,[2] and Ingall and Norins.[3]

considerations in the differential of early and late congenital syphilis.

In summary:

Infants should be evaluated for syphilis if they were born to seropositive (nontreponemal test confirmed by treponemal tests) women who:

1. Have untreated syphilis;
2. Had syphilis that was treated in pregnancy but (a) less than 1 month before delivery, or (b) with a nonpenicillin regimen, or (c) with the appropriate penicillin regimen but without subsequent expected decrease in nontreponemal antibody titers;
3. Do not have a well-documented history of syphilis treatment; or
4. Have a well-documented history of syphilis treatment before pregnancy but had insufficient serologic follow-up during pregnancy to assess disease activity.

An infant should not be released from the hospital until the serologic status of his or her mother is known.

The evaluation of children born to women in any of the categories above should include:

1. A thorough physical examination for evidence of congenital syphilis;
2. Testing for nontreponemal antibody titers;
3. CSF analysis for cells, protein, and VDRL test;
4. Long bone x-ray films;
5. Other tests as clinically indicated (e.g., chest x-ray films); and
6. If possible, an FTA-ABS test on the purified 19-S IgM of serum.

TABLE 31-2. Differential Diagnosis of Infant Congenital Syphilis

	Other causes
Vesiculobullous eruption	Toxic epidermal necrolysis
	Staphylococcal infection (Ritter's disease)
	Pseudomonas sepsis
	Sepsis due to *Listeria,* group B streptococci, *Haemophilus influenzae* type B
	Viral infection: herpes simplex, varicella, vaccinia, cytomegalovirus (CMV)
	Candidiasis
	Hereditary: epidermolysis bullosa, urticaria pigmentosa, porphyria, Letterer-Siwe, dermatitis herpetiformis
Hepatosplenomegaly (with or without lymphadenopathy, cutaneous hematopoiesis, and hematologic abnormalities)	Erythroblastosis
	Other congenital infections: sepsis, CMV, rubella, herpes simplex, toxoplasmosis, varicella, hepatitis
	Biliary atresia, choledochal cyst
	Metabolic disorders: galactosemia, cystic fibrosis, mucopolysaccharidosis
Hydrops fetalis	Erythroblastosis
	α-Thalassemia
	Congestive heart failure
	Neuroblastoma
	Congenital nephrotic syndrome: lupus, microcystic disease, renal vein thrombosis
	Congenital infection: CMV, toxoplasmosis, hepatitis
Pseudoparalysis of Parrot	Erb's palsy
	Osteomyelitis
Wimberger's sign (focal metaphyseal defects)	Osteomyelitis
	Infantile generalized fibromatosis
Metaphyseal lesions	Hyperparathyroidism
Celery stick diaphysis	Rickets, rubella, CMV, tuberculosis
Higoumenakis' sign	Rubella
Pathologic fractures	Healed clavicular fracture
Periostitis	Battered child syndrome
	Melorheostosis, Caffey's infantile cortical hyperostosis

TREATMENT

Ideally, all pregnant women with syphilis should be treated with penicillin, as prenatal penicillin therapy usually prevents congenital disease. Desensitization of women with penicillin allergy is highly recommended because the efficacy of erythromycin is likely to be

TABLE 31-3. Differential Diagnosis of Late Congenital Syphilis

Syndrome	Features
Ectodermal dysplasia (Marshall's syndrome)	Conical pointed incisors, saddle nose, frontal bossing, sparse hair or alopecia, cataracts, sensorineural deafness
Enamel hypoplasias	Defects of incisors consist of deep horizontal grooves; small hypoplastic teeth, sometimes with apical notching
Rubella	Dental hypoplasia with small, peg-shapped teeth
Erythroblastosis	Enamel hypoplasia, but predominantly affects deciduous crowns
Dental fusion	Developmental fusion of adjacent incisors may produce a round notched tooth resembling Hutchinson's incisor
Cogan's syndrome	Interstitial keratitis and vestibuloauditory symptoms
Rickets	Periostitis and deformities; anterior bowing of tibia, frontal bossing

poor, and tetracycline administration during pregnancy is relatively contraindicated.

Infants should be treated if they have:

1. Any evidence of active disease (physical examination or x-ray),
2. A reactive CSF-VDRL test,
3. An abnormal CSF finding (WBC > 5/mm³ or protein concentration greater than 50 mg/dl) irrespective of CSF serologic results,
4. Quantitative nontreponemal serologic titers which are fourfold (or greater) higher than those of their mother,
5. Positive test for FTA-ABS 19-S IgM antibody, if performed, or
6. A mother who has untreated syphilis or relapse or reinfection after treatment.

Recommended treatment: 100,000 to 150,000 units/kg of aqueous crystalline penicillin G daily (administered as 50,000 units/kg IV every 8 to 12 h) or 50,000 units/kg of procaine penicillin daily (administered once IM) for 10 to 14 days. If more than 1 day of therapy is missed, the entire course should be restarted. All symptomatic neonates should also have an opthalmologic exam. Infants who require evaluation but do not meet the criteria for intensive therapy may be treated with a one-time dose of 50,000 units/kg of benzathine penicillin G if close follow-up cannot be ensured.

Seropositive untreated infants must be closely followed at 1, 2, 3, 6, and 12 months. Nontreponemal antibody titers should decrease by 3 months of age and should disappear by 6 months of age. If these titers are found to be stable or increasing, the child should be reevaluated and fully treated. Treponemal antibodies may be present up to 1 year of age. If they are present beyond 1 year, the infant should be treated for congenital syphilis.

Treated infants should also be followed to ensure decreasing nontreponemal antibody titers. Infants with documented CSF pleiocytosis should have CSF reexamined every 6 months or until the cell count is normal. If the cell count is still abnormal after 2 years, or if a downward trend is not present at each examination, the infant should be re-treated. The CSF-VDRL should also be checked at 6 months; if it is still reactive, the infant should be re-treated.

PREVENTION

The first line of defense against congenital syphilis is treating primary and secondary syphilis cases and effective contact tracing. The fewer the total number of cases of primary and secondary syphilis, the fewer the number of cases that joins the pool of early and late latent syphilis, and therefore the fewer latent syphilitic patients among women in the childbearing age group. Because women may acquire syphilis during pregnancy, high-risk women should be rescreened in the third trimester. High-risk women generally include those attending public clinics or those who are of low income, single, or report more than one STD.

Routine prenatal screening is the second major line of defense, but as noted earlier, a substantial proportion of women who give birth to children with congenital syphilis receive little or no prenatal care. Clearly, a major challenge for public health is to extend prenatal care to all pregnant women. Such an achievement, if combined with case investigation, reactor follow-up, and targeted screening, could eradicate congenital syphilis as well as reduce infant and maternal mortality from many causes.

REFERENCES

1. Colby RA et al: *Color Atlas of Oral Pathology.* Philadelphia, Lippincott, 1971
2. Kaufman RE et al: Questionnaire survey of reported early congenital syphilis. *Sex Transm Dis* 4:135, 1977
3. Ingall D, Norins L: Syphilis, in *Infectious Diseases of the Fetus and Newborn Infant,* J Remington, JO Klein (eds). Philadelphia, Saunders, 1976

ADDITIONAL READING

Dunn RA, Zenker PN: Why radiographs are useful in evaluation of neonates suspected of having congenital syphilis. *Radiology* 182:639, 1992
Greenberg MS et al: The association between congenital syphilis and cocaine/crack use in New York City: A case-control study. *Am J Public Health* 81:1316, 1991

Greenberg SB, Bernal DV: Are long bone radiographs necessary in neonates suspected of having congenital syphilis? *Radiology* 182:637, 1992

Ikeda MK, Jenson HB: Evaluation and treatment of congenital syphilis. *J Pediatr* 117:843, 1990

Minkoff HL: Preventing fetal damage from sexually transmitted diseases. *Clin Obstet Gynecol* 34:336, 1991

Zenker P: New case definition for congenital syphilis reporting. *Sex Transm Dis* 18:44, 1992

For a more detailed discussion, see Schulz KF, Murphy FK, Patamasucon P, Meheus AZ: Congenital Syphilis, Chap. 67, p 821, in STD-2.

Child sexual abuse occurs commonly. Although its exact incidence and prevalence are unknown, it is estimated that at least 1 in 4 girls and 1 in 10 boys will be molested before age 16. Over 50,000 cases are reported each year in the United States. Statistics from other countries show similar frequencies of occurrence.

When sexually transmitted diseases (STDs) occur in children, sexual abuse must be ruled out. Since sexual abuse is deleterious to the psychological health of children, cases of STD in children should be carefully investigated to determine how the child acquired the infection.

In children who are known to be abused, estimates of the prevalence of STD vary depending on the criteria and microbiological tests used for diagnosis, the age range of the children examined, and the underlying prevalence of disease in the community where the children were studied. Table 32-1 lists STDs found in surveys of sexually abused children and their frequencies of occurrence.

HISTOLOGY AND PHYSIOLOGY OF THE GENITAL TRACT IN CHILDREN

The genital tract of prepubertal girls provides a different microenvironment for STD pathogens than that of postmenarchal females. The vagina of young girls is lined with a thin, atrophic columnar epithelium. The pH is 6.5 to 7.5, higher than that found in adults. The cervix does not have active mucus-secreting glands, and the normal female child does not have a demonstrable vaginal discharge.

After puberty, the vaginal wall is lined with a thick, stratified squamous epithelium containing glycogen. The vagina is normally acidic (pH less than 4.5), and cervical glands secrete varying amounts of mucus. The epithelium of the cervical canal is columnar.

Because of the presence of columnar epithelium in the child's vagina, some STD pathogens such as *Neisseria gonorrhoeae* and *Chlamydia trachomatis* that infect the cervix of adult women will cause vaginitis in children. The high vaginal pH may also increase a child's susceptibility to infection.

Similar differences in the histology of the genital tract of boys compared with adult males have not been reported. STD in male children probably occurs less frequently than in female children because male children have less exposure to STD pathogens due to their lower incidence of sexual abuse.

378

TABLE 32-1. STDs Reported in Surveys of Sexually Abused Children

Reference	Ages	Number of subjects	Disease*	Number tested	No. (%) positive
Tilelli[1]	2–16 yr	130	GC	103	3 (2.9%)
DeJong[2]	6 mo–17 yr	142	GC	142	2 (1.4%)
Rimsza[3]	2 mo–17 yr	311	GC	285	21 (7.4%)
			TP	104	0 (0%)
Groothuis[4]	< 13 yr	16	GC	11	5 (45.4%)
Khan[5]	< 13 yr	113	GC	71	14 (19.7%)
White[6]	< 13 yr	409	GC	176	47 (26.7%)
			TP	108	6 (5.5%)
			TV	21	4
			HPV		3
Grant[7]	8 mo–17 yr	157	GC		12
			HPV		2
			HSV		1
DeJong[8]	6 mo–13 yr	532	GC	532	25 (4.7%)
			BV		3
			HPV		3
			HSV		1
			TP	532	1 (0.2%)
Fuster[9]	1–12.5 yr	50	CT	47	8 (17%)
			GC	49	0 (0%)

*GC = *N. gonorrhoeae*
TP = *T. pallidum*
TV = *T. vaginalis*
HPV = human papilloma virus (anogenital warts)

HSV = herpes simplex virus (genital)
BV = bacterial vaginosis
CT = *C. trachomatis*

MODES OF TRANSMISSION OF STD IN CHILDREN

Four factors make it difficult to determine modes of transmission of STD in children:

1. The magnitude of the problem of child sexual abuse has only recently been recognized by practitioners and researchers.
2. Often children are reluctant to report sexual abuse because of fear of retaliation from the abuser or because of feelings of guilt or embarrassment. In addition, they may be unable to report because of a lack of verbal skills. Histories given by caretakers may be unreliable because the child has not informed them of the abuse, or because of the caretaker's involvement in the abuse. A high percentage of abused children are abused by family members.
3. It is conceivable that diseases which are transmitted only by sexual contact in adults may be nonsexually transmitted in

children. Even in normal, healthy families, children have much more intimate contact with family members than most adults would ever have with people who are not their sexual partners. Young children frequently sleep and bathe with their parents and share household objects such as towels and toothbrushes with others. This degree of intimacy in normal, nonabusive households raises the possibility that STDs are not necessarily sexually transmitted in all instances.

4. Some STDs in children can be acquired before birth, during birth, or through breast feeding. It is often difficult to differentiate perinatal infection from infection acquired through sexual abuse.

Accurately determining the mode of transmission of STD pathogens in children requires the examiner to have an open mind and willingness to consider the possibility of either sexual or nonsexual transmission.

Sexual versus Nonsexual Transmission of STD in Children

Neisseria gonorrhoeae

Although *N. gonorrhoeae* can infect an infant during birth, asymptomatic infection seldom if ever persists after the neonatal period.

In children diagnosed with gonococcal pharyngeal, genital, and anorectal infections, histories of sexual abuse are commonly obtained. When gonorrhea is diagnosed in a child, it is important to culture household contacts for the disease. Other infected adults and children are commonly found in the child's environment.

Chlamydia trachomatis

Chlamydia trachomatis infects infants during vaginal delivery, causing conjunctivitis during the neonatal period and pneumonia during the first few months of life. Occasionally, infected infants do not manifest positive cultures until several weeks after birth, perhaps because of the suppression of infection by maternal antibody. Carriage in infants has been documented for greater than 6 months in the conjunctiva, nasopharynx, and oropharynx—and more than 1 year in the rectum and vagina.

Acquisition of *C. trachomatis* infection during childhood is suggested by an increasing prevalence of antibody to the organism between birth and 15 years of age. However, this has not been a consistent finding in all studies of antibody prevalence and in part could be due to cross-reacting antibody to *Chlamydia pneumoniae.*

Alternatively, acquisition of chlamydial antibody during childhood could reflect sexual abuse. The prevalence of culture-proven *C. trachomatis* vaginal and rectal infections has been found to be significantly more common in sexually abused children than in controls. Since *C. trachomatis* infections of the adult genitalia and rectum are clearly sexually transmitted, a similar mode of transmission probably occurs in children.

Trichomonas vaginalis

Trichomonas vaginalis has been found in the nasopharynx and vagina of newborns born to infected mothers. Sexual transmission in prepubertal children has been infrequently reported. The prepubertal vagina does not provide a favorable environment for the organism.

Although acquisition of *T. vaginalis* by adults through fomites has been suspected in some instances, there are no documented cases of adults becoming infected from fomites. Since trichomonal infections in children are so uncommon, the possibility of easy spread through fomites is unlikely.

Herpes Simplex Virus (HSV)

The acquisition of genital HSV infection by children should raise the possibility of sexual abuse. Infection by either type 1 or type 2 virus can occur in the genital area.

Although HSV can survive in certain fomites for a number of hours, fomite transmission of the disease is unlikely. Transmission requires direct contact of viable virus with either a mucous membrane or an abraded skin surface on the individual who becomes infected.

Children have been shown to transmit HSV from symptomatic or asymptomatic infections in their mouths to their genital areas. Sexual transmission through child abuse is also well documented.

Other viruses and bacteria can cause lesions in the genital area of children which resemble genital herpes. Any herpes virus found should be typed as 1 or 2. Viral cultures may not detect the virus after crusting of vesicles occurs. Obtaining sera for HSV-1 and HSV-2 antibodies acutely and 6 weeks after the infection can be helpful in documenting the acquisition of HSV. However, most serologic tests for HSV-2 in current clinical use do not differentiate well between antibodies to HSV-1 and HSV-2. Newer, specific tests are necessary (see Chap. 11, Genital Herpes).

Condyloma Acuminatum

Genital and anal warts are caused by certain types of human papillomavirus (HPV). Common warts on other parts of the body are caused by other types of HPV and seldom cause anal or genital warts by autoinoculation. When this does occur in adults, the appearance is said to be that of common warts on other parts of the body, rather than acuminate (filiform) in appearance. Condyloma acuminata in children have been shown to be caused by the same types of HPV which cause anal or genital warts in adults.

The sexual transmission of condyloma acuminata is well documented. However, transmission of nongenital (e.g., planter) warts is thought to occur often through fomite contact, and a possible role of fomites in transmission of genital HPV infection is conceivable. Skin-to-skin contact between individuals is thought to be necessary for transmission of infection in adults, and this may well be true for children also. Perinatal transmission of HPV also occurs, resulting in laryngeal papillomatosis; and perinatal transmission to genital or anal sites is also possible, but requires further study. Condyloma acuminatum in the first year of life in the absence of sexual abuse probably can result from infection through contact with the virus during delivery, but the efficacy of perinatal transmission, and the time after birth at which the onset of lesions can no longer be attributed to perinatal infection, are undefined. In adults, most genital HPV infections are not associated with visible lesions.

The frequency with which subclinical genital HPV infection occurs in children who have been sexually abused is not yet well studied. Of children with anal or genital warts, at least 50 percent have histories of sexual abuse. The presence of warts should thus raise the suspicion of abuse.

Gardnerella vaginalis

Gardnerella vaginalis is considered a sexually transmitted bacterium in adults. The organism is more prevalent among adolescent males and females who are sexually active. It is also more commonly found in sexually abused children than in controls. Clinical evidence of bacterial vaginosis, a mixed infection of *G. vaginalis* and other microorganisms, has also been described in abused children.

Most studies of *G. vaginalis* in children and adolescents show that a small proportion of the nonabused or non–sexually active subjects also carry the organism. Nevertheless, the presence of this organism should raise the index of suspicion that abuse might have occurred.

Human Immunodeficiency Virus (HIV)

HIV infection has been reported as a sequela of sexual abuse. The frequent occurrence of microtrauma from abusive sexual activities with children could lead to a portal of entry for the virus from infected adults. As with adults, it is likely that anorectal penetration would lead to particularly efficient transmission; the susceptibility of the preadolescent vagina to HIV inoculation is unknown.

Syphilis

Syphilis is rarely reported as a complication of sexual abuse. Occurrence of syphilis in children beyond the first year of life is likely to be caused by sexual contact, especially if peripartum serologic tests of mother or newborn were negative.

Molluscum Contagiosum

Although molluscum contagiosum has been identified as a sexually transmitted disease in adults, the frequent occurrence and location of the disease in young children indicates it is easily spread by casual nonsexual contact. In many children with genital molluscum, a careful history and exam reveal that lesions existed on other parts of the body before genital lesions are noted.

DIAGNOSIS AND TREATMENT OF STD WITH SUSPECTED CHILD ABUSE

Screening for STD in Abused Children

Confirmation of the diagnosis of abuse requires a careful review of the child's history, physical examination, and social situation. If the diagnosis of sexual abuse is made, laws in most jurisdictions mandate reporting to child protection agencies. The safety, health, and welfare of the child should be the practitioner's primary concern. The following general considerations should guide the evaluation:

1. Many institutions have a service that is particularly skilled in the interview and examination of children suspected of having experienced sexual abuse. This service may be offered by the pediatric or gynecology departments and, if available, should be provided in the evaluation from the first contact.
2. If the child is symptomatic, all available and appropriate cultures and examination should be completed without delay before the child is begun on therapy.
3. All culture and examination samples must be thoroughly and clearly labeled, and delivery to the appropriate laboratory must be ensured by personal delivery if necessary. The results may be required for legal proceedings.
4. If sexual abuse is documented by the presence of spermatozoa, an STD, or social history, the child must be placed in a secure environment pending investigation and social and legal disposition.
5. The majority of children who have been the victims of sexual abuse do not have specific physical findings to confirm the diagnosis. Subtle findings such as bruising may be present, but the physical examination is likely to reveal no abnormality. However, the absence of abnormalities on physical examination does not make a diagnosis of sexual abuse unlikely. Oral sexual contact is a common form of abuse, as are fondling and external genital contact.
6. The presence of multiple STDs in a child may indicate that the child has been abused by multiple persons.

Recommended evaluation

Since a child's report of assault may not be complete, specimens for culture for *N. gonorrhoeae* and *C. trachomatis* should be collected from the pharynx and rectum as well as from the vagina (girls) or urethra (boys).

Internal pelvic examinations usually should not be performed unless indicated by the presence of a foreign body or by trauma.

Follow-up visits should be scheduled so as to minimize trauma to the child; for asymptomatic children, an initial visit and one at 8 to 12 weeks may be sufficient.

In cases of continuing abuse, the alleged offender may be available for medical evaluation. In such instances, care for the child may need to be modified when results of the evaluation of the offender are known.

Test Selection and Specimen Handling

When a sexually transmitted agent is identified from a sexually abused adult or child, that laboratory result may be required for use in subsequent legal action. For cultivable pathogens, culture diagnosis is most appropriate. Nonculture tests for such agents are not recommended at any time in the evaluation of sexual assault or sexual abuse in children, other than for diagnosis of HIV infection. Isolation of *N. gonorrhoeae* and *C. trachomatis* by culture, and their confirmation by recognized techniques, is the necessary standard. Exceptions may include the serologic diagnosis of syphilis, and demonstration of HSV-2 seroconversion.

Table 32-2 outlines recommended laboratory procedures for evaluation of sexually abused children. All presumptive isolates of *N. gonorrhoeae* from children should be confirmed by at least two tests that use different principles, e.g., biochemical, enzyme substrate, or serologic. A false-positive diagnosis of gonorrhea because of the misidentification of nonpathogenic *Neisseria* species can cause unnecessary difficulties for children and their families. Culture should also be used to screen for *Chlamydia,* as monoclonal antibodies in direct immunofluorescent stains or enzyme-linked immunoassays are not sensitive enough in low-risk populations to be used for diagnosis of *Chlamydia* in sexually abused children. Isolates should be stored at −70°C for possible future studies, and the use of a reference laboratory should be considered. Expert laboratory consultations are recommended for testing as well as for chain-of-evidence issues.

Treatment

Treatment prior to diagnosis is usually not indicated, unless there is evidence that the assailant is infected. The infection rate in children is sufficiently low that prophylactic treatment will

TABLE 32-2. Recommended Laboratory Procedures at Initial and Follow-up Evaluation of Sexually Abused Children (Prepubertal)

Gram's stain of any genital or anal discharge*
Culture for *N. gonorrhoeae*†
Culture for *C. trachomatis*†
Wet preparation of vaginal secretion for trichomonads, clue cells, and the presence of an amine odor when mixed with KOH‡
Culture of lesions for herpes simplex virus (HSV)
Serologic test for syphilis
Serologic test for human immunodeficiency virus (HIV)§
Frozen serum sample

Note: Syphilis and HIV serologic tests should be repeated in 12 weeks. All other tests should be repeated 10 to 14 days after the initial examination.
*Care should be taken in the interpretation of results of any Gram's stain of anal discharge.
†Cultures of pharynx, rectum, and vagina/urethra should be done.
‡Vaginal pH testing is not recommended because of a lack of known standard in children.
§Testing for HIV should be based upon the prevalence of infection and suspected risk.

prevent few infections. In addition, the risk of complications from STD in children is low. Very few cases of pelvic inflammatory disease or peritonitis in prepubertal children have been documented, perhaps because the immature cervix presents a barrier to the ascending spread of infection. Presumptive treatment following assault may be given, however, if the victim or victim's family requests it, or if follow-up examination of the child cannot be ensured.

REFERENCES

1. Tilelli JA et al: Sexual abuse of children. *N Engl J Med* 302:319,1980
2. DeJong AR et al: Sexual abuse of boys. *Am J Dis Child* 136:990,1982
3. Rimsza ME, Niggemann EH: Medical evaluation of sexually abused children: A review of 311 cases. *Pediatrics* 69:8, 1982
4. Groothuis JR et al: Pharyngeal gonorrhea in young children. *Pediatr Infect Dis* 2:99,1983
5. Khan M, Sexton M: Sexual abuse of young children. *Clin Pediatr* 22:369,1983
6. White ST et al: Sexually transmitted diseases in sexually abused children. *Pediatrics* 72:16,1983
7. Grant LJ: Assessment of child sexual abuse: Eighteen months' experience at the Child Protection Center. *Am J Obstet Gynecol* 148:617,1984
8. DeJong AR: Sexually transmitted diseases in sexually abused children. *Sex Transm Dis* 13:123,1986
9. Fuster CD, Neinstein LS: Vaginal *Chlamydia trachomatis* prevalence in sexually abused prepubertal girls. *Pediatrics* 79:235,1987

ADDITIONAL READING

Anon: American Academy of Pediatrics Committee on Child Abuse and Neglect: Guidelines for the evaluation of sexual abuse of children. *Pediatrics* 87:254, 1991

Bell TA et al: Chronic *Chlamydia trachomatis* infections in infants *JAMA* 267:400, 1992

Desenclos JC et al: Pediatric gonococcal infection, Florida, 1984 to 1988. *Am J Public Health* 82:426, 1992

Gutman LT et al: Human immunodeficiency virus transmission by child sexual abuse. *Am J Dis Child* 145:137, 1991

McCann J: Use of the colposcope in childhood sexual abuse examinations. *Pediatr Clin North Am* 37:863, 1990

Paradise JE: The medical evaluation of the sexually abused child. *Pediatr Clin North Am* 37:839, 1990

Schwarcz SK, Whittington WL: Sexual assault and sexually transmitted diseases: Detection and management in adults and children. *Rev Infect Dis* 12 (suppl 6):S682, 1990

For a more detailed discussion, see Jenny C: Child Sexual Abuse and STD, Chap. 72, p. 895, in STD-2.

Patient Education and Counseling
and Other Strategies for Prevention
of Sexually Transmitted Diseases

INTRODUCTION AND DEFINITIONS

The term *counseling* has been used rather loosely in the STD field
to include informing and educating patients about test results and
STDs, encouraging compliance with medication and follow-up
appointments, initiating sex partner referral, promoting condom
use, and promoting other risk-reduction strategies. More rigorous
definitions of counseling would include questioning and listening to
identify the needs and concerns of the patient and helping the patient
decide what *to do* in response to his or her own concerns—what
future actions to take. Counseling of patients with HIV infection
has begun to take on a more narrow meaning in some circles, having
specifically to do with long-term assistance with stress reduction
and coping.

Approaches to informing, educating, and counseling patients vary
greatly from one country to another, and from one clinical setting
to another within individual industrialized countries. In many
developing countries, the huge clinical load and limited resources
have inhibited development of any informing, education, or counseling for STD-HIV infection. Even in industrialized countries,
many clinicians have inadequate training, motivation, or time to
inform, educate, or counsel, and there is a widespread belief that
only paramedical professionals can or will provide these services.
This is one of the most rapidly evolving areas in clinical management
and public health approaches to STD-HIV infection.

Our view is that in the STD-HIV field, as in most other areas of
medicine, a primary care team approach is needed, which requires
clinician participation in patient education and counseling at the
outset, with periodic reinforcement, together with participation of
specially trained individuals—who currently are called *disease
intervention specialists* in the United States but at other times and
other places have been called contact tracers, social workers, public
health nurses, community health nurses, counselors, health assis-
tants, etc. Although some aspects of this work, such as contact
tracing, have been fairly well defined in the STD field, other aspects
of the work remain primitive. This chapter addresses issues of
general concern in informing, educating, and counseling patients
with traditional STDs. Chapter 35 focuses on special issues in HIV
counseling and testing. Much work remains to be done in improving
the conceptual framework in this area, and this is certainly not the
last or definitive chapter to be written on this subject.

GENERAL STD EDUCATION AND COUNSELING

A major goal of patient education and counseling about STDs is patient compliance with several important behaviors. Compliance is defined as the extent to which the patient follows through with prescribed treatment regimens and other instructions for the management or cure of a disease or infection and with advice on changing sexual behavior leading to the prevention of infection and disease. This implies the transfer of knowledge as well as the added dimension of inducing, persuading, or otherwise motivating patients to prevent the future risk of infection, and responding to concerns and questions raised by the patient in connection with this episode of STD, and future related issues.

Effective education and counseling are not easy for many medical conditions, even under the best of circumstances. However, it may be even more difficult with STD patients because much of the burden of morbidity is borne by poorer and less well educated members of society. These groups often feel alienated and powerless over events in their lives and frequently are made up of minority racial and ethnic groups. The probability that a patient will comply with treatment- and prevention-related recommendations is generally recognized to be determined by a complex range of factors, including health beliefs, psychological characteristics, and social conditions.

Although many behavioral messages may be given to patients within the context of STD counseling, the five principal messages are as follows:

1. Take oral medication as directed (when applicable).
2. Return for follow-up tests (when applicable).
3. Ensure examination of sex partners.
4. Reduce risk by
   a. Abstaining from any sexual activity until follow-up test.
   b. Abstaining from any sexual activity whenever symptoms appear.
   c. Using condoms in risky or unknown settings.
5. Respond immediately and appropriately to infection or disease suspicion.

Counselors can address these matters in whatever order best fits the needs of the patient as long as they consider (1) which message is most important *to* the patient, (2) which message is most important *for* the patient, (3) how much time is available, and (4) how the time can be most effectively used to achieve the best results. Logically, patients may respond first to messages most pertinent to their own cure, next to the cure of those closest to them, and finally to their longer-term health status and the health of others. The most successful counselors tailor the messages to the expressed needs and concerns of the patient. Specific sample messages to stress for each STD are listed in Table 33-1.

TAKE MEDICATION AS DIRECTED

The difference between the oral medication regimen the clinician prescribes and the one the patient actually follows may be distressingly great. In general, clinicians not only overestimate patient compliance but often cannot reliably predict which of their patients will comply. However, research on compliance indicates that one simple way of predicting is to ask the patient if he or she understands what has been prescribed, is able to repeat it, and expects to be able to comply.

Reasons for noncompliance are side effects, complexity of the regimen, and communication failure between health care provider and patient. The most obvious potential consequence of noncompliance is treatment failure resulting in further spread of the infection as well as complications for the patient.

The quality of the clinician-patient relationship has been judged to be a critical factor in compliance. Satisfaction with treatment and resulting compliance are greater when patients' expectations have been fulfilled, the clinician has responded to their concerns, responsive information about their conditions has been provided, and sincere concern and empathy have been shown. Compliance improves if the health care staff pays more attention to the instructions provided to patients.

When new or complex information is offered, the clinician should evaluate comprehension by asking the patient to repeat essential elements of the message, particularly the specific actions required by the treatment plan. Written instructions should be provided whenever possible in order to reinforce oral communication. The written instructions should be individualized and include information about both the benefits and the side effects of medications.

The following key points should be included in the patient–health care provider interaction to ensure that medication is taken as prescribed:

1. Emphasize the need for taking all the medication, regardless of symptoms and even after they resolve, and why the medication should not be shared with others.
2. Establish a specific medication schedule:
   a. What time the patient is to take the oral medication.
   b. What the patient is to do if a dose is missed.
   c. What to do if the patient feels the medication is not working or is causing side effects.
3. Review contraindications and potential side effects.
4. Identify and discuss potential compliance problems.

TABLE 33-1. Sexually Transmitted Disease Counseling Summary*

Disease and biological agents	Behavioral messages to emphasize
Chlamydial infections, nongonococcal urethritis (NGU), and mucopurulent cervicitis (MPC)	Understand how to take any prescribed oral medications. If tetracycline is prescribed, take it 1 h before or 2 h after meals and avoid dairy products, antacids, iron- or other mineral-containing preparations, and sunlight. Return if symptoms persist or recur. Refer sexual partner(s) for examination and treatment. Avoid sex until patient and partner(s) are cured. Then use condoms to prevent future infections.
Gonorrhea	Same as for NGU
Pelvic inflammatory disease (PID)	Same as for NGU, except return 2 to 4 days after initiation of therapy for progress evaluation, and periodically as necessary until symptoms have resolved.
Vaginitis	Understand how to take or use any prescribed medications. Avoid alcohol until 24 h following completion of metronidazole therapy. Continue taking vaginally administered medications even during menses. Women with trichomoniasis: refer partners for treatment. Return if problems persist or recur. Use condoms to prevent trichomonas infections.
Genital warts	Return for weekly or biweekly treatment, and follow up until lesions have resolved. Abstain from sex or use condoms during therapy.
Genital herpes	Understand how to take or use any prescribed medications. Keep involved area clean and dry. Since both initial and recurrent lesions shed high concentrations of virus, abstain from sex while symptomatic. An undetermined but presumably small risk of transmission also exists during asymptomatic intervals. Condoms may offer some protection. Pregnant women: make obstetricians aware of any history of herpes.

*SOURCE: Centers for Disease Control: Sexually Transmitted Diseases Summary 1986. Department of Health and Human Services Publication 00-3380, Atlanta

TABLE 33-1. Sexually Transmitted Disease Counseling Summary
(Continued)

Disease and biological agents	Behavioral messages to emphasize
Syphilis	Same as for NGU, and also return for follow-up serologic tests 3, 6, 12, and 24 months after therapy.
Chancroid	Same as for NGU, and also return weekly or biweekly for evaluation until the infection is entirely healed.
Pediculosis pubis	Use topical medication as prescribed. Disinfect clothing and linen by washing them in hot water, by dry cleaning them, or by removing them from human exposure for 1 to 2 weeks. Avoid sexual or close physical contact until after treatment. Ensure examination of sexual partners as soon as possible. Return if problem persists or recurs.
Scabies	Same as for pediculosis.
Hepatitis B	The frequency of clinical follow-up is determined by symptomatology and the results of liver function tests. Hepatitis B vaccine is available to susceptible individuals.

RETURN FOR FOLLOW-UP TESTS

The importance of follow-up tests [test of cure (TOC)] in the management of specific STDs varies with the pathogen. TOCs are evolving as a control effort for several STDs. TOC is most important for syphilis, chancroid, and pelvic inflammatory disease; important for following unreliable patients who must fill a prescription and/or take multiple dose therapy; less important when treatment regimens are used that are very highly effective (e.g., ceftriaxone for gonorrhea), and when compliance is very likely (e.g., reliable patient taking doxycycline for chlamydial infection); and least important when the main goal of treatment is symptomatic benefit rather than cure (e.g., treatment of genital warts or genital herpes). In clinics where resources are limited, posttreatment cultures for all patients are not feasible and policies for TOC evaluations must be based on cost-effectiveness analysis. In clinics that are already unable to serve all new patients seeking treatment, TOC policies should be carefully prioritized and limited to those that are truly essential. In areas where TOC evaluations can be encouraged, clinicians can enhance the likelihood of improving patient return rates as follows:

1. Review the medical purpose of TOC evaluations.
2. Negotiate appointment date and time.
3. Emphasize the need to avoid unprotected sex until the retest is negative.
4. Identify and discuss potential compliance problems.
5. Provide in written form information detailed above (items 1 to 3).

ENSURE EXAMINATION OF SEX PARTNERS

Identification and timely referral of sex partners for examination, and treatment when indicated, can reduce reinfection rates among STD patients since reinfections in a large portion of men and women can be traced to the person who was the source of the original infection; prompt treatment of sex partners also prevents further spread of infection in the community and can prevent complications in the infected partner. Attempts must be made to capitalize on patients' knowledge of, and influence with, their own sex partners. Three commonly used methods of partner referral counseling are outlined in Table 33-2.

Self-referral is an economical method for the referral of sex partners in relatively low priority situations. The patient assumes full responsibility for notifying all sex partners in need of medical assessment. The health professional gathers no identifying information.

Contact referral assumes that patients can effectively communicate referral messages for medical evaluation to at least some sex partners. This system is recommended for "priority" situations which require monitoring of sex partner referral efforts by health provider staff. Patients can elect the option of referring some or all of their sex partners; the remaining partners are contacted by health provider staff. The counselor assists patients in deciding how to present information to sex partners to elicit the desired results. The clinic staff helps patients understand why they can and should participate in the process, as well as emphasizing that partners must be examined promptly (usually within 24 to 48 h). Patients must be aware that action by health personnel remains an option for ineffective referrals. The staff of the medical facility elicits identifying and locating information on each sex partner to monitor examination and preventive treatment of sex partners and to contact sex partners who do not comply with the referral. Allowing patients to refer sex partners to appropriate medical care affords patient and partners the opportunity to discuss the disease. Such discussions allow a patient to know when consorts have had a medical assessment and thus avoid the potential for reinfection.

In the *health provider referral* option, a medical facility staff member elicits from the patient identifying and locating information

TABLE 33-2. Referral Options for the Examination of Sexual Partners

Procedure	Description	Advantages	Disadvantages
Self-referral	Total patient responsibility; no identification of sex partners. Appointment cards are provided to patient for distribution to sex partners.	Reduces cost. Requires less personnel time.	Difficult to evaluate. Some patients may be disinterested, lack communication skills, or be hostile toward some sex partners.
Contact referral	Health care professional provides patient the option of having partners referred by health care personnel or by themselves within specified time period. Option is provided only if the patient appears to be interested, responsible, and able. Identification of sex partners required.	A monitoring system ensures that epidemiologic treatment is applied. Reduces cost. Encourages patient participation.	Lacks anonymity. Patient may not comply, requiring health department to intervene and lose time in the referral process.
Health provider referral	Health care provider assumes total responsibility for referral of sex partners.	Maintains patient anonymity. Permits monitoring by health department. Ensures application of epidemiologic treatment.	Increases cost. Discourages patient participation.

on all sex partners and assumes full responsibility for referring these persons for medical assessment. This staff member is currently termed a *disease intervention specialist* in the United States. The patient is not involved in the process and is not advised of the outcome of the effort. This approach provides a high degree of confidentiality as well as accountability for measuring the success of individual referrals and can be an efficient way of locating patients and/or individuals who are at risk of infection. However, it is expensive, and patients who assume no responsibility for solving their own health problems gain no experience for subsequent situations.

In summary, health provider staff involved in the process of partner referral should

1. Assess the patient's response and determine the patient's concern regarding sex partners.
2. Determine the patient's capability of participating in sex partner referral.
3. Describe the methods of sex partner referral that are available.
4. Determine the method of referral for each sex partner.
5. Establish time limits for the referral of sex partners by the patient.
6. Recommend that the patient abstain from any sexual activities with previous partners until they are medically assessed and counseled. As an adjunct, reinforce this final item by restating it in any written material provided to the patient.

REDUCE RISK

Risk reduction is one of the most important parts of the counseling process, as it can prevent infected patients from transmitting their infection to others and from acquiring new STDs.

Barrier methods of prophylaxis, such as the condom, when used properly appear to be highly effective in preventing the transmission of many STDs including HIV infection. Latex condoms should be promoted for STD prevention rather than natural membrane condoms, which have tiny pores through which some smaller viruses conceivably might pass. Spermicides which contain nonoxynol-9 may be a useful protective adjunct to condoms since this substance has been shown to inactivate HIV and several other STD pathogens, although the use of spermicides as an STD prevention agent with condoms has not been evaluated as such in people. To maximize their effectiveness, explicit information on condoms and how to use them, as outlined in Table 33-3, should be provided. Clinicians, counselors, and other staff members must be taught how to persuade patients to recognize their risk for acquiring or transmitting STDs and how to use condoms regularly.

In addition to condom use, patients need to know which sexual

TABLE 33-3. Instructions for Condom Users

For maximum protection, condoms must be used correctly. Health
workers should not assume that people know how to use condoms. All
condom users should receive very clear and explicit instructions:

Keep a condom with you.

Use a condom every time you have intercourse.

Always put the condom on the penis before intercourse begins.

Put the condom on when penis is erect.

Do not pull the condom tightly against the tip of the penis. Leave a small
empty space—about 1 or 2 cm—at the end of the condom to hold
semen and reduce risk of breakage. Some condoms have a nipple tip
that will hold semen.

Unroll the condom all the way to the bottom of the penis.

If the condom breaks during intercourse, withdraw the penis
immediately and put on a new condom.

After ejaculation, withdraw the penis while it is still erect. Hold onto the
rim of the condom as you withdraw so that the condom does not slip off.

Use a new condom each time you have intercourse. Throw used
condoms away.

If a lubricant is desired, use water-based lubricants such as
contraceptive jelly. Lubricants made with petroleum jelly may damage
condoms. Do not use saliva because it may contain virus.

Store condoms in a cool, dry place if possible.

Condoms that are sticky or brittle or otherwise damaged should not be
used.

SOURCE: Instructions for condom users. Population Reports Series L: 6, xiv:3,
p L-274, 1986. The Johns Hopkins University, Baltimore

TABLE 33-4. Gradient from Higher to Lower Risk of HIV Transmission by
Sexual Contact with an Infected Sexual Partner

High	Unprotected receptive anal intercourse
	Unprotected receptive vaginal intercourse
	Unprotected insertive vaginal intercourse
	Unprotected insertive anal intercourse
	Any type of sexual intercourse with correct use of a condom
	Oral contact (penile, vaginal, anal)
Low	"Wet" kissing (deep or tongue kissing)

SOURCE: World Health Organization: Prevention of sexual transmission of
human immunodeficiency virus (HIV): Management and counseling.
Geneva: World Health Organization, 1990

practices reduce the potential risk of infection (Table 33-4). Patients
should be educated and counseled on such social skills as negotiating
sexual limits with their partners and clarifying unsafe and safer sex
practices. Counselors need to adopt a nonjudgmental attitude in
discussing lifestyles and lifestyle changes. Recommendations for

making abrupt, unrealistic changes may produce only short-term results. The patient must find these messages acceptable and attainable. Patients should be provided with an opportunity to consider alternative lifestyles that reduce their risk of future infection. Clinicians and other staff members should stress the following key points:

1. Present options tailored to the patient's sexual lifestyle.
2. Emphasize reducing future risk by:
   a. Abstaining from any sexual activity until follow-up test.
   b. Abstaining from any sexual activity whenever symptoms appear.
   c. Using condoms in any risky or unknown settings.
3. Provide written information detailed above (item 2).

RESPOND TO DISEASE SUSPICION

Unfortunately, a common response to illness—even STDs—is to "wait and see" if the symptoms persist or subside. Persons who continue sexual activity while having symptoms contribute substantially to the spread of STDs. Moreover, the symptoms of many STDs can be inconspicuous or mild, especially for women. Health providers should encourage patients to seek medical evaluation after having unprotected sex (intercourse without a condom) with someone who is known to have or is suspected of having an STD. Although patients should be taught to recognize symptoms as a signal to seek immediate medical care, it is even more important to stress that STDs in both men and women may be asymptomatic. Because lack of symptoms is an unreliable guide to freedom from infection, periodic examinations should be encouraged for persons involved in repeated high-risk practices.

For their future reference, health providers should ensure that patients

1. Recognize the major signs and symptoms of common STD
2. Understand that asymptomatic infections are common
3. Pursue prompt medical evaluation of signs and symptoms or of exposure to known or suspected STD
4. Abstain from sexual activity while symptoms are present or while suspicion of infection exists
5. Bring or refer sex partner(s) for evaluation and counseling
6. Retain this information by reinforcement, through the provision of the information above (items 1 to 5) in written form

CONCLUSION

As noted earlier, the main reasons for the high incidence rates of STD are behavioral. There is growing recognition of the value of using knowledge from the social and behavioral sciences in influencing lifestyle choices, reinforcing positive health habits, and promoting the adoption of healthy behavior. More than ever, change of the patient's sexual behavior is now regarded as an essential element in the prevention and ultimate control of STD.

ADDITIONAL READING

Boekeloo BO et al: Frequency and thoroughness of STD/HIV risk assessment by physicians in a high-risk metropolitan area. *Am J Public Health* 81:1645, 1991

Holtedahl KA et al: Patients with sexually transmitted disease: A well-defined HIV risk group in general practice? *Fam Pract* 8:42, 1991

Roter DL et al: Routine communication in sexually transmitted disease clinics: An observational study. *Am J Public Health* 80:605, 1990

Vinson RP, Epperly TD: Counseling patients on proper use of condoms. *Am Fam Physician* 43:2081, 1991

Washington AE et al: Assessing risk for pelvic inflammatory disease and its sequelae. *JAMA* 266:2581, 1991

Wenger NS et al: Reduction of high-risk sexual behavior among heterosexuals undergoing HIV antibody testing: A randomized clinical trial. *Am J Public Health* 81:1580, 1991

Zenilman JM et al: Effect of HIV posttest counseling on STD incidence. *JAMA* 267:843, 1992

The importance of patient counseling is dramatically evident with HIV infection. In the absence of safe and effective treatment or vaccine, the best hope today for controlling the AIDS epidemic is to educate the public about the seriousness of the threat, the ways the virus is transmitted, and the practical steps each person can take to avoid acquiring or spreading it. Counseling persons who are at risk of acquiring HIV infection and offering HIV antibody testing are important components of that strategy. The primary public health purpose of counseling is to induce behavior changes to minimize the risk of HIV infection and transmission. This can best be achieved not only by motivating individuals to modify their behavior, but by creating social acceptance for safe behavior and reinforcing it whenever possible.

GENERAL CONSIDERATIONS

Table 34-1 outlines persons who should be offered HIV counseling and testing.

Reasonable guidelines for HIV antibody testing and counseling are that

1. They are recommended routinely to clients or patients by knowledgeable health professionals when indicated for medical or public health purposes.
2. They are available to persons seeking self-initiated testing.
3. The testing is done after appropriate counseling and receipt of information that allows specific consent to be given.
4. Specific verbal or written consent is obtained.
5. The procedures are conducted confidentially or anonymously.
6. Posttest counseling increases the person's understanding of the significance of HIV infection, or how to avoid transmission to others, if infected.

In addition, patient counseling may require more than just addressing the immediate crisis. Ancillary referral resources (medical, psychosocial, social, and/or supportive) should also be made available to the individual to assist in the long-term adjustment to infection.

In general, for STD counselors to become HIV counselors does not require learning an entirely new set of skills, but it does differ in the following ways:

1. *Population counseled.* Counseling services provided to STD patients are usually limited to persons already diagnosed with an STD listed as reportable in the state where the diagnosis is made. Counseling at HIV antibody testing sites, however, is provided

TABLE 34-1 Persons Who Should Be Offered HIV Counseling and Testing

Men who have had sex with other men

Injecting drug users (IDUs)

Heterosexuals with multiple sexual partners

Patients who are evaluated or treated for sexually transmitted diseases

Persons who received transfusions of blood, blood products, or clotting factor between 1977 and 1985

Sexual partners of persons in the above categories

Tuberculosis patients

Patients whose signs and symptoms suggest a differential diagnosis which includes HIV infection

Rape victims

Persons who experience parenteral or mucous membrane exposure to blood or body fluids with a high likelihood of HIV contamination

to at least four categories of persons: (a) persons voluntarily requesting the test, (b) persons in the posttesting phase, including those found to be HIV-negative, (c) persons diagnosed with HIV infection, and (d) the family members, friends, or sex partners of the HIV-positive person.

2. *Supportive counseling.* HIV and other STD counseling both depend heavily on exposure and risk-reduction counseling as a primary public health goal. However, HIV counseling also aims to maintain the social, emotional, and physical health of the infected person. As a result, AIDS counselors must develop a wide range of skills and be prepared to arrange specific referrals and patient care services.

PRETEST COUNSELING

Counseling before testing is essential, since a person requesting this service should have a reasonable understanding of the medical and social implications of HIV infection before providing consent. The benefits and potential consequences of testing should be explored with each individual wishing to be tested.

Although pretest counseling is performed before determination of whether the individual is in fact infected, pretest counseling can emphasize that the sexual transmission of HIV can be prevented if precautions are taken. The need for precautions, however, depends on whether the individual or his or her sex partners are infected. If neither is infected, no precautions are needed as long as each can be certain that the relationship is exclusively monogamous. A single negative test should not be interpreted as evidence that the patient is not infected if high-risk behavior has occurred within the previous 6 months, and counseling should emphasize continued prevention measures until any necessary follow-up testing is completed. If one partner is infected, the most certain way to avoid transmission is to abstain from sexual intercourse. If both are infected, it is not known whether continued reexposure to the virus causes the disease to progress more rapidly in persons infected with HIV. Finally, if the infection status of a sex partner is unknown, it is wise to assume that the partner could be infected and thus avoid sexual contact where mucous membranes may be exposed to bodily fluids. In general, the same methods that prevent passing the virus on to others also prevent infection from occurring in a person who is not infected.

The ability of health departments, hospitals, and other health care providers to ensure confidentiality of patient information and the public's confidence in that ability are crucial to increasing the number of persons requesting or willing to undergo counseling and testing for HIV antibody. Most U.S. public health agencies concur it is possible to conduct antibody testing with reasonable assurance that confidentiality can be maintained. If, however, confidentiality cannot be ensured, procedures allowing anonymity should be available as an option for persons who would otherwise not be tested.

Finally, persons need to consider what means of social support they will have if they are infected. Will they be able to obtain sufficient support from family members or friends? And who among these will keep the information confidential? They may wish to establish contact with community support groups after receiving the test results.

In summary, pretest counseling should

1. Establish the patient's risk behaviors for HIV infection
2. Provide risk-reduction counseling
3. Provide details on the meaning and implication of test results
4. Help the patient prepare a plan for dealing with the information provided by the test, including assessing the patient's support system and coping resources and informing the patient of community resources for seropositive and seronegative persons

DIAGNOSIS OF HIV INFECTION

HIV infection can be diagnosed by isolation of the virus from viral cultures, but the most widely used method of diagnosis is serologic testing. Immunodiagnosis of HIV infection is made by performance of two types of antibody tests in sequence. The first is an enzyme-linked immunosorbent assay (ELISA), which detects antibodies to multiple viral proteins. If positive, the test is repeated. Repeatedly positive tests are confirmed by performance of a Western blot for antibody detection. HIV antibody tests should not be reported as positive until samples that are repeatedly reactive by ELISA testing have been confirmed as positive with a Western

people; unfortunate consequences have resulted from disclosure, especially when too many, or thoughtless, people were told.

Seropositive women of childbearing age should understand the risks and implications of mother-to-infant transmission of HIV. Evidence indicates the high risk (approximately 30 percent) of fetal transmission and infant infection, although the transmission may depend on the timing of the mother's HIV infection, the mother's immunologic status, and other possible factors. Infected women should be advised of means to avoid pregnancy and should be referred for family planning services. The identification of HIV-infected pregnant women as early in pregnancy as possible is important to enable optimal management of the pregnancy, to plan medical care for the infant, and to provide counseling about family planning and future pregnancies.

Seropositive people should be counseled to prevent further transmission of HIV by taking the following steps:

1. They should inform prospective sex partners of their own infection with HIV. Sexual abstention is the only option that would eliminate all risk of sexually transmitted HIV infection.
2. They should take appropriate precautions (e.g., avoiding, in particular, anal sex) to prevent the sexual partner from coming into contact with the infected person's blood, semen, or cervical or vaginal secretions. Although the efficacy of using condoms to prevent infection with HIV is still under study, consistent use of condoms should reduce HIV transmission.
3. They should inform previous sex partners and any persons with whom needles were shared of their potential exposure to HIV and encourage them to seek counseling or testing.
4. Injection drug users should never share needles and other equipment.
5. Seropositive people should refrain from sharing toothbrushes, razors, or other items that could become contaminated with blood.
6. Seropositive people should not donate blood, plasma, body organs, breast milk, tissues, or semen.
7. They should avoid pregnancy and use family planning services.
8. They should clean and disinfect contaminated surfaces properly.

COUNSELING OF PERSONS WITH AIDS

AIDS is the most severe manifestation of HIV infection; it occurs in adults typically after about 10 years of infection have passed. Ideally, persons diagnosed with AIDS will have known of the risk of developing this syndrome for some time, although even then the emotional implications of a potential future diagnosis for these patients can be enormous. Physicians should inform the patient directly as soon as possible after the diagnosis is confirmed, providing a clear, frank, and sensitive explanation of what the patient can expect. Although wide variation in the progression has been observed in patients with the same clinical diagnosis, meeting the criteria for an AIDS diagnosis as defined by CDC has resulted in death in at least three-quarters of reported cases within 2 years of diagnosis.

Persons with AIDS will feel uncertain about the future and wonder how this condition will affect the way they live, the risk they may pose to others, and the risk others may pose to them. Risk-reduction advice concerning safer sex and infection control is essential in counseling persons diagnosed as having AIDS just as it is for all other HIV-infected persons. Although patients may need to face the future with a hopeful outlook, they should be encouraged to consult with their physicians rather than seeking out unproved "miracle" cures. The patient should be told that massive efforts are underway to find an effective treatment. Information concerning how to learn about available treatment and experimental drug trials should be provided to the patient.

Even for counselors accustomed to discussing serious or fatal diseases with patients, the differences between AIDS and most other diseases need to be considered:

1. HIV is potentially transmissible throughout the time a person is infected; moreover, it appears the older the infection, the greater the likelihood of transmission. Permanent lifestyle changes can eliminate or reduce the potential for infecting others. These changes, although difficult, must be encouraged, and the patient must be assured that some personal control over the future is possible by avoiding unsafe sexual practices and injection drug use.

2. Because of ignorance, a diagnosis of AIDS can result in fear of abandonment or outright rejection by loved ones, family friends, and even health professionals, resulting in social isolation and leaving the patient without the emotional or financial support required during this important period. Guilt may even cause the patient to attempt to terminate important social and/or familial linkages, creating unnecessary social and domestic disruption. The patient may suffer from fear about infecting others or of being infected with opportunistic organisms by others. These anxieties may be manifested in sexual dysfunction and social withdrawal or even hostility. Persons who have recently been diagnosed with HIV infection or AIDS require psychological support, and the many community support groups that have been formed to meet this need may prove of great benefit. Initially, however, these persons may find joining a support group too

frightening. Instead, more informal social settings may provide the structures needed for the patient to resist the tendency to remain isolated.

3. The natural history of AIDS is frequently marked by intermittent development of unusual and severe illnesses. As a result, each new illness represents a major psychological stress. This pattern of illnesses is often progressive and additive, leading to the physical and emotional exhaustion of the patient.

A person diagnosed with AIDS must be made aware of and encouraged to adopt guidelines for sexual behavior that avoid HIV transmission as well as reduce the risk of subsequent opportunistic diseases. In addition, these guidelines should reduce the potential for other STDs which may be much more serious than usual because of existing immunodeficiency.

In summary, counseling of persons with AIDS should

1. Encourage limiting sexual activity to an established and informed partner, avoiding any practices which entail the exchange of semen, vaginal or cervical secretions, or blood, especially insertive anal sex
2. Inform the patient, as well as any partner, of the necessity for fidelity
3. Provide information on cleaning and disinfection procedures
4. Provide referral services to community support groups established to meet the needs of persons with AIDS
5. Include information on how to learn about experimental drug trials
6. Provide, in written form, information detailed above (items 1 to 5)

COUNSELING OF FAMILY, PARTNERS, AND FRIENDS

As with any potentially terminal illness or condition, AIDS and HIV infection create a crisis not only for the patients but also for those close to them. At a minimum, patients must be strongly encouraged to notify their sex or needle-sharing partners of their potential exposure. These individuals should be counseled and encouraged to be tested. If the HIV antibody test is negative, recent sex partners may be advised to repeat the test within several months to allow time for the antibodies to be detected. In addition, the partners should be encouraged to monitor their own health status by consulting their physicians, especially if they choose not to be tested, if they are seropositive, or if they continue to engage in sex with the patient. This is true even if safer sex practices are continued, since these may still carry some risk of infection.

The patient's family and friends who have neither had sexual contact nor shared needles with the patient should be reassured that they could not have become infected as a result of casual contact with the patient. Indeed, they should be made aware that the patient is likely to be extremely sensitive to indications that these family members and friends are withdrawing and are afraid of close contact. Fear of abandonment and isolation is frequently extremely pronounced in terminally ill patients and can be even further exaggerated in AIDS patients because of the stigma attached not only to the disease but to certain population groups associated with it. In fact, the attitudes of some health care providers toward these groups may constitute a major barrier to the provision of optimal care.

In most instances, the partners, family members, and friends will react to the news of the patient's diagnosis with grief. Most people have come to recognize that an AIDS diagnosis will almost certainly result in death. Despite this, the counselor should try to forestall a premature initiation of the mourning process by keeping the family and patient focused on prevention and treatment issues. The availability of treatments and experimental protocols and the possibility of extending the patient's survival time should all be discussed.

However, the family, partners, and friends will eventually need to be prepared for the patient's functional and cognitive decline. As death nears, referral for more intensive grief counseling may be appropriate. Agencies offering support groups for caretakers of AIDS patients can be a particularly valuable resource.

Because of the continuous growth and change in our understanding of HIV-associated conditions, the continually changing treatment options, and the extensive (often sensational) media coverage of AIDS, the counselor will need to ensure that some arrangement for continuing communication with the patient, the family, partners, and friends about these issues is available. Support groups, community voluntary organizations, and AIDS information services can serve this purpose.

In summary, the counseling of family, partners, and friends should

1. Encourage abstinence or the adoption of sexual practices between the established partner and the AIDS patient that do not entail the exchange of semen, vaginal or cervical secretions, or blood
2. Inform the established partner of the necessity for abstinence or fidelity
3. Reassure family and friends that infection is not possible through casual contact with the person with AIDS
4. Provide information on cleaning and disinfection procedures
5. Provide referral services to community programs established to meet the needs of persons with AIDS

6. Include information on how to learn about experimental drug trials
7. Provide, in written form, information detailed above (items 1 to 6)

CONCLUSION

Many authorities have stressed that education will be the primary means of AIDS prevention in the 1990s. Counseling is an emotionally charged and psychologically challenging intervention strategy. When one discusses AIDS with HIV-infected persons and those at risk, major life events and issues, such as sex, love relationships, family, and death, are involved. Many people, particularly young adults, are not accustomed to dealing with some of these issues or even discussing them. The counselor will be indispensable in helping people discuss these issues while maintaining the primary goal of counseling: modification of behavior to decrease the risk of disease transmission.

Although AIDS-prevention counseling contains elements familiar to experienced STD counselors, it requires greater depth, sensitivity, and skills. Training will be needed by many to improve their capacity to provide counseling to troubled individuals. Training will also be needed to increase the quality of and the opportunities for counseling services. The ultimate control of AIDS and prevention of HIV infection will depend in large part on how widely available counseling services are and how well counselors meet their challenges.

ADDITIONAL READING

Boekeloo BO, et al: Frequency and thoroughness of STD/HIV risk assessment by physicians in a high-risk metropolitan area. *Am J Public Health* 81:1645, 1991

Centers for Disease Control: Interpretation and use of the Western blot assay for serodiagnosis of human immunodeficiency virus type 1 infections. *MMWR* 1989: 38 (No. S-7)

DiClemente RJ, et al: Determinants of condom use among junior high school students in a minority, inner-city school district. *Pediatrics* 89: 197, 1992

Dock NL, et al: Human immunodeficiency virus infection and indeterminate Western blot patterns. Prospective studies in a low prevalence population. *Arch Intern Med* 151:525, 1991

Giesecke J, et al: Efficacy of partner notification for HIV infection. *Lancet* 338: 1096, 1991

Higgins DL, et al: Evidence for the effects of HIV antibody counseling and testing on risk behaviors. *JAMA* 266: 2419, 1991

Landis SE, et al: Impact of HIV testing and counseling on subsequent sexual behavior. *AIDS Educ Prev* 4: 61, 1992

Landis SE, et al: Results of a randomized trial of partner notification in cases of HIV infection in North Carolina. *N Engl J Med* 326: 101, 1992

Makadon HJ: Assessing HIV infection in primary care practice. *J Gen Internal Med* 6:52, 1991

Marks G, et al: HIV-infected men's practices in notifying past sexual partners of infection risk. *Public Health Rep* 107: 100, 1992

Mason J, et al: Incorporating HIV education and counseling into routine prenatal care: A program model. *AIDS Educ Prev* 3: 118, 1991

Perry S, et al: Suicidal ideation and HIV testing. *JAMA* 263:679, 1990

Rugg DL, et al: Evaluating the CDC program for HIV counseling and testing. *Public Health Rep* 106: 708, 1991

Rutherford GW, et al: Partner notification and the control of human immunodeficiency virus infection. Two years of experience in San Francisco. *Sex Transm Dis* 18: 107, 1991

Wenger NS, et al: Reduction of high-risk sexual behavior among heterosexuals undergoing HIV antibody testing: A randomized clinical trial. *Am J Public Health* 81: 1580, 1991

Zenilman JM, et al: Effect of HIV posttest counseling on STD incidence. *JAMA* 267: 843, 1992

For a more detailed discussion, see Parra W, Drotman DP, Siegel K, Esteves K, and Baker T: Patient Counseling and Behavior Modification, Chap. 88, p. 1057, in STD-2.

Sexual assault is defined as an act of sexual intimacy performed without the consent of the victim through use or threat of use of force, or when the victim is unable to give consent because of physical or mental disability.

Sexually transmitted diseases (STDs) are the most common medical problems complicating sexual assault. STD has been identified in more than half of female victims at their initial or follow-up visits. STD diagnosed at the time of a sexual assault can add to the emotional problems experienced by victims, whether or not the disease was acquired as a result of the assault. In addition, victims often express severe anxiety about the possibility of contracting an STD from the assailant. This anxiety can exacerbate the emotional trauma they experience, aggravate posttraumatic stress, and delay their recovery.

Because sexual assaults occur commonly, medical practitioners who treat STD are likely to see sexual assault victims in their practices.

SPECIAL ISSUES IN THE MANAGEMENT OF SEXUAL ASSAULT VICTIMS

Several factors make the diagnosis and treatment of STD in victims of sexual assault different from diagnosis and treatment in other sexual relationships. Although sometimes well known to the victim, often the assailant is a stranger or casual acquaintance. Since the health status of the offender is likely to be unknown, it is difficult to estimate the risk of contracting an STD in any individual case.

Often, sexual assault victims are seen after a single episode of sexual contact. Although the relative infectivity of some organisms has been determined, little is known about the infectivity of many STDs after a single episode of intercourse. This makes it difficult to estimate the risk of contracting an STD after assault.

In addition, it is difficult to determine if an STD diagnosed after a sexual assault predated the attack or was a result of it. Even if a positive culture is obtained shortly after the assault, it is possible that the results represent bacteria or viruses found in infected semen rather than a previously undiagnosed asymptomatic infection of the victim. With some organisms such as herpes simplex virus (HSV), changes in antibody levels to the organism in the victim's sera can be monitored to determine whether or not the infection was recently acquired. However, reliable tests for immune responses to many sexually transmitted organisms do not exist, as in the case of *Neisseria gonorrhoeae*. With other tests, such as serologic tests for *Chlamydia trachomatis*, it can be difficult to differentiate newly acquired infection from previous infection.

The site of the assault may also affect the likelihood of contracting an STD. For example, because of their predisposition for cervical columnar epithelium, *N. gonorrhoeae* and *C. trachomatis* are more readily transmitted by vaginal intercourse than by oral intercourse, while human immunodeficiency virus (HIV) would be more likely to be transmitted by anal intercourse than by vaginal or oral intercourse.

Finally, whether or not the male assailant ejaculates during a sexual assault will affect the likelihood of the victim's contracting an STD. Many sex offenders are sexually dysfunctional. Sexual problems prohibiting intromission and ejaculation decrease the victim's risk of certain STDs or pregnancy resulting from the assault.

EPIDEMIOLOGY OF SEXUAL ASSAULT

Sexual assault victims are more likely to be young, single, female members of minority groups who have a low income. The highest incidence occurs in older adolescents and young adults. Many of the same factors have been identified as risk factors for STD. These epidemiologic factors reinforce the need for careful evaluation for STD as part of the medical care of sexual assault victims.

RISK OF SPECIFIC DISEASES AFTER VAGINAL SEXUAL ASSAULT OF FEMALES

Any sexually transmissible agents, including HIV, may be transmitted during an assault, but the risk of acquiring gonococcal and/or chlamydial infections and vaginal infections (trichomoniasis, bacterial vaginosis) appears to be highest. Syphilis and viral STDs are rarely reported after assault. Genital herpes and HIV infections are not likely to be contracted during a sexual assault, but the threat of these infections creates severe anxiety for victims. Inferences about STD risk may be based on the known prevalence of these diseases in the community. If the suspected assailant is identified, that individual should be evaluated for STD to the extent possible under the law. STD after assault is common enough to warrant a thorough diagnostic workup for STD as part of a sexual assault evaluation.

EVALUATION

The initial evaluation of the victim for STD should be performed, if possible, within 24 h of the assault and should include the following:

Cultures for *N. gonorrhoeae* and *C. trachomatis* from specimens from any sites of penetration or attempted penetration.

Collection of a blood sample for a serologic test for syphilis and for storage of a serum sample for possible future testing. Serologic testing for HIV and hepatitis B infection should be considered.

For women, examination of vaginal specimens for *T. vaginalis* and for evidence of bacterial vaginosis.

Pregnancy tests.

Follow-up evaluations should be performed 14 to 21 days after the assault, to repeat studies other than those for syphilis and viral STDs. A third visit may be scheduled at 8 to 12 weeks to repeat initial serologic studies, including tests for antibodies to *Treponema pallidum,* hepatitis B virus, and/or HIV.

Test Selection and Specimen Handling

When a sexually transmitted agent is identified from a sexually abused person, that laboratory result may be required for use during subsequent legal action. Isolation of *N. gonorrhoeae* and *C. trachomatis* organisms by culture, and their confirmation by recognized techniques, is the necessary standard. All presumptive isolates of *N. gonorrhoeae* from children should be confirmed by at least two tests that use different principles, e.g., biochemical, enzyme substrate, or serologic. Where culture diagnosis is possible (e.g., gonorrhea, chlamydial infection, genital herpes), direct specimen antigen detection tests or DNA probe tests are not recommended for use on specimens from a victim of sexual abuse. These tests may be used to diagnose *C. trachomatis* in adult victims only in those areas where culture is not available. Results of nonculture tests may be used to guide medical management but should not be used for forensic purposes. The potential for an inaccurate result is greatest in children, and in general nonculture tests are not recommended at any time as an alternative to culture in the evaluation of sexual assault or sexual abuse in children. Exceptions include serologic diagnosis of HIV infection and syphilis. Also, if HSV-2 specific serologic testing is available from a reference lab, demonstration of HSV-2 seroconversion in paired sera may be useful. Isolates should be stored at $-70°C$ for possible future studies, and the use of a reference laboratory should be considered. Expert laboratory consultations are recommended for testing as well as for chain-of-evidence issues.

TREATMENT

Treatment should be given for an infection identified on examination, and preventive treatment is advisable for any infection identified in the assailant. Although the risk of infection is frequently low, use of presumptive treatment is controversial. Some clinicians recommend presumptive treatment for all victims of sexual assault, while some reserve presumptive treatment for special circumstances, for example, when follow-up examination of the victim cannot be ensured, or when treatment is specifically requested by the patient. Although no regimen provides coverage for all potential pathogens, the following regimens should be effective against gonorrhea, chlamydia, trichomonal infections, bacterial vaginosis, and, most likely, syphilis.

Empirical regimen for victims of sexual assault:

Ceftriaxone, 125 mg, given IM, and Metronidazole, 2g, orally, *to be followed by either*

Doxycycline 100 mg orally 2 times a day for 7 days *or*

Tetracycline HCl 500 mg orally 4 times a day for 7 days.

ADDITIONAL READING

Glaser JB et al: Sexually transmitted diseases in postpubertal female rape victims. *J Infect Dis* 164:726, 1991

Hillman R et al: Adult male victims of sexual assault: An underdiagnosed condition. *Int J STD AIDS* 2:22, 1991

Jenny C et al: Sexually transmitted diseases in victims of rape. *N Engl J Med* 322:713, 1990

Lacey HB: Sexually transmitted diseases and rape: The experience of a sexual assault centre. *Int J STD AIDS* 1:405, 1990

Ross JD et al: Rape and sexually transmitted diseases: Patterns of referral and incidence in a department of genitourinary medicine. *J R Soc Med* 84:657, 1991

Schwarcz SK, Whittington WL: Sexual assault and sexually transmitted diseases: Detection and management in adults and children. *Rev Infect Dis* 12 (suppl 6): S682, 1990

For a more detailed discussion, see Jenny C: Sexual Assault and STD, Chap. 95, in STD-2.

Index

Abortion, spontaneous: and
STDs, 335
(*See also* Pregnancy)
Acquired immunodeficiency
syndrome (*see*
HIV/AIDS)
Acyclovir: for HSV, 130,
149–150, 151t–152t
anorectal, 295
in pregnancy, 153
Adenovirus: neonatal
pneumonitis, 360
AIDS (*see* HIV/AIDS)
Alcohol use, 3, 4–5
Amebiasis:
donovanosis vs., 97
and HIV/AIDS, 120
Amoxicillin:
for chlamydial infections, 344
for gonorrhea, 36
Anaerobic bacteria: and
vaginosis, 245–246
Anal intercourse and
infections, 11, 12t, 13t,
291
chlamydial proctitis, 46, 291
CMV, 156
donovanosis, 96, 96f, 97
genital ulcers, 310
(*See also* Genital ulcer
adenopathy syndrome)
gonococcal, 26, 28, 32, 33t,
35t, 291, 293–294
treatment, 36–37
HIV, 106, 291
HPV warts, 163, 165, 291
HSV proctitis, 145–146, 291
LGV, 57t, 58t, 60–61, 296,
297
proctitis, 291, 293–295
syphilis, 65, 71, 295–296
Anal warts (*see* Human
papillomavirus
infection)

Anilingus:
STD association, 13t
(*See also* Oral-anogenital
sex)
Anogenitorectal syndrome:
differential diagnosis, 60–61
LGV, 60–61, 296–297, 311t
Anorectal anatomy, 292f
Antibiotics: and VVC risk, 225
Antiretroviral therapy: for
HIV/AIDS, 127–129
Aortic syphilis, 82–84
Argyll Robertson pupil, 80t, 81
Arthritis, STDs and, 319–334
differential diagnosis,
330–333, 332f
gonococcal
in children, 356
disseminated infection
(DGI), 31–32, 38,
328–329, 329t, 331
in neonates, 353
HBV, 329
HIV, 330
LGV, 330
management, 333
Mycoplasma hominis, 330
Reiter's syndrome, 319–328
syphilis, 330
Atopic dermatitis: scabies
and, 204, 208
Autonomic nervous system
dysfunction: in HSV
infection, 142
Azithromycin:
for chlamydial infections, 53
for NGU, 277
AZT (zidovudine): for
HIV/AIDS, 127–128

Bacterial cystitis (*see* Cystitis)
Bacterial infections:
in HIV/AIDS, 131
(*See also* specific bacteria)

Bacterial vaginosis (*see* Vaginosis, bacterial)
Bacteroides, 246
  and PID, 255
  urethritis, 272
  vaginosis in pregnancy, 338
Balanitis, 17
  in Reiter's syndrome, 323, 325f
Balanoposthitis: candidal, 227
Bartholin glands, 21
Bartholinitis: chlamydial, 48
Blacks: STDs in, 7, 63, 136
Brain abscesses: in HIV/AIDS, 117
Bubonulus (LGV), 58–59
Butoconazole: for vulvovaginal candidiasis, 230
BV (*see* Vaginosis, bacterial)

Calymmatobacterium granulomatosis, 93
  (*See also* Donovanosis)
Campylobacter:
  and HIV/AIDS, 120, 133
  proctocolitis/enteritis, 298
  and Reiter's syndrome, 319
Candida albicans, 223
Candidiasis:
  ectocervicitis, 239
  female specimen collection, 22–23
  and HIV/AIDS, 110, 115, 119, 122, 158
    management, 122, 131
  and trichomoniasis, 219
  vulvovaginal (VVC), 223–232, 238
    antibiotics and, 225
    BV coexisting with, 245
    clinical manifestations, 226–227
    diabetes and, 224–225
    diagnosis, 227–229, 228f, 229f, 242t–243t

epidemiology, 223
  oral contraceptives and, 224
  pathogenesis, 224–226
  pregnancy and, 224
  treatment, 230–231, 242t–243t
Cardiovascular syphilis, 82–85
CD4 cells: and HIV/AIDS, 103, 108t, 109, 110, 125
  treatment, 119
CDC on HIV/AIDS:
  case definition, 110, 111t–113t
  classification, 107t, 107–110
Cefixime: for gonorrhea, 36
Cefoxitin: for PID, 264
Ceftizoxime: for gonorrhea, 38
Ceftriaxone:
  for cervicitis, 240
  for chancroid, 91
  for DGI, 333
  for epididymitis, 289
  for gonorrhea, 36, 37, 38, 294
    in newborns and children, 356, 357
    in pregnancy, 343
  for PID, 264
  for sexual assault victims, 411
  for syphilis, 73
Cerebrovascular syphilis, 76–77
Cervical cancer:
  and AIDS, 110, 125
  HPV and, 166, 168–169, 240, 348
Cervicitis, 238–240
  BV coexisting with, 245
  chlamydial, 46–47, 52t, 141
  diagnosis, 239–240
  differential diagnosis, 140–141, 240–241
  ecto-, 239–240
  endo-, 238–240

gonococcal, 28, 29f
  treatment, 36–37
herpetic, 140–141
mucopurulent, 238–239
  counseling on, 390t
  and PID, 259
  treatment, 240
prevention, 241, 244
treatment, 240
Cesarean section: and
  postpartum infection,
  338–339
Chancre, syphilitic, 65f,
  65–66, 66f, 71, 148,
  309, 311t
Chancroid, 87–92, 309
  clinical manifestations,
    88–90, 89f, 90f, 311t
  complications, 312
  counseling on, 391t
  diagnosis, 90–91, 313t, 314,
    317f
  differential diagnosis, 89,
    148
  dwarf, 89
  epidemiology, 87
  groove sign, 312
  HIV and, 87, 90, 106
  LGV vs., 60
  microbiology, 88
  pathogenesis, 88
  treatment, 91, 315
Charcot's joints, 80, 81
Children:
  chlamydial infections in,
    380–381
  condylomata acuminata in,
    381–382
  Gardnerella vaginalis in, 382
  gonococcal infections in,
    354–356, 357, 380
  HIV/AIDS in, 382
  HSV in, 381
  molluscum contagiosum in,
    383
  sexual abuse of, 378–386

  diagnosis and treatment,
    383–385
  (*See also* Sexual abuse of
    children)
  STD transmission in: sexual
    vs. nonsexual, 380–383
  syphilis in, 382
  trichomoniasis in, 381
  (*See also* Infants)
Chlamydial infections, 41–55
  bartholinitis, 48
  cervicitis, 46–47, 238–239,
    240
  in children, 380–381, 384,
    385
  clinical manifestations, 45
    in infants, 359–360,
      380–381
  counseling on, 390t
  diagnosis, 49–53
    in children, 384, 385t
    in infants, 361
    in men, 51t
    in women, 52t
  endometritis, 48
    postpartum, 339
  epidemiology, 42–45, 43t,
    44f
    in infants, 359
  epididymitis, 46, 281
  female specimen collection,
    22–23
  and Fitz-Hugh-Curtis
    syndrome, 267
  gonococcal infections
    compared with, 43t
  and HIV transmission, 106
  inclusion conjunctivitis: in
    infants, 352, 359–360,
    361–363, 380
  in infants, 359–364, 380–381
    clinical manifestations,
      359–360, 380–381
    inclusion conjunctivitis,
      352, 359–360, 361–363,
      380

pneumonitis, 360, 361, 362, 380
LGV, 41, 56–62, 309
   (*See also*
      Lymphogranuloma
      venereum)
in men, 45–46
   diagnosis, 51t
microbiology, 41–42, 42t
and other STDs, 4
perihepatitis, 49, 52t
and PID, 254, 255, 257, 262, 266, 355
   treatment, 264
pneumonitis: in infants, 360, 361, 362, 380
postpartum pelvic, 339
in pregnancy, 340t, 343–344, 350, 358
prevention, 54
proctitis, 43, 43t, 46, 51t, 291, 296–297
   treatment, 297, 305
proctocolitis, 51t, 56, 60–61, 291
prostatitis, 46
Reiter's syndrome, 46, 319, 320
salpingitis, 48
   in pregnancy, 337, 344
sexual assault and, 410, 411
therapy, 53–54, 264
   in infants, 361–362
   in pregnancy, 344
   proctitis, 297
urethritis
   female, 47–48, 52t, 233, 235
   male, 42–43, 43t, 45, 51t, 218, 271, 272t, 273–279
in women, 46–49
   diagnosis, 52t
Chlamydia pneumoniae, 42t
Chlamydia psittaci, 42t
Chlamydia trachomatis, 41–55

(*See also* Chlamydial
   infections)
Chloramphenicol: for
   donovanosis, 97
Chorioamnionitis, 337–338
   BV and, 246
   cervicitis and, 238, 241
Ciprofloxacen: for gonorrhea, 36
Circumcision:
   and genital ulcers, 308
   and HIV transmission, 106
Clindamycin:
   for bacterial vaginosis, 250–251
   for PID, 264
Clinical and laboratory
      approach, 10–24
   follow-up tests, 391–392
   history taking, 10–11
   in HIV/AIDS, 116–117
   physical examination of
      genital tract, 11–24
      female, 18–24
      male, 11–18
   sexual partner examination, 392–394, 393t
Clostridium difficile: and
      HIV/AIDS, 120, 133–134
Clotrimazole: for vulvovaginal
      candidiasis, 230, 243t
CMV (*see* Cytomegalovirus)
CNS infections:
   in HIV/AIDS, 117–118
   (*See also* Meningitis;
      Neurosyphilis)
Cogan's syndrome, 375t
Colpitis macularis, 239
Colposcopy, 23
Compliance with treatment, 389
   (*See also* Counseling on
      STDs)
Condoms, 3, 5, 170, 241, 394–395
   instructions for use, 395t

Endocervical infections,
        gonococcal, 28, 29f
    treatment, 36–37
Endocervicitis, 238–240
    salpingitis, 238, 241
Endometrial biopsy: for PID,
        262
Endometritis:
    bacterial vaginosis and, 246
    chlamydial, 48
        postpartum, 338, 344
    endocervicitis and, 238, 241
    GBS, 344
    and PID, 254, 257, 258, 259
    puerperal, 338
Endovaginal ultrasonography
        (EVUS): for PID, 262
Entamoeba histolytica,
        299–300, 302f–303f
Enteritis, 297–304
    bacterial, 297–299
    CMV, 304
    defined, 292–293
    in HIV/AIDS, 120
    management, 304–308
    parasitic, 299–303
    (*See also* Proctitis)
Enterobacter: and cystitis,
        233
Enterobius vermicularis, 303
    and PID, 255
Epidemiology, 1–9
    BV, 245
    chancroid, 87
    chlamydial infections,
        42–45, 43t, 44f
        in infants, 359
    CMV, 155–157
    contraception, 5
    demographics and social
        correlates, 6–8
    donovanosis, 93, 95
    drug use and STDs, 4–5
    epididymitis, 281–282, 283t
    future challenges, 8–9
    genital herpes, 135–136

genital ulcer adenopathy
        syndrome, 309
    gonococcal infections, 26
    HAV, 182–183
    HBV, 189–192
        in homosexuals, 190, 191t
    HIV, 104–106
    HPV infection, 162–163
    LGV, 56, 309
    lice, 200
    molluscum contagiosum, 175
    Reiter's syndrome, 320–322,
        321f
    risk factors and risk
        markers, 2t, 2–6
    scabies, 204–205
    sexual assault, 410
    sexual behavior, 5–6
    STDs as risk factors for
        other STDs, 4
    syphilis, 63–64
        in infants, 365–366
    transmission dynamics, 1–2
    trichomoniasis, 212–214
    urethritis, nongonococcal
        (NGU), 273
    vulvovaginal candidiasis, 223
Epididymis, 18, 281–290
Epididymitis:
    chlamydial, 46, 51t
    clinical manifestations,
        283–285
    complications, 285, 288
    diagnosis, 283–285,
        288t–289t
    epidemiology and etiology,
        281–282, 283t
    gonococcal, 30
    Pseudomonas, 281, 282, 283
    treatment, 286f–287f,
        288–290
    trichomonal, 218
Epstein-Barr virus (EBV), 135
    arthritis, 330
Erythromycin:
    for chancroid, 91

for chlamydial infections,
53, 344
in infants, 361, 362, 363
for donovanosis, 98
for gonorrhea, 343
for LGV, 61, 297
for NGU, 277
for ophthalmia neonatorum
prophylaxis, 358
Escherichia coli:
and cystitis, 233
in infants, 360
and PID, 255
Esophagitis: in HIV/AIDS,
119, 122–124

Fellatio:
gonorrhea, 30
and HSV-1, 136
STD association, 11, 12t–13t
(*See also* Oral-anogenital sex)
Female genital tract:
examination, 18–24, 19f–23f
external genitalia and
perineum, 20–21
rectovaginal, 24
vagina, cervix, uterus,
and adnexal structures,
20f–22f, 21–24
in pregnancy, 335–337
prepubescent, 378
Fetal transmission (*see*
Maternal transmission)
Fever: in HIV/AIDS, 133
Fitz-Hugh-Curtis syndrome
(FHC), 49, 52t, 266–269
clinical manifestations,
267–268
diagnosis, 268–269
(*See also* Pelvic
inflammatory disease)
Fluconazole: for candidiasis,
131
Foscarnet:
for CMV, 160
for HSV, 153

Fusobacterium: vaginosis in
pregnancy, 338

Ganciclovir: for CMV, 131,
159–160, 303
Gardnerella vaginalis, 245–246
in children, 381–382
and PID, 255
in pregnancy, 345
trichomoniasis concurrent
with, 219
Gastrointestinal tract infections:
and HIV/AIDS, 119–120
(*See also* Diarrhea)
GBS (*see* Group B
streptococci)
Genital herpes, 135–154
aseptic meningitis, 141–142
atypical, 145
cervicitis, 140–141
clinical manifestations,
137t, 137–141, 138t
complications, 141–143
counseling on, 390t
diagnosis, 148–149,
316f–317f
differential diagnosis, 89,
148–149
disseminated, 143
epidemiology, 135–136, 309
extragenital lesions, 142–143
in HIV-infected patient, 147
transmission, 106
treatment, 152
HSV-1, 136, 137, 137t, 138t
HSV-2, 135–138, 137t, 138t
neonatal exposure, 340t,
346–348
pathogenesis, 136–137
pharyngeal, 141
in pregnancy, 153, 340t,
346–348
prevention, 153
primary, 138–140, 139t, 140f
summary of clinical
course, 143–144

recurrent, 144t, 144–145,
  145t, 147–148
  therapy, 150, 151t
  superinfection, 143
  therapy, 149–153, 151t–152t
    in pregnancy, 153,
      347–348
  virology, 135
Genital tract examination:
  female, 18–24 (*See also*
      Female genital tract)
  male, 11–18 (*See also* Male
      genital tract)
Genital tract infections, lower,
    in women, 233–244
    (*See also* Cervicitis; Cystitis;
      Urethritis; Vaginitis)
Genital ulcer adenopathy
    syndrome, 309–318
  clinical manifestations,
    310–312, 311t
  complications, 312
  definition, 309
  diagnosis, 312–315, 313t
  differential diagnosis, 315,
    316f–317f
  epidemiology, 309
  etiology, 309–310
  treatment, 315
Genital ulcers:
  differential diagnosis, 71,
    89, 148–149
  and HIV transmission, 106
Genital warts (*see* Human
    papillomavirus
    infection)
Gentamicin:
  for epididymitis, 287f
  for PID, 264
Giardiasis, 299, 300f–301f
  and HIV/AIDS, 120
Gingivitis: and HIV/AIDS,
    119
GI tract infections:
  in HIV/AIDS, 119–120
  (*See also* Diarrhea)

Gonococcal infections, 25–40
  antimicrobial susceptibility,
    25–26
  arthritis
    in children, 356
    DGI, 31–32, 38, 328–333
    in neonates, 353
  in children, 354–356, 380
    sexual abuse and, 352,
      356, 380, 384, 385t
    treatment, 357
  chlamydial infections
    compared with, 43t
  clinical manifestations,
    27–30
  complications
    local, 30
    systemic, 31–32
  counseling on, 390t
  culture, 32–33, 33t
  disseminated (DGI), 31–32,
    328–333
    diagnosis, 330–333, 332f
    in pregnancy, 342
    treatment, 38, 333
  endocarditis, 32
    treatment, 38
  endocervical, 28, 29f,
    238–239
    treatment, 36–37
  epidemiology, 26
  epididymitis, 281
    treatment, 289
  female specimen collection,
    22–23
  and Fitz-Hugh-Curtis
    syndrome, 267
  and HIV transmission, 106
  in infants, 342–343, 352–354
    treatment, 356–357
  laboratory diagnosis, 32–35
  meningitis, 32
    treatment, 38
  microbiology, 25
  ophthalmia neonatorum,
    352–353, 361

prevention, 358
treatment, 38–39
and other STDs, 4
pharyngeal, 28, 30, 32, 37
treatment, 37
and PID, 30, 254, 255, 257, 262, 266
in children, 355
in pregnancy, 342
treatment, 264
postpartum pelvic, 339
in pregnancy, 340t, 342–343, 350
treatment, 37–38, 343, 358
prevention, 39
proctitis, 293–294
rectal, 28, 293–294
treatment, 36–37, 305
and Reiter's syndrome, 319, 320
salpingitis, 30
in children, 355, 356t
in pregnancy, 337
sexual assault and, 410, 411
stained smears, 33–35, 34f, 35t, 294
treatment, 35–39
anorectal, 36–37, 305
in children, 356–357
DGI, 38, 333
epididymitis, 289
ophthalmia neonatorum, 38–39
in pregnancy, 37–38, 343, 389
urethritis, 36–37, 278
and trichomoniasis, 214
urethritis, 26, 27f, 27–28, 233, 271, 272t, 273–279
in children, 355–356
diagnosis, 274–276
male, 272t, 273–276, 2721
postgonococcal, 271–272
treatment, 36–37, 278
vaginitis in children, 354–355

Gonococcemia, 31–32, 38
Granuloma inguinale (*see* Donovanosis)
Granuloma venereum (*see* Donovanosis)
Group B streptococci infections: in pregnancy, 340t, 344–345
Gummas, syphilitic, 84–85, 370
Gynecologic complications: of lower genital tract infections, 241

Haemophilus ducreyi, 87, 88, 309
(*See also* Chancroid)
Haemophilus influenzae:
and HIV/AIDS, 118, 131, 132
in infants, 360
and PID, 255
Hairy leukoplakia: and HIV/AIDS, 110, 119
HBV (*see* Hepatitis B virus)
Headache: in HIV/AIDS, 133
Hepatitis, viral, 180–199, 181t
management of acute, 198
serologic diagnosis, 193t
(*See also specific viruses*)
Hepatitis A virus (HAV), 180–185, 181t
clinical manifestations, 183–184
epidemiology, 182–183
immunity, 182, 182f
prevention, 184–185
Hepatitis B immunoglobulin, 195
Hepatitis B virus (HBV), 181t, 185–195
arthritis, 329, 333
clinical manifestations, 192
counseling on, 391f
diagnosis, 192–194, 193t
epidemiology, 189–192
in homosexuals, 190, 191t

and HIV/AIDS, 117, 118
pathobiology and
        immunity, 185–189,
        186f, 188f
prevention, 180, 194t,
        194–195
sexual assault and, 411
Hepatitis C virus (HCV),
        181t, 197
Hepatitis D virus (HDV),
        181t, 195–197
and HBV, 187, 195–197
Hepatitis E virus (HEV), 180,
        181t
Hepatitis, non-A non-B
        (NANB), 181t, 197–198
Hepatocellular carcinoma:
        HBV and, 187–188
Herpes simplex virus (HSV):
anorectal, 295
arthritis, 330
asymptomatic infection, 146
cervicitis, 238–239, 240
in children, 381
and conjunctivitis in
        infants, 381
endocervicitis, 238–239
genital infection, 135–154,
        233, 309, 311t (See also
        Genital herpes)
    diagnosis, 313t, 315
    in HIV patient, 147
    in immunocompromised,
        147
    prevention, 153
    recurrence, 147–148
    therapy, 149–153
and HIV/AIDS, 115, 122,
        124, 147, 152
anorectal, 295
management, 130, 131,
        152
in immunocompromised
        host, 147, 152t
neonatal, 340t, 346–348
and other STDs, 4

in pregnancy, 340t, 346–348
proctitis, 145–146, 151t,
        291, 295
    treatment, 305
resistance, 152–153
type 1, 135–138, 143–144
type 2, 135–138, 143–144,
        145
    (See also Genital herpes)
urethritis, 272–273, 274, 278
High-frequency transmitters, 6
Hispanics: STDs in, 7
Histoplasmosis: and
        HIV/AIDS, 114
History taking, 10–11
and HIV/AIDS, 116
HIV/AIDS, 99–123, 124–134
acute primary syndromes,
        107
antiretroviral therapy,
        127–129
arthritis, 330
asymptomatic infection, 109
bacterial infection
        management, 131
CDC case definition, 110,
        111t–113t
CDC classification, 107t,
        107–110
chancroid and, 87, 90
in children, 382
clinical manifestations,
        107t, 107–110, 108t
CMV and, 109, 115t, 116,
        119, 120–122, 121f,
        130, 155, 156, 157, 160,
        304
CNS infections, 117–118
counseling, 387, 398–408,
        399t
    in advanced
        infection/disease,
        403–405
    for family, partners, and
        friends, 405–407
    negative test, 401–402

positive test, 402–403
posttest, 401–403
pretest, 399–400
diagnosis, 400–401
diarrhea
management, 133–134
parasitic, 303
didanosine for, 128–129
encephalitis, 117
enteritis, 120
epidemiology, 104–106
esophagitis, 119
fever and headache, 133
GI tract infections, 119–120
HPV infection and, 4, 169,
173
HSV infection, 115, 122,
124, 147, 152
anorectal, 295
and transmission, 147
treatment, 130, 131, 152
initial clinical evaluation,
124–125
from injected drug use, 105
interventions (general),
126–127
laboratory tests and
diagnostic procedures,
125, 400–401
malignancies, 120
meningitis, 118
and molluscum contagiosum,
115, 177, 179
mucocutaneous
manifestations, 110,
114, 114t
management, 130
neonatal, 106, 348–349
neuropsychiatric
manifestations, 131–132
neurosyphilis and, 82
treatment, 82
ocular infections, 120–122,
121f
odynophagia management,
130–131

oral infections, 119
P. carinii pneumonia and,
115t, 115–117, 158
management, 132–133
prophylaxis, 129–130
pathogenesis, 100–104, 103f
patient history, 10, 124
perinatal transmission, 106
persistent generalized
lymphadenopathy, 109
physical exam, 124
pneumonia management,
132–133
in pregnancy, 348–349
pretest counseling, 399–400
primary care, 124–134
proctitis, 120, 291
pulmonary complications,
115t, 115–116
risk factors for acquisition
and transmission, 106
salmonellosis and, 120, 131,
133
sexual assault and, 411
sexual transmission, 104–105
sinusitis management, 131
symptomatic infection,
109–110
syphilis and, 106, 126
treatment, 73, 82
T cells and, 100–104, 107,
108t, 109, 125, 127
count and management
decisions, 127
testing guidelines, 398–399,
399t
from transfusions, 105
trichomoniasis and, 219
viral replication, 99–100,
102f
viral structure, 99, 100f, 101f
virology, 99–100, 100f, 101f,
102f
Walter-Reade staging
classification, 108t
zalcitabine for, 129

zidovudine (AZT) for, 127–128
Hodgkin's disease: LGV vs., 60
Homosexuals:
  chlamydial infections in, 43, 44f, 50
  CMV in, 156
  Entamoeba histolytica in, 299–300
  epididymitis in, 281
  genital ulcers in, 309, 310
  gonorrhea in, 28, 32–33, 33t, 293–294
  HAV in, 183
  HBV in, 190, 191t, 194
  HDV in, 195
  HIV/AIDS in, 104, 127
  HPV warts in, 163, 169
  HSV proctitis in, 145–146, 295
  intestinal and anal infections in
    etiology, 294t
    evaluation and management, 306f, 307f, 308
    prevention, 308
  LGV in, 56, 60–61
  molluscum contagiosum in, 177
  parasitic infections in, 299–303
  patient history taking, 10
  proctitis in, 291, 293
  shigellosis in, 297–298
  syphilis in, 63, 65, 295–296
HPV (*see* Human papillomavirus)
Human immunodeficiency virus (*see* HIV/AIDS)
Human papillomavirus (HPV) infection, 162–174
  anal, 163, 165
  and cervical neoplasia, 240
  in children, 381–382

clinical manifestations, 163–165
counseling on, 390t
diagnosis, 169–170
epidemiology, 162–163
giant, 165
HIV and, 4, 169, 173
and intraepithelial neoplasia, 166, 168–169, 240, 348
in men, 164f, 164–165, 166f
molluscum contagiosum vs., 170, 177
neonatal, 172–173, 348, 349
in pregnancy, 172–173, 348
treatment, 170–173
in women, 165, 167f
Hutchinson's teeth, 370, 371f
Hydrocele: vs. epididymitis, 285–286, 288t–289t
Hypertrophic ectopy, 46

Idomoeba butschlii, 301
Immunocompromised host:
  CMV in, 157, 158
  genital HSV infection, 147, 152t
  HBV carriage, 187
  (*See also* HIV/AIDS)
Immunofluorescent antibody: for HIV, 109
Indomethacin: for Reiter's syndrome, 333
Infants:
  chlamydial infections in, 359–364
    inclusion conjunctivitis, 352, 359–360, 361–363, 380
    pneumonitis, 360, 361, 362, 380
  gonococcal infections in, 342–343, 352–354
    arthritis, 353
    ophthalmia neonatorum, 352–353, 358, 361
    treatment, 356–357

syphilis in, 365–377
  clinical manifestations,
    366–370
  diagnosis, 371–374,
    373t–375t
  epidemiology, 365–366
  treatment, 374–376
  (*See also* Neonatal
    infections; Children)
Infertility: from PID, 265
Inguinal syndrome: LGV, 57t,
  58t, 58–60, 59f, 311t
Intrauterine devices (IUDs):
  and PID, 255
Isoniazid: for tuberculosis, 118
Isosporiasis: and HIV/AIDS,
  120, 303

Jarisch-Herxheimer reaction,
  72

Kaposi's sarcoma: and
  HIV/AIDS, 115t, 128
Keratoacanthomas:
  molluscum
    contagiosum vs., 177
Keratodermia blennorrhagica:
  in Reiter's syndrome,
    323, 325, 326f–327f
Ketoconazole:
  for candidiasis, 131
  for vulvovaginal
    candidiasis, 231
Klebsiella pneumoniae:
  and cystitis, 233
  in infants, 360

Labia: examination of, 20–21
Laboratory approach (*see*
  Clinical and laboratory
  approach)
LGV (*see* Lymphogranuloma
  venereum)
Lice, 200–203, 201f
  counseling on, 391t

epidemiology, 200
management, 202–203
Lindane:
  for lice, 203
  for scabies, 210
Lymphadenopathy:
  and genital ulcers, 310, 312
  HIV infection, 108t, 109
Lymphogranuloma venereum
  (LGV), 41, 56–62
  anogenitorectal syndrome,
    60–61, 296–297, 311t
  arthritis, 330
  clinical manifestations, 57t,
    57–60, 311t, 312
  diagnosis, 50, 51t, 61, 313t,
    314, 315
  differential diagnosis, 60, 89
  epidemiology, 56, 309
  groove sign, 312
  inguinal syndrome, 57t, 58t,
    58–60, 59f, 311t
  pathogenesis, 56–57
  primary lesion, 58, 58t, 309
  treatment and prevention,
    61–62, 315
Lymphomas: in HIV/AIDS, 120

Male genital tract:
  examination, 11–18, 15t, 16f
    groin, 15–17
    penis, 17
    rectum and pelvic organs,
      18
    scrotum, 17–18
  prepubescent, 378
Malignancies:
  cervical (*see* Cervical cancer)
  in HIV/AIDS, 120
Marshall's syndrome, 375t
Maternal transmission,
  338–350
  bacterial vaginosis, 345
  chlamydial infections, 340t,
    343–344

CMV, 156, 157, 340t, 345–346
genital mycoplasmas, 345
gonorrhea, 340t, 342–343
group B streptococci, 340t, 344–345
HBV, 190
HIV/AIDS, 106, 348–349, 403
HPV warts, 172–173, 348
HSV, 340t, 346–348
syphilis, 64, 339, 340t, 341
Trichomonas vaginalis, 349
(*See also* Neonatal infections; Pregnancy)
Medication counseling, 389
Meningitis:
differential diagnosis of aseptic, 142
gonococcal, 32
treatment, 38
herpetic, 141–142
in HIV/AIDS, 118
management, 133
syphilis, 75–76
Meningovascular syphilis, 76–77
Metronidazole:
for bacterial vaginosis, 243t, 249–250
for giardiasis, 299
toxicity, 221–222
for trichomoniasis, 221, 243t, 349
Miconazole: for vulvovaginal candidiasis, 230, 243t
Microsporidium: and HIV/AIDS, 303
Mobiluncus, 245–246
Molluscum contagiosum, 175–179
in children, 383
clinical manifestations, 175–177, 176f
diagnosis, 177, 178f

differential diagnosis, 170
epidemiology, 175
and HIV/AIDS, 115, 177, 179
HPV vs., 170, 177
treatment and prevention, 179
Molluscum dermatitis, 177
Mononucleosis: CMV, 157
Mucocutaneous disorders:
in HIV/AIDS, 110, 114, 114t
management, 130
in Reiter's syndrome, 323, 325f, 325–326
Mycobacterium avium complex: and HIV/AIDS, 115t, 116, 133
Mycobacterium tuberculosis:
and HIV/AIDS, 115t, 116, 117, 118, 133
and PID, 255
Mycoplasma genitalium:
urethritis, 272
Mycoplasma hominis, 245–246
arthritis, 330
and PID, 255, 355
postpartum pelvic infection, 339
in pregnancy, 345
Myelitis, transverse: in HSV infection, 142

Neisseria gonorrhoeae, 25
(*See also* Gonococcal infections)
Neisseria meningitidis: in infants, 360
Neonatal infections:
bacterial vaginosis, 345
chlamydial, 340t, 343–344, 359–364, 380–381
CMV, 156, 157, 340t, 345–346, 360
genital mycoplasmas, 345

gonococcal, 352–354
  ophthalmia neonatorum,
    38–39, 352–353, 358,
    361
  treatment, 38–39, 356–357
gonorrhea, 340t, 342–343
group B streptococci, 340t,
    344–345
HBV, 190
HIV/AIDS, 106, 348–349
HPV warts, 172–173, 348
HSV, 340t, 346–348
inclusion conjunctivitis,
    352, 359–360, 361–363,
    380
maternal transmission,
    338–350
syphilis, 64, 339, 340t,
    341–342, 365–377
  clinical manifestations,
    366–370
  diagnosis, 371–374, 374t
  epidemiology, 365–366
  pathogenesis, 366
  treatment, 374–376
Trichomonas vaginalis, 349
(*See also* Infants; Maternal
    transmission)
Neoplasia, cervical
    intraepithelial (CIV):
and HIV/AIDS, 110, 125
and HPV infection, 166,
    168–169, 240, 348
Neuropsychiatric
    manifestations: in
    HIV/AIDS, 131–132
Neurosyphilis, 74–82
asymptomatic, 74–75
cerebrovascular, 76–77
classification, 74t
HIV infection and, 82, 118
meningeal, 75–76
meningovascular, 76–77
parenchymatous, 77–79,
    78t, 79t

pathogenesis, 74
tabes dorsalis, 79–81, 80t
treatment, 81–82
  HIV-infected patients, 82
(*See also* Syphilis)
NGU (*see* Urethritis,
    nongonococcal)
Norfloxacin: for gonorrhea,
    36
Nystatin: for vulvovaginal
    candidiasis, 243t

Ocular infections:
chlamydial, 352, 359–360,
    361–363
CMV, 120–122, 121f, 158,
    160
gonococcal, 38–39, 352–353,
    361
in HIV/AIDS, 120–122, 121f
Reiter's syndrome, 326
Odynophagia: in HIV/AIDS,
    130–131
Ofloxacin: for gonorrhea, 36
Oophoritis: and PID, 254
Ophthalmia neonatorum,
    352–353, 361
prevention, 358
treatment, 38–39
(*See also* Conjunctivitis)
Opportunistic infections: and
    HIV/AIDS, 115
(*See also* specific infections)
Oral-anogenital sex, 291
gonococcal infections, 28, 30
and HIV transmission, 106
HSV transmission, 136, 146
STD association, 11, 12t–13t
Oral contraceptives:
and PID, 256
and VVC risk, 224
Oral mucosa infections: in
    HIV/AIDS, 119
Osteochondritis: in congenital
    syphilis, 369, 370

Pap smear, 21–22
Parametritis: and PID, 254
Parasitic infections: sexual transmission of, 299–303
Paresis, general, 77–79, 78t
Partner recruitment, 6
Patient education on STDs, 387–397
    summary, 390t–391t
    (*See also* Counseling on STDs)
Pelvic examination, 18–24, 19f–23f
    and HIV/AIDS, 117
Pelvic inflammatory disease (PID), 10, 52t, 254–270
    acute-phase reactants and, 259–260
    atypical, 266
    BV and, 245, 254, 255
    cervicitis and, 241
    chlamydial, 254, 255, 257, 262, 266, 355
        treatment, 264
    clinical manifestations, 257–260, 261t
    counseling on, 390t
    diagnosis, 257–262, 258t, 261t
    differential diagnosis, 263, 263t
    etiology, 254–255
    Fitz-Hugh-Curtis syndrome, 266–269
    gonococcal, 30, 254, 255, 257, 262, 266
        in children, 355
        in pregnancy, 342
    iatrogenic, 256
    infertility from, 265
    mycoplasmal, 255, 355
    postpartal, 257
    prevention, 265–266
    prognosis, 265

risk factors, 256–257
salpingitis and, 254, 259, 260, 261t, 262, 263, 265
treatment, 263–265
Pelvis, coronal section:
    female, 255f
    male, 282f
Penicillin G:
    for gonorrhea: in infants, 357
    Jarisch-Herxheimer reaction, 342
    for syphilis, 72
        congenital, 375
        late benign, 85
        neuro-, 72
        in pregnancy, 341
Penis: examination of, 17
Pentamidine: for PCP prophylaxis, 121–122
Peptostreptococcus:
    PID in children, 355
    vaginosis in pregnancy, 338
Perihepatitis:
    chlamydial, 49, 52t
    and Fitz-Hugh-Curtis syndrome, 266–269
Perinatal transmission (*see* Maternal transmission)
Peritonitis, pelvic: and PID, 254, 266
Permethrim: for lice, 203
Pharyngeal infection:
    gonococcal, 28, 30, 32, 37
        treatment, 37
    herpetic, 141
Phimosis, 17
Pneumocystis carinii pneumonia (PCP) in HIV/AIDS, 115t, 115–117, 158
    management, 132–133
    prophylaxis, 129–130
Pneumonia:
    in HIV/AIDS, 132–133

Pneumocystis carinii, 115t,
115–117, 129–130,
132–133, 158
Pneumonitis, chlamydial: in
infants, 360, 361, 362,
380
Pregnancy:
BV in, 246, 251, 338, 345
chlamydial infections in,
340t, 343–344, 350, 358
treatment, 344
chorioamnionitis, 337–338
BV and, 246
cervicitis and, 238, 241
CMV in, 340t, 345–346
ectopic, 337
from PID, 265
genital mycoplasmas in, 345
gonococcal infections in,
340t, 342–343, 350
treatment, 37–38, 343, 358
HIV in, 348–349
host-parasite relationships
in, 335–337, 336f
HPV in, 172–173, 348
HSV in, 340t, 346–348
management, 347–348
intrauterine infection,
337–338
lower genital tract
infections and, 241
maternal puerperal
infection and antenatal
STDs, 338–339
mucus plug, 337
Mycoplasma hominis in, 345
STDs in, 335–351
management, 350
(*See also specific STDs*)
streptococci B infections in,
340t, 344–345
syphilis in, 339, 340t, 341, 350
treatment, 341–342,
374–375
(*See also* Syphilis,
congenital)

trichomoniasis in, 219, 221,
349
and VVC risk, 224
(*See also* Maternal
transmission; Neonatal
infections)
Probenecid: for gonorrhea, 36
Proctitis, 291–308
chlamydial, 43, 43t, 46, 51t,
291, 296–297
definitions, 291–293
differential diagnosis, 146
gonococcal, 293–294
herpetic, 145–146, 151t,
291, 295, 305
in HIV/AIDS, 120, 291
management, 304–308
syphilitic, 295–296
Proctocolitis, 297–304
bacterial, 297–299
chlamydial, 51t, 56, 60–61,
291
CMV, 304
defined, 291, 292
differential diagnosis, 146
management, 304–308
parasitic, 299–303
(*See also* Proctitis)
Prostate gland: examination, 18
Prostatitis:
chlamydial, 46
trichomonal, 218
Proteus mirabilis: and cystitis,
233
Protozoan infections, 299–301
Pruritus: and HIV/AIDS, 110,
122
Pseudomonas: epididymitis,
281, 282, 283
Pubic lice, 200–203, 201f
counseling on, 391t
Pulmonary infections:
in HIV/AIDS, 115t, 115–124
management, 131, 132–133
(*See also* Pneumonia;
Pneumonitis)

Quinacrine: for giardiasis, 299

Rape (*see* Sexual assault)
Reactive arthritis (*see* Reiter's syndrome)
Receivers, 6
Rectal intercourse and infections (*see* Anal intercourse and infections)
Rectovaginal examination, 21f, 23, 24
Rectum, male: examination of, 18, 304
Referrals on STDs, 392–394, 393t
Reiter's syndrome, 46, 310, 319–328
  arthritis, 322–323, 324f
  clinical manifestations, 322–328, 323t
  differential diagnosis, 330–333, 332f
  epidemiology, 320–322, 321f
  etiology and pathogenesis, 319–320
  HLA-B27 haplotype and, 320
  management, 333
  mucocutaneous, 323, 325f, 325–326
  and NGU, 46
  ocular, 326
  salmonellosis and, 319
  systemic, 326–327
Retinal hemorrhages: in HIV/AIDS, 121
Retinitis: CMV, 120–122, 121f, 158, 160
Rickets, 375t
Risk assessment, 11
Risk factors:
  for HIV acquisition and transmission, 106
  for STDs, 2t, 2–6
Risk markers, 2t, 2–6

Risk reduction counseling, 394–396, 395t
  in HIV/AIDS, 399–400, 404, 405
Romberg's sign, 80t, 81
Rubella, 375t

Sadomasochism: STD association, 14t
Salmonellosis, 298–299
  and HIV/AIDS, 120, 131, 133
  and Reiter's syndrome, 319
Salpingitis:
  chlamydial, 48
    in pregnancy, 337, 344
  differential diagnosis, 263t
  and ectopic pregnancy, 337
  endocervicitis and, 238, 241
  and Fitz-Hugh-Curtis syndrome, 266–269
  gonococcal, 30
    in children, 355, 356t
    in pregnancy, 337
  and PID, 254, 259, 260, 261t, 262, 263, 265
Sarcoptes scabiei, 204
Scabies, 204–211
  classic, 205–206
  clinical manifestations, 205–208
  counseling on, 391t
  crusted (Norwegian), 207–208
  diagnosis, 206t, 208–210
  differential diagnosis, 208
  epidemiology, 204–205
  nodular, 207
  treatment, 210–211
Schistosoma: and PID, 255
Scrotum: examination of, 17–18
Seborrheic dermatitis: and HIV/AIDS, 110, 114, 122

Serology:
  for CMV, 158–159
  for HBV, 192–193, 193t
  for syphilis, 69–70, 71,
      74–75, 76, 77, 78–79,
      81, 97, 314–315,
      372–373, 374t–375t
Sexual abuse of children, 352,
      378–386
  chlamydial infections,
      380–381
  condyloma acuminatum
      and, 381–382
  diagnosis and treatment,
      383–385
  Gardnerella vaginalis and,
      381–382
  gonococcal infections and,
      352, 356, 380, 384, 385t
  HIV/AIDS and, 382
  HPV and, 381–382
  HSV and, 381
  molluscum contagiosum
      and, 383
  reportage, 379t
  screening, 383–384
  and STDs, 379–386
  syphilis and, 382
  trichomoniasis, 381
Sexual assault:
  epidemiology, 410
  and STDs, 409–412
    evaluation, 410–411
    management, 409–410
    risk, 410
    treatment, 411–412
Sexual behavior, 2, 3, 5–6
Sexual history, 10–11
Sexual orientation, 3
Sexual partners:
  number of, 6
  referral and examination of,
      392–394, 393t
Sexual practices risks,
      394–395, 395t

disease association, 12t–14t,
      124
  (*See also* Risk factors)
Shigellosis, 297–298
  and HIV/AIDS, 120, 133
  and Reiter's syndrome, 319
Silver nitrate: for ophthalmia
      neonatorum
      prophylaxis, 358, 360
Sinusitis: in HIV/AIDS, 131
Social correlates, 6–8
Spectinomycin: for gonorrhea,
      36, 37, 38, 294
  in children, 357
  in pregnancy, 343
Spermatocele: vs.
      epididymitis, 288t–289t
Spermicides, 394
Spinal cord syphilis, 77
Staphylococcus aureus:
      conjunctivitis in
      infants, 352, 360
Staphylococcus saprophyticus:
      and cystitis, 233
Strawberry cervix, 239
Streptococci B infections: in
      pregnancy, 340t,
      344–345
Streptococcus pneumoniae:
      and HIV/AIDS, 115, 118,
      131, 132
  in infants, 360
Sulfisoxazole:
  for chlamydial infections, 53
  for LGV, 61, 297
Syphilis, 63–86
  anorectal, 65, 71, 295–296
    management, 305
  arthritis, 330
  cardiovascular, 82–84
    treatment, 84–85
  cerebrovascular, 76–77
  chancre, 65f, 65–66, 66f, 71,
      148, 309, 311t
  in children, 382

congenital, 64, 339,
 341–342, 365–377, 380t
 clinical manifestations,
  366–370
 diagnosis, 371–374
 differential diagnosis, 374t
 early, 366–370
 epidemiology, 365–366
 late, 370, 375t
 pathogenesis, 366
 treatment, 374–376
counseling on, 391t
dark field microscopy, 68,
 70, 314, 372
direct fluorescent antibody
 test, 68–69, 372
and donovanosis, 97
early, 64–73
 clinical manifestations,
  65–68
 diagnosis, 70–71, 312,
  313t, 316f–317f
 differential diagnosis,
  71–72
 laboratory tests, 68–70
 pathogenesis, 64–65
 treatment, 72–73
epidemiology, 63–64, 309
and HIV, 106, 126
 treatment, 73, 82
in infants (*see* congenital
 above)
laboratory tests, 68–70,
 314–315, 372–374
late benign, 84
 treatment, 84–85
latent infection, 71, 72
LGV vs., 60
meningeal, 75–76, 118
meningovascular, 76–77
microbiology, 63
neuro-, 74–82
 (*See also* Neurosyphilis)
in pregnancy, 339, 340t,
 341, 350

treatment, 341–342,
 374–375
 (*See also* congenital *above*)
primary, 65f, 65–66, 66f, 70
 differential diagnosis, 71,
  89, 148
 treatment, 72
 (*See also* chancre *above*)
proctitis, 295–296
secondary, 66–68, 67f, 70–71
 differential diagnosis,
  71–72
 treatment, 72
serology for, 69–70, 71,
 74–75, 76, 77, 78–79,
 81, 97, 314–315,
 372–373, 374t–375t
sexual assault and, 411
stages, 64
transmission, 64
treatment
 anorectal, 305
 cardiovascular, 84–85
 congenital, 374–376
 early, 72–73
 epidemiologic, 73
 in HIV patients, 73, 82
 Jarisch-Herxheimer
  reaction, 72
 late, 84–85
 in pregnancy, 374–375

Tabes dorsalis, 79–81, 80t
T cells: and HIV/AIDS,
 100–104, 107, 108t,
 109, 125, 127
 count in management
  decisions, 127
Terconazole: for vulvovaginal
 candidiasis, 230
Testes: examination of, 17–18
Testicular abscess, 285
Testicular cancer: epididymitis
 vs., 285, 286f–287f,
 288t–289t

Testicular infarction, 285
Testicular torsion:
    epididymitis vs.,
      284–285, 286f–287f,
      288t–289t
Test of cure (TOC), 391–392
Tetracycline:
    for chlamydial infections, 49
    contraindication in
      pregnancy, 341
    for cystitis, 235
    for donovanosis, 97
    for epididymitis, 289
    for LGV, 61, 297
    for NGU, 277, 278
    for ophthalmia neonatorum
      prophylaxis, 358
    for sexual assault victims,
      411
    for syphilis, 72
Thrush, candidal: and
    HIV/AIDS, 108t,
    118–119
Tinidazole: for trichomoniasis,
    243t
Tobramycin:
    for epididymitis, 287f
    for PID, 264
Toxic shock syndrome, 238
Toxoplasmosis: and
    HIV/AIDS, 117–118,
    133
Transfusions:
    CMV from, 157
    HIV from, 105
Transmission dynamics, 1–2
Treponemal tests, 69–70, 71,
    76, 77, 78–79
    congenital infections,
      371–374
Treponema pallidum, 63
    (*See also* Syphilis)
Trichomonas vaginalis, 212,
    213f
    and urethritis, 273

Trichomoniasis, 141, 212–222,
    238
    asymptomatic, 214, 215
    BV coexisting with, 245
    in children, 381
    clinical manifestations,
      216–219
    complications, 219
    diagnosis, 219–221,
      242t–243t
    ectocervicitis, 239
    epidemiology, 212–214
    in men, 218–219, 220–221
    nonvenereal transmission,
      214
    pathogenesis, 214–216
    perinatal, 214
    in pregnancy, 219, 221,
      349
    prostatitis, 218
    sexual transmission, 214
    treatment, 221–222,
      242t–243t
    in women, 216–218, 217t,
      219–220
Trimethoprim-
    sulfamethoxazole:
    for chancroid, 91
    for epididymitis, 287f, 289
    for PCP, 129–130,
      132–133
Tuberculosis:
    and HIV/AIDS, 110, 115t,
      116, 117, 118, 133
    and PID, 255

Ureaplasma urealyticum:
    arthritis, 319, 330
    in pregnancy, 338, 345
    urethritis, 272
Urethra: coronal section of
    male, 282f
Urethral syndrome, 233
Urethritis:
    chlamydial

female, 47–48, 52t, 233, 235
male, 42–43, 43t, 45, 51t, 218, 271, 272t, 273–279
female, 233–238
  characteristics of, 234t
  chlamydial, 47–48, 52t, 233, 235
  gonococcal, 26, 27f, 27–28, 233, 271, 272t, 273–279
  in children, 355–356
  clinical manifestations, 273–274
  differential diagnosis, 275–276
  male, 271, 272t, 273–274
  treatment, 36–37, 278
male, 17, 271–280
  chlamydial, 42–43, 43t, 45, 51t, 271, 272t, 273–279
  clinical manifestations, 273–274
  differential diagnosis, 275–276
  etiology, 271–273, 272t
  gonococcal, 271, 272t, 273–276
  management, 276t, 277–279
  nongonococcal (NGU), 271–280
  postgonococcal (PGU), 271–272
  nongonococcal (NGU), 233, 271–280
  clinical manifestations, 273–274
  counseling on, 390t
  diagnosis, 274–276
  epidemiology, 273
  etiology, 272–273
  nonvenereal, 273
  treatment, 277–279
Reiter's syndrome, 322
trichomonal, 218

Uterus: examination of, 21f, 21–24

Vaccination: HBV, 194–195
Vaginal atrophy, 238
Vaginal discharge: differential diagnosis and management, 240–241
Vaginal examination, 20f, 21f–22f, 21–24
Vaginal flora: and STDs, 4
Vaginal infections:
  prevalence of, 238
  (See also specific infections)
Vaginal speculum, 19, 20f
Vaginitis:
  counseling on, 390t
  desquamative inflammatory, 238
  gonococcal: in children, 354–355
  nonspecific (see Vaginosis, bacterial)
  ulcerative, 238
Vaginitis, candidal (see Candidiasis, vulvovaginal)
Vaginosis, bacterial (BV), 22, 238, 245–253
  asymptomatic, 251
  in children, 382
  and chorioamnionitis, 338
  complications, 246
  diagnosis, 242t–243t, 247–249
  epidemiology, 245
  etiology, 245–246
  and PID, 245, 254, 255
  postpartum, 339
  in pregnancy, 246, 251, 338, 345
  prevention, 251–252
  treatment, 242t–243t, 249–251

Varicella zoster virus (VZV), 135
 and HIV/AIDS, 114
 management, 122
VDRL test, 69, 70, 75, 76, 77, 79, 81
Verruca vulgaris (*see* Human papillomavirus infection)
Viral hepatitis, 180–199, 181t
 (*See also* Hepatitis)
Viral urethritis, 272–273
Vulvar vestibulitis, 238
Vulvitis: characteristics of, 234t
VVC (vulvovaginal candidiasis) (*see* Candidiasis, vulvovaginal)

Walter Reed HIV staging classification, 107, 108t
Warts, genital (*see* Human papillomavirus infection)
Western blot: for HIV, 400–401

Yersinia enterocolitica: and arthritis, 319

Zalcitabine: for HIV/AIDS, 129
Zidovudine (AZT): for HIV/AIDS, 127–128